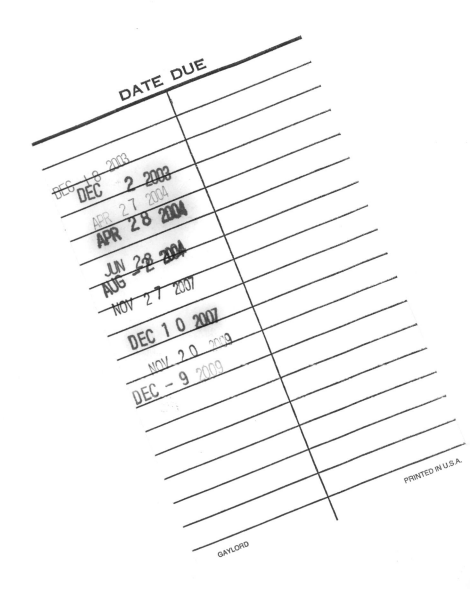

DATE DUE

DEC 1 8 2003
DEC 2 2003
APR 27 2004
APR 28 2004
JUN 28 2004
AUG
NOV 27 2007
DEC 1 0 2007
NOV 20 2009
DEC - 9 2009

PRINTED IN U.S.A.

GAYLORD

THE POLITICAL LIFE OF MEDICARE

AMERICAN POLITICS AND POLITICAL ECONOMY
A SERIES EDITED BY BENJAMIN I. PAGE

THE

POLITICAL

LIFE OF

MEDICARE

JONATHAN OBERLANDER

THE UNIVERSITY OF CHICAGO PRESS

CHICAGO AND LONDON

Jonathan Oberlander is assistant professor of social medicine at the
University of North Carolina at Chapel Hill, where he teaches health policy
in the School of Medicine and Department of Political Science.

The University of Chicago Press, Chicago 60637
The University of Chicago Press, Ltd., London
© 2003 by The University of Chicago
All rights reserved. Published 2003
Printed in the United States of America

12   11   10   09   08   07   06   05   04   03   1   2   3   4   5
ISBN: 0-226-61595-2 (cloth)
ISBN: 0-226-61596-0 (paper)

Library of Congress Cataloging-in-Publication Data
Oberlander, Jonathan.
The political life of Medicare / Jonathan Oberlander.
p. ; cm.—(American politics and political economy)
Includes bibliographical references and index.
ISBN 0-226-61595-2 (cloth : alk. paper)—ISBN 0-226-61596-0
(paper : alk. paper)
1. Medicare—Political aspects—United States.
[DNLM: 1. Medicare. 2. Financing, Government—United States. 3. Health
Care Costs—United States. 4. Health Policy—United States. 5. Politics—
United States. WT 31 O115m 2003] I. Title. II. Series.
RA412.3 .O24 2003
368.4'26'00973—dc21
2002014255

To my family,
Barbara, Herb, and Beth Oberlander,
and Krista Perreira

CONTENTS

ACKNOWLEDGMENTS

My interest in health politics began when I was an undergraduate at the University of North Carolina at Chapel Hill. That interest was generated by my studies with Professor Joel Schwartz. After failing to get into Professor Schwartz's popular class on politics in the Soviet Union, I settled for a class he taught on health care politics. I did not take the class expecting very much. I knew absolutely nothing about the subject, and in 1987, health care reform was hardly a significant issue in American politics. But the class opened my eyes, and I eventually dropped my previous concentration in Middle Eastern politics to study health policy. In recent years, I have had the pleasure of coteaching that same class here at the University of North Carolina at Chapel Hill with Joel. He and his wife Myrna are special friends. I am indebted to Joel for setting me on this path and for sharing his passion both for teaching and reforming American medical care.

My greatest intellectual and professional debt is to Ted Marmor. I arrived as a graduate student at Yale University not knowing much about Medicare and even less about squash (Ted's real passion). I still don't know anything about squash, but thanks to Ted, I have managed to learn about Medicare. Ted has read this manuscript countless times at every stage, from my first scribblings to the final draft, always with critical suggestions for revisions and an editor's eye for clarity (I am resisting the temptation to therefore hold him responsible for all the mistakes contained herein). Ted has taught me a tremendous amount about health politics, Medicare policy, the welfare state, and most importantly, not to lose sight of why I got into this field. He is both a close friend and a frequent collaborator, and I am fortunate to have him as both. This book never would have happened without Ted's encouragement and guidance.

I have greatly benefited from the expertise and commentary of Larry Brown and Joe White. I have learned much from their scholarship on health politics and both of them offered extensive comments on the penultimate draft of the book. Timothy Jost and two reviewers for the University of Chicago Press read the entire manuscript with care and provided a number of useful suggestions for revision. David Mayhew, James Morone, and Mark Schlesinger also provided close readings and extensive comments on earlier drafts. I owe each of them a special debt: David Mayhew for teaching me about Congress, James Morone for turning me on to the historical movement in political science, and Mark Schlesinger for sharing his understanding of Medicare policy. The book is much better for the time and effort that all of these people have taken to share their thoughts with me.

At the University of North Carolina, I have been fortunate to be in the Department of Social Medicine, where I have enjoyed the company of a terrific group of colleagues: Larry Chuchill, Giselle Corbie-Smith, Alan Cross, Arlene Davis, Gordon DeFriese, Sue Estroff, Gail Henderson, Nancy King, Bill Lachicotte, Don Madison, Joe Morrissey, Tom Ricketts, Des Runyan, Barry Saunders, Sohini Sengupta, Jeffrey Sonis, Ron Strauss, and Keith Wailoo. I have also had the assistance of a number of members of a wonderful administrative staff over the years: Judy Benoit, Allan Christman, Leslie Cornell, Becky Eatmon, Jackie Jones, Terri McGowan, and Lisa Perry. Social Medicine has always provided an intellectually exciting, warm, and personal environment. In return, I promise to clean my office one day (really!).

I want to give special thanks to Kathy Griggs, my current administrative assistant, who provided much-needed emergency aid in preparing the manuscript for publication during the frenzied final months. I also wish to thank two wonderful research assistants, Laura Sutton and Rebecca Matteo, for all of their work on this project. Becca got me out of numerous quagmires as the final deadline approached, and her research efforts were invaluable.

The Robert Wood Johnson Foundation supported me as a Scholar in Health Policy at the University of California, Berkeley. I thank them, and the Robert Wood Johnson program at Berkeley, for providing me with the time and resources to pursue this and other projects. I also benefited greatly from a research fellowship in governmental studies at the Brookings Institution.

A number of friends helped me though graduate school and beyond, among them Terri Bimes, Simon Evenett, Paul Frymer, Bowen Garrett, Laurie Goldsmith, Leon Jourolmon, Lucia Kerpel, Andrew Levy, Ed Pickens, Michael Schoenbaum, David Solar, Andrew Solares, Xin Sun, Sinan Utku, Mort Webster, Daniel Weissman, Gerald Williams, and Lareef Zubair. I thank everyone for making life interesting and for being dependable accomplices in distraction.

This book is dedicated to my family. My parents, Herb and Barbara Oberlander, deserve special thanks; without their never wavering support, I would not have been able to do this. My sister, Beth Oberlander, has always been there for me, and I am eternally grateful. And my wife, Krista Perreira, has been a patient, loving, and caring partner. She has made my life a joy.

Finally, the University of Chicago Press has been a wonderful partner in shepherding me through the publication process. I want to thank Ben Page, the series editor, for his trenchant observations and suggestions for revision. Special thanks as well to John Tryneski, my editor, for his support, insights, and exhortations, and to Erik Carlson for his copyediting expertise.

Introduction

On September 14, 1995, Republican congressional leaders unveiled their plan to overhaul Medicare, the federal health insurance program for elderly and disabled Americans. Emboldened by their first congressional majority in four decades and early legislative successes, the Republican leadership proposed the most sweeping changes in the program's history.[1] They sought to end Medicare's status as a budgetary entitlement by imposing a cap on program spending. They called for a reduction in Medicare expenditures of $270 billion over seven years, a 30% decrease that represented the largest spending cut in Medicare's history. And they proposed transforming Medicare into a competitive market by expanding beneficiaries' options to leave the traditional Medicare system for private health insurance plans.

Newt Gingrich, Speaker of the House of Representatives, promoted Medicare reform as a centerpiece of the Republican legislative agenda, "the heart of this fight" to balance the federal budget.[2] In so doing, he ignored the advice of Republican National Committee chairman Haley Barbour. Barbour warned that Medicare was "the Achilles heel" of the Republican revolution and urged the party to leave it alone until after the 1996 national elections.[3] Gingrich instead launched a full-scale public campaign—complete with pretested communication strategies devised by political consultants—to enact Medicare reform.[4] Having witnessed, and indeed helped to orchestrate, the demise of the Clinton administration's health plan during 1993–94, Gingrich took care not to repeat the admin-

1

istration's perceived mistakes in "losing" health care reform. He moved to neutralize opposition from interests adversely affected by the Medicare changes while securing unanimity on the issue in his own party, both aims that had eluded President Clinton during his failed quest for health reform.[5] The speaker's political acumen in organizing the Medicare campaign was widely praised.[6] California congressman Bill Thomas, chair of the influential Subcommittee on Health of the House Ways and Means Committee, touted the Gingrich plan as "bold, innovative . . . and radical" and confidently declared that transforming Medicare was part of the Republican "mandate of the year."[7]

No amount of legislative bravado or advice from political consultants, though, could temper the inevitable controversy that followed the proposals to change the course of one of the nation's most popular social programs. President Clinton, who had been grasping for political relevance after the humbling Democratic losses in the 1994 congressional elections, seized on the issue. The president vowed he would "not let . . . [the Republican party] destroy Medicare."[8] Congressional Democrats similarly found a unified opposition voice in decrying the Republican Medicare proposal as turning back "30 years of trust and 30 years of hope that our parents and our grandparents will always have the health care they need."[9] The usually gentlemanly Sam Gibbons, the ranking Democratic member of the Ways and Means Committee, personified the intensity of the Medicare reform debate. Upset with strict limits on the time Republican leaders allocated for congressional debate over their Medicare plan, Gibbons angrily confronted subcommittee chair Bill Thomas in a House hallway and grabbed him by the necktie.[10]

Democrats charged the $270 billion cut in program spending would devastate Medicare. Such a sizable and rapid decrease in program spending, they claimed, would inevitably erode the access of the elderly to physicians and hospitals, harm the quality of medical care for Medicare beneficiaries, and ultimately drive both patients and physicians out of the traditional Medicare program and into private insurance plans. Senate minority leader Tom Daschle warned that, if implemented, the Republican proposals would trigger a "Medicare meltdown."[11] Moreover, Democratic politicians charged, the large Medicare spending cuts were not required by the program's financial condition. Instead, the Republicans were using Medicare savings to fund tax cuts for the wealthy.[12] Some Democrats also argued Republican proposals went too far in pushing program beneficiaries into HMOs and in opening up Medicare to private insurance companies more interested in making profits than in providing health care. Senator Edward Kennedy, a longtime Democratic leader on health issues, acerbically remarked that "the Republican Medicare plan may be heaven for the health insurance industry, but it is hell on senior citizens."[13] One Democratic congressman explained that the Republican party's traditional label, GOP (Grand Old Party), now stood for "Get Old People."[14]

Republicans responded that the sweeping changes were necessary to restore Medicare's financial solvency and keep pace with innovations in the private health care system. They accused Democrats of launching a "Medi-scare" campaign that stirred seniors' anxieties while ignoring the imperatives of program reform. In the absence of corrective action, they noted, federal actuaries predicted the Medicare hospitalization insurance trust fund would "be exhausted," and thus unable to cover all benefit payments, as early as 2002.[15] Republicans argued their reforms were critical to avoid the impending trust fund "bankruptcy crisis." Congress had to "save" Medicare, Congressman Bill Thomas warned, "because if we do nothing, Medicare will go broke."[16] The view that reform was both necessary and beneficial to Medicare was embodied in the title Republicans chose for the 1995 legislation: the Medicare Preservation Act.

Republican lawmakers also contended that substantial reductions in program spending could be achieved without harming beneficiaries if Medicare embraced the managed care strategies of the private market. The Republican leadership portrayed Medicare as an outdated insurance model that reflected the health care system of 1965 rather than 1995, even invoking the movie *Jurassic Park* to warn about the dangers of not modernizing the programmatic "dinosaur."[17] They pointed to rates of growth in program spending exceeding those in the private sector during the mid-1990s. And they asserted opening Medicare up to private insurance plans would not, as Democrats charged, destroy the program but instead improve it by increasing the range of choices available to Medicare enrollees and enhancing quality and innovation in delivery of medical services.

The flurry of charges and countercharges left the press scrambling to figure out who was right and who was guilty of demagoguery. Many journalists found both sides of the debate to be misleading. Linda Killian captured the conventional wisdom, writing that "neither the Democrats nor the Republicans were telling the whole truth. Most of what was going on was political posturing aimed at "scaring old people" and winning political points."[18] Others simply confessed confusion about the true impact of the proposed changes.[19] In the meantime, some health policy analysts accused both Democrats and Republicans of ignoring the real issue: how to absorb the baby boom generation retiring into Medicare beginning in 2010. For these analysts, the baby boomers were a "fiscal tsunami" threatening to overwhelm the program and the federal budget.[20] The elderly population in the United States was projected to increase from thirty-two million in 1990 to seventy million in 2030, with an accompanying decline in the ratio of workers per retiree. A growing number of observers warned these demographic trends made Medicare "unsustainable in its current form."[21] Reforms even more sweeping than the Republican legislative proposals—such as transforming Medicare into a full-fledged voucher system for private health insurance—were said to be required if the program was to remain viable into the twenty-first century. Without such changes, these analysts concluded, Medicare was destined to face an unappealing future of staggering increases in payroll taxes on workers or draconian cuts in benefits for retirees.[22]

Other analysts rejected such projections as far too gloomy. The baby boomers could be absorbed into Medicare, as well as Social Security, without radical reform. They pointed out that European countries had successfully dealt with similar demographic pressures without the dire socioeconomic consequences forecast for the United States by some observers.[23] Moreover, these nations had successfully controlled health spending for older populations without resort to market solutions such as vouchers.[24] There was no reason, they argued, Medicare could not similarly cope with the medical care costs of the baby boom while preserving its programmatic structure.

THE MEDICARE CONSENSUS

Lost in the political din surrounding the Republican proposals and the contested demographic assessments of policy experts was a simple, and yet stunning, historical fact. The debate over federal health insurance for the aged that had ended with Medicare's enactment in 1965 had been reopened.

During the late 1950s and early 1960s, Medicare emerged as a polarizing issue in American politics. Its legislative history bore the markings of a deeply ideological and partisan debate that reflected persistent divisions over the failed national health insurance proposals of the Truman administration.[25] The conflict was settled only by the decisive results of the 1964 elections, which generated broad liberal Democratic majorities in both the House of Representatives and the Senate. The new majorities enabled President Lyndon Johnson to sign Medicare legislation into law after a decade of stalemate.

What made the events of 1995 so extraordinary is that in the three decades following the program's enactment, the polarizing politics of

Medicare's beginnings had largely disappeared. Medicare had become a cherished institution in American political life, broadly popular with the public as one of the few acknowledged successes of the American welfare state.[26] The popularity of Medicare was due in no small part to the substantial number of American families it helped. By 1995, the program provided health insurance to thirty-three million elderly and four million disabled Americans, as well as coverage for kidney dialysis to 230,000 patients with end-stage renal disease.[27] The reach of Medicare, though, extended far beyond these beneficiaries, as the program touched children and grandchildren who were spared the burden of paying for much of their parents' or grandparents' medical care. Moreover, unlike other government programs serving only the poor, such as Aid for Families with Dependent Children (AFDC), Medicare's constituency had a middle-class identity, since all retirees were eligible for the program regardless of income.

As a consequence, the controversy surrounding Medicare's enactment disappeared once the program began operation. Political opponents learned if not to like the program, then at least to accommodate to its popularity. Members of Congress, as well as presidential administrations, vied to be seen as program friends and, more crucially, to avoid being seen as threatening Medicare, lest they pay a heavy price at election time. The policy world similarly accommodated to Medicare's popularity. Health care analysts focused mainly on incremental proposals to make Medicare's existing structure more efficient and equitable.[28] Improving Medicare, rather than replacing or fundamentally restructuring it, defined the agenda for both policymakers and analysts.

The central thesis of this book is that from 1966 to 1994 Medicare was governed by the politics of consensus. Medicare politics in this period was consensual in three key respects. First, policymaking took on a predominantly bipartisan character, with Democrats and Republicans generally agreeing on the direction of program reform even as that direction changed substantially over time. Second, bipartisanship produced a quiescent politics, in which Medicare policymaking rarely triggered large-scale public debates. Third, and most critically, with no debate over ideology or programmatic first principles, from 1966 to 1994 a de facto consensus prevailed in favor of maintaining Medicare as a universal, federally operated government health insurance program. That consensus was liberal at its core. Consequently, programmatic stability meant that, over time, the Medicare consensus continued to embody a liberal vision of the program's structure, philosophy, and goals.

I argue that the Medicare consensus fractured in 1995, in the midst of a

Central thesis of this Book.

radically altered political environment and a changing health system, leading to the rise of a new politics of Medicare. The difference was not merely substantive, though the consensus that Medicare should operate as a universal public program eroded substantially. In 1995, Medicare entered (or more precisely, reentered) a different *type* of politics. Bipartisanship gave way to sharp partisan differences, quiescence was replaced by controversy, and political conflicts were played out against the backdrop of a public debate as Medicare moved from the margins to the center of American politics. The scope of conflict in Medicare after 1995 thus differed fundamentally from the politics of 1966–1994.[29] It was wider, with an engaged public, and the very nature of the program was at stake, echoing in important ways the political contest over Medicare's enactment. As consensus fractured, then, Medicare moved in 1995 from a politics of program management (low-visibility, low-conflict, low-ideology politics that focuses on program administration and efficiency with limited public involvement) to a politics of program transformation (high-visibility, high-conflict, ideological politics that centers around efforts to change—or enact—a program's basic structure and philosophy with a greater role for the public).[30]

How Medicare politics operated during the era of relative consensus and stability, as well as the fracturing of that consensus in 1995 and its aftermath, is the subject of this book. To be sure, the politics of consensus in Medicare was far from absolute. There have always been opponents of Medicare in Congress.[31] During the era of consensus (1966–94) there were important disagreements between Democrats and Republicans on particular issues—for instance, in deciding who should bear the financial burden of rising Medicare costs. Republicans generally were more willing to impose higher costs on elderly beneficiaries, while Democrats looked first to physicians and hospitals as targets of spending cuts. There were also some instances where Medicare politics sparked public controversy, such as the repeal of catastrophic health insurance in 1989 and, despite strong protests from the medical profession, the introduction of professional standard review organizations in 1972 to monitor the medical care delivered to Medicare beneficiaries. And during the program's first three decades, there were substantial changes in program policy, including the transformation of Medicare's regulation of health care providers.

Yet Medicare's congressional enemies were few in number and their political impact negligible. And differences between Democrats and Republicans were tightly contained within the bipartisan consensus that favored maintaining Medicare as a federally operated health insurance program. Medicare's popularity created a political boundary few politicians were willing to cross to challenge its fundamental purposes or organization. In the end, the common ground between Republicans and Democrats on Medicare policy during 1966–1994 was far more impressive and consequential than their differences. The policy changes adopted in Medicare reform were generally supported by both parties. And public controversy over Medicare was an exception to a norm of quiet politics and policy-making that operated far from the public eye. In a political environment bounded by consensus, policy reforms of tremendous importance, such as the introduction of hospital and physician payment reforms during the 1980s, were enacted with little controversy and scant public notice.[32]

It is also crucial to recognize that in key respects the Medicare consensus, throughout both periods of maintenance and fracturing, was an elite rather than public phenomenon. As I will show, the public did not support critical elements of the consensus that federal policymakers held strongly, such as the limits on Medicare benefits. And the unraveling of consensus in 1995 with the rise of the market as a model for Medicare reform occurred as a result of changes among policymakers and politicians, not the mass public. Chapter 6 examines the significance of this split between the public and political elites for democratic accountability in Medicare politics.

MEDICARE: THE THREE TENSIONS

My intent is not to write a comprehensive history of Medicare. There are many subjects and events of significance not treated here. Rather, the aim is to analyze Medicare's political development from 1965 to 2002. I therefore selectively highlight patterns and episodes representing central themes in Medicare politics. It is my hope that these themes will provide a useful framework for the reader to consider the politics of Medicare.[33]

Despite its prominence in American politics and health care policy, there has been relatively limited scholarly attention to the politics of Medicare after 1965. A substantial literature on Medicare policy has developed, produced predominantly by economists, but it has little to say about program politics.[34] Political scientists have conducted important research on particular periods and issues in Medicare politics.[35] Yet there is currently no work that comprehensively investigates Medicare politics across all three decades of its operation and the different dimensions of program policy.[36] This book is intended to redress that void. I weave together existing studies of Medicare with my own research in a new synthesis in order to tell the story of the program's political development. I also seek to illuminate areas of Medicare politics remarked upon only rarely—in particular, the dynamics surrounding program financing and benefits (previous studies of Medicare have by and large focused on the politics of cost control). My analysis therefore relies extensively on primary sources, including government documents, congressional hearings, and interviews.[37]

I believe Medicare's political development can be understood as the working-out of a series of tensions that were embedded in the program's structure at its inception. The story of Medicare's first three decades is how these tensions played out in program politics. The first tension was a gap between the promise of Medicare (as understood by the public) to protect the elderly against the potentially devastating costs of medical care and the actual performance of the program in delivering on that promise.[38] From the beginning, Medicare had substantial gaps in its coverage that left elderly, and later disabled, beneficiaries vulnerable to the high costs of health care. As medical care inflation in the United States marched steadily upward, and as Medicare's benefit coverage failed to expand to keep pace with the standard in the private insurance market, the gap between promise and performance widened. Still, despite the reputed political power of the elderly, there were no significant expansions of Medicare benefits for two decades. Medicare quickly acquired a political reputation after its enactment as a financially "uncontrollable" program. That stigma defused pressures for enhancing Medicare benefits. The rise of a private supplemental insurance market for Medicare beneficiaries further weakened pressures to expand program benefits. And when expansion finally came in 1988 with the addition of catastrophic health insurance, it proved remarkably short-lived. Congress repealed catastrophic insurance in 1989, only sixteen months after its celebrated passage.

A second tension stemmed from the commitment of the federal government to pay the medical bills of Medicare beneficiaries while simultaneously relinquishing control over the total bill for the program and abdicating any authority to regulate payments to medical providers. In large part, this represented a compromise born of the political circumstances of Medicare's enactment. Program architects sought to assuage the opposition of the medical profession to federal health insurance and secure its cooperation in implementing Medicare. They consequently forswore any government intention to intervene in or regulate private medical practice. As Medicare costs rose and consumed an increasing proportion of the federal budget, and as government deficits worsened, the compromise proved untenable. During the 1980s, federal policymakers reasserted control over payment policies at the expense of hospitals and physicians through the adoption of a new Medicare regulatory regime. Yet the new regulations did not impose an aggregate budgetary cap on Medicare spending or alter the budgetary entitlement status of the program. As a result, the federal government still found itself with an open-ended commitment to Medicare spending, helping set the stage for the political turbulence that hit Medicare in the mid-1990s.

Finally, the third tension was produced by a social insurance financing system adopted to assure Medicare's political success, but that proved to be ill suited to a health insurance program. In their efforts to create a politically strong program, the architects of Medicare looked to an established American model of a successful welfare state program: Social Security. Social Security politics was marked by high levels of public support, a history of benefit and eligibility expansions, and a reputation for administrative efficiency. Much of Medicare's structure, including its payroll tax and trust fund financing arrangements, was therefore copied from old-age insurance.[39] These social insurance arrangements have played an important role in generating Medicare's public popularity and political stability.

However, in contrast to customary assumptions about the immense political advantages shared by universal social insurance programs, Medicare did not follow the expansionary course of Social Security.[40] From the beginning, its political and financial fortunes were more troubled than those of Social Security. The logic of social insurance, including universal eligibility and contributory financing through payroll taxes, produced different patterns in Medicare from the ones it produced in Social Security. In large part, this was because Social Security's financing arrangements had an unexpected effect on Medicare. Adapting a financing system for pensions premised on stable actuarial projections of future costs to the highly uncertain world of medical care insurance turned out to be much more difficult than anticipated. Consequently, the unintentional effect of Medicare's financing arrangements was to trigger a series of intermittent financial shortfalls in the program, culminating in the widely publicized bankruptcy crisis of 1995–96. These financing arrangements created a recurrent pattern in Medicare's development, as moments of financial shortfall were accompanied by political efforts to change the direction of program policy. Yet while earlier financing shortfalls were dealt with through bipartisan, consensual policy remedies, the 1995 shortfall generated considerable controversy and partisan acrimony. Medicare's financing arrangements, particularly its actuarial forecasts, have influenced political debate by focusing attention on the program's long-term financial condition. As a result, much of the present indictment against Medicare is in fact based on predictions about its future performance. The foundation of Medicare's stability has now become the object of programmatic conflict.

The bulk of this book is devoted to tracing these themes in the politics of benefits, regulation, and financing across Medicare's development and within the broader contexts of national politics and medical care policy in the United States. During the past three decades, there have been substantial changes in the political environment of federal health insurance. The federal deficit became a national preoccupation and the balanced budget a prominent rallying cry, and in 2000 the budget returned, albeit temporarily, to surplus.[41] The Democratic Party first lost its hold on the presidency that had begun with Franklin Roosevelt, and then its control of Congress. The liberalism of Lyndon Johnson's Great Society gave way to the conservative revolution of Ronald Reagan and Newt Gingrich. Support for the welfare state and federal activism in social policy was shaken by economic anxiety and ideological skepticism about the limits of government.[42] The private health care system was transformed by the rise of managed care, and market-based reform has become an influential model for health policy. How these changes in American politics and the health care system have shaped Medicare is a vital part of my story.

Medicare also offers a window through which to view the policy dilemmas presently confronting American medical care: the tension between guaranteeing an individual right to medical care and constraining the social costs of that care, the proper balance between government and private sector responsibility in organizing and delivering medical care, the choice between competitive and regulatory visions for health care cost containment, and the potential and limits of managed health care. Nor are these issues simply a road map to the past. The future of American medical care, as well as Medicare, will be determined by how public and private policymakers reconcile these dilemmas.

THE POLITICS OF MEDICARE POLICY

In addition to providing a historically informed account of Medicare's policy development, a second objective of this study is to analyze the politics of Medicare policy: that is, to identify the patterns of political influences on Medicare policymaking and the political sources of stability and change in Medicare and to explain who gets what in program policy and why. The study of Medicare's development also has much to contribute to our understandings of the character of health care and welfare state politics in the United States. This book, then, is a work of political analysis as well as policy history.

Scholarship on Medicare frequently separates policy from politics.[43] Economists writing about Medicare usually ignore politics altogether, analyzing Medicare reform without any reference to ideology, political institutions, or normative issues. And when they do write about politics, they often portray it as an unwelcome guest that ruins the best-laid plans of researchers who formulate rational, objective Medicare policy. There is palpable frustration among many policy analysts that the political world does not accept the expert advice that the policy world offers it. This leads some analysts to the technocratic conclusion that the program would be better off if Medicare policy were quarantined from political influence, for instance, by adopting cost controls that are determined by automatic formulas rather than by politicians.[44] I do not believe that this disjunction between policy and politics is intellectually defensible. The technocratic perspective ignores the role that politics plays in highlighting the values inherent in public policy choices, which are objective only in textbook accounts of the policy process.[45] In addition, useful policy analysis ultimately depends on political analysis of feasibility and implementation, just as good political analysis depends on policy knowledge. This book makes the case that understanding Medicare requires attention both to policy and politics.

concept

Some readers will look to this book for a single, overarching theory of Medicare politics. They will be disappointed—and they should be. Political scientists generally divide into two intellectual camps. The first, monotheorists, believe that diverse political behavior can be explained by a single elegant and coherent theory, and that case studies offer the opportunity to verify the explanatory power of their chosen model. Political analysis is for them the search for a grand unifying theory.[46] Polytheorists draw on multiple theories to explain political behavior and commonly find that there is no single politics of public policy. Rather, different policies are associated with different politics. This book falls squarely in the camp of polytheorism, a well-established tradition in policy studies.[47] I believe that Medicare provides strong support for the necessity of theoretical pluralism. Given the size, complexity, and diversity of a program like Medicare, it would be surprising indeed to discover a single theory that explained everything. I have not found such a theory, nor do I believe one exists. The richness of Medicare politics defies such artificial simplification. In fact, an important argument of this book is that the program has three main types of politics: the politics of benefits, the politics of regulation, and the politics of financing. Each of these policy arenas has generated its own political patterns, with variations in interest group power, government authority, the scope of conflict, and the direction of program reform. Consequently, multiple theoretical lenses are necessary if Medicare's political picture is to be properly developed.

There is no shortage of assertions about how various forces influence democratic policymaking and how American political institutions operate.[48] Scholars variously contend that public policy is dominated by pressure groups, responds to the preferences of citizen opinion, or reflects the dictates of national political culture.[49] Each of these schools of thought provides a different explanatory lens through which to view Medicare politics. Here I highlight two key lenses. *Interest group* theorists argue that the permeability of American political institutions to social interests, the dependence of politicians and political parties on campaign funds, and the indifference of the mass public to many issues in which pressure groups have a concentrated stake make interest groups the primary influence on policymaking.[50] In Medicare, interest group explanations predict that Medicare policy should follow the political preferences of the major groups representing elderly beneficiaries as well as hospitals and physicians: the American Association for Retired Persons, the American Medical Association, and the American Hospital Association.

In contrast, *public opinion* theorists assert that the public governs public policy. These scholars point to the prevalence of polling in contemporary politics as a source of pressure on policymakers.[51] Polls reinforce electoral incentives for politicians to respond to or anticipate public opinion; otherwise, they risk being seen as ignoring the public's will. In Medicare, public opinion explanations predict that program policy should conform to the public's preferences, with popular reforms adopted in response to citizen pressure and measures lacking public support blocked for fear of incurring public wrath.

Medicare offers an inviting opportunity to investigate the validity of public opinion and interest group claims against evidence from one of the nation's most significant public programs. To what extent are the hypotheses generated by these theories supported by the Medicare case? Readers can make their own judgments throughout the narrative. Chapter 6 offers my analysis of how these and other political forces have influenced Medicare.

MEDICARE AND THE WEAK AMERICAN STATE

I also draw on the Medicare case to challenge conventional assumptions about American politics and public policy. It is widely held that American government is weak. The foundations of this assumption are familiar. The

United States is commonly viewed as a nation with "less structural basis for [government] autonomy than in any other modern [democracy]."[52] Political power in the American system is fragmented and dispersed through a system of checks and balances, separation of powers, and federalism.[53] There is no guarantee a president's proposals will gain congressional approval. Not only may the opposition party control Congress, but members of the president's own party may also act independently, and often in defiance, of the president's agenda.[54] State governments pursue their own policy initiatives, often absent coordination with other states or federal policymakers. At the national level, opponents have ample opportunities to block legislation, which in order to become law must pass through a gauntlet of legislative committees and subcommittees, votes in both the House and Senate, conference committees, presidential approval, and constitutional sanction from the Supreme Court.[55] By international standards, American political parties are impotent.[56] They cannot control which candidates run for office under their banner and do not consistently produce party discipline on votes in Congress. Bureaucrats, a critical source of policy expertise and innovation, enjoy much less standing and independence in the United States than in other countries.[57] As the authors of a standard health politics textbook ruefully conclude: "The American system is designed to default to inaction. A decentralized Congress, an overrated and weakened presidency, budget deficits, distrust of bureaucracies, erosion of state budgets, and federal preemption of state regulation . . . dictate policy gridlock."[58]

Finally, American political culture is said to be characterized by a deep-rooted suspicion of government and centralized power that traces back to the American revolution against British rule.[59] Americans are viewed as inherently distrustful of the national government's power and authority, a "polity suspicious of its own state"[60] with a citizenry that "fears public power as a threat to liberty."[61] Americans cling to the paramount values of individualism and freedom, putting their faith in the market rather than government institutions. Proposals to expand the government's authority and social responsibilities run into an ideologically reflexive fear of public power trampling individual rights. The political scientist Samuel Huntington speaks of an American creed whose "distinctive aspect is its antigovernment power. Opposition of power, and suspicion of government as the most dangerous embodiment of power, are the central themes of American political thought."[62] In contrast to European nations that recognize the necessity and virtue of strong government action, the United States is characterized by an "ideology of statelessness."[63]

As a result of this weakness and fragmentation, American politicians are often alleged to be incapable of pursuing policies that reflect the public interest or concentrate public authority. Interest groups fill the void left by political parties to influence legislators.[64] Private interests take advantage of the fragmented policy process to advance their own agendas. Policymaking responds to the electoral resources of powerful groups and the calculations of politicians seeking reelection, rather than rational and objective analysis of social problems. Congress is said to be uninterested in or incapable of substantive policymaking[65] And the boundaries of political culture as well as the absence of an established bureaucracy severely limit the scope of policy options available to government actors.[66]

This image of American government has been influential in thinking about health policy. Both scholars and journalists frequently claim, for example, that national health insurance is not feasible in the United States. American political institutions, they argue, are simply incompatible with the political conditions necessary to operate a government-administered health insurance program. American government lacks the political capacity and administrative competence that parliamentary regimes rely on to manage health programs effectively. These institutional barriers are said to be reinforced by an individualist, antigovernment political culture that will not permit a national health insurance system similar to those in other industrial democracies.[67]

In the case of Medicare, however, the stereotype of American government does not fit the facts. I argue here that Medicare provides substantial evidence contradicting simplistic notions of a "weak" government in the United States. Federal policymakers have often acted independently and pursued policies against the interests of private groups associated with the program. Contrary to conventional thinking, neither interest groups representing the elderly nor hospitals and doctors have consistently dominated Medicare policy. Furthermore, Congress has been an important source of Medicare policy innovation, contradicting the prevailing image of the national legislature. Medicare policymaking has often resembled "congressional government," a neglected story for those in search of the American state. And the success of Medicare regulatory reforms in slowing the growth in program costs during the 1980s and 1990s belies assertions that American political institutions are incompatible with effective management of government health insurance.[68] While critics were busy explaining why cultural and institutional barriers meant the United States would never adopt the centralized cost containment mechanisms common in European and Canadian health systems, Medicare was busy adopting many of the same mechanisms.

This is not to argue that American health politics is identical to those in other countries, or that Medicare precisely resembles other national health programs. There are critical differences between Medicare's programmatic arrangements and the "international standard."[69] As I will explain, these differences may grow even larger over time. And the character of American health politics is obviously exceptional; the United States remains the only industrialized democracy without universal health insurance. Yet careful analysis of Medicare's experience does suggest that American political institutions and culture are compatible with a broader array of policy responses than is usually assumed. It also suggests analysts have seriously underestimated the political capacity of U.S. government. Standard assumptions about what is feasible in American health policy, which are currently structuring debate over Medicare reform, require fundamental rethinking.

A ROAD MAP

My story begins with the origins of Medicare. Chapter 2 traces Medicare's roots in the struggles over national health insurance during the early decades of the twentieth century. I then review the emergence of the Medicare strategy and the legislative battles over Medicare's enactment during the 1950s and 1960s. Finally, I highlight Medicare's political foundations and the tensions embedded in its programmatic structure. The next three chapters analyze how these tensions played out in Medicare politics during its era of consensus, from 1966 to 1994. Chapter 3 explores the politics of Medicare benefits. I explain why the dominant pattern has been the absence of benefit expansions despite substantial gaps in Medicare insurance coverage. I then examine the rise and demise of the largest attempted benefit expansion in Medicare's history: catastrophic health insurance. Chapter 4 examines the dynamics of Medicare financing. The focus is on the political effects of the program's social insurance funding arrangements, including trust funds and actuarial forecasts. I explain how these arrangements have influenced program politics and explore their relationship to changing directions in Medicare reform. Chapter 5 examines the politics of Medicare regulation. I trace how the initial compromise prohibiting federal activism in regulating Medicare payments to hospitals and doctors gave way to a more aggressive regulatory regime during the 1980s.

For much of the program's history, the politics of benefits, regulation, and financing was consensual. Chapter 6 analyzes the politics of consensus in Medicare, summarizing the patterns in the previous chapters and investigating the major influences on program policymaking. As noted earlier, the era of consensus in Medicare politics ended abruptly in 1995. The core principles of Medicare—government health insurance, federal administration, universal entitlement—that have remained stable since 1965 are now subject to serious challenge. Chapter 7 explains why consensual politics broke down and analyzes the fight over Medicare reform. I discuss how the political foundations supporting the program have changed during the past three decades, examine the state of Medicare politics in the 2000 elections and beyond, and conclude by speculating on Medicare's future and the potential emergence of a new program consensus.

TWO

Medicare's Roots

THE ELUSIVE SEARCH FOR NATIONAL HEALTH INSURANCE

Medicare is unique among international health insurance programs. "No other industrial democracy," Theodore Marmor observes, "has compulsory health insurance for its elderly citizens alone, and none started its program with such a beneficiary group."[1] This peculiarity raises a series of critical questions regarding Medicare. Why did the United States enact federal health insurance for the aged? What were the objectives of those who crafted the Medicare strategy? And why has Medicare not developed into a broader system of national health insurance similar to those in other countries? This chapter examines the origins of Medicare in earlier campaigns for national health insurance, the rise of health insurance for the elderly as an issue in American politics, the legislative battle over Medicare's enactment, and the program that emerged in 1965 as a result of that battle. The aim is to provide the reader with sufficient historical background to evaluate the subsequent changes and continuities in program politics that are the focus of this book. An extensive literature already exists on the history and politics of Medicare's enactment.[2] This chapter is intended only as a summary for those unfamiliar with the story. Readers who are already familiar with Medicare's origins may wish to skip ahead to the chapter's last section, "Medicare as Law: Programmatic Foundations and Assumptions," which connects themes in Medicare's beginnings and program structure to its subsequent political development. There I elaborate on the core elements of the Medicare consensus that I argue governed program politics for the next three decades.

THE LOST REFORM: NATIONAL HEALTH
INSURANCE 1912–52

Medicare represented the fourth wave in the campaign for national health insurance in the United States.[3] That campaign commenced during the Progressive Era. Government health insurance had already arrived in Europe, with Germany, in 1883, the first European country to introduce compulsory sickness insurance for its workers.[4] England followed several other European nations in 1911 with its own health insurance program. These developments came at "a moment when American politics was peculiarly open to foreign models and imported ideas."[5] The German and English programs drew the attention of American Progressives, who regarded illness as a prime cause of poverty and dependence, as well as a consequence of the inevitable strain of working life in industrial society. Though some workers received coverage through fraternal societies and unions, the vast majority of Americans lacked adequate protection against the costs of illness, and blacks, women, and the elderly were commonly excluded from existing plans.[6] Moreover, while scientific advances were creating a growing demand for modern medicine, the cost of new advances put medical services increasingly beyond the reach of workers.[7] As a solution, Progressive reformers proposed compulsory health insurance in conjunction with a cash sickness benefit to replace lost wages, hoping to make medical care affordable for industrial workers and to provide protection from the financial costs of illness.

In 1912, Theodore Roosevelt ran for president as the nominee of the Progressive Bull Moose Party on a platform that included support for compulsory health insurance for industrial workers. Roosevelt, however, lost to Woodrow Wilson, depriving national health insurance of the executive-level political sponsorship it had enjoyed in Germany and England.[8] Instead, pressure for compulsory health insurance in the United States was generated from outside the government.[9] The American Association for Labor Legislation (AALL), founded in 1906 as a Progressive political group of academic social scientists, labor activists, and lawyers, led the movement for health insurance. The AALL combined the Progressive aspiration for scientific study of social problems with an ambitious political agenda to ameliorate the impact of industrialization. Within its first decade, the group successfully pressed states to adopt workmen's compensation legislation. When the AALL had secured reforms covering industrial accidents and was "flushed with a seemingly easy victory . . . Medical care insurance was selected as the next logical step for action."[10]

Since social welfare provision in the United States remained the province of the states, the AALL focused its energies on a state-by-state campaign. In 1915, the organization drafted a model bill for compulsory health insurance to submit to state legislatures and initiated a "public education" campaign, replete with data demonstrating the need for medical care coverage, to mobilize popular support for health insurance. Most surprising, in view of the subsequent history of American health politics, the AALL's efforts initially drew support from the primary organization of the medical profession, the American Medical Association (AMA). Many AMA leaders at the time were supportive of public health reforms and sympathetic to the Progressive cause. They believed compulsory health insurance would inevitably come to the United States, as it had to Europe. The AMA's Committee on Social Insurance reasoned that physicians' "blind opposition, indignant repudiation, bitter denunciation of these [compulsory health insurance] laws is less than useless; it leads nowhere and it leaves the profession in a position of helplessness as the rising tide of social development sweeps over it."[11] And in a 1916 editorial that echoed the thinking of much of the medical establishment, the *Journal of the American Medical Association* praised national health insurance, gushing that "no other social movement in modern economic development is so pregnant with benefit to the public."[12] The appointment of I. M. Rubinow—a former physician and the preeminent American scholar as well as advocate of social insurance—as executive secretary of the AMA's Committee on Social Insurance symbolized its leadership's enthusiasm for government health insurance.[13]

Buoyed by the cooperation of the medical profession, the AALL believed its campaign for health insurance legislation would follow the same quick path to enactment as workmen's compensation. Yet though the AALL's model bill was introduced in fifteen states and commissions to study health insurance were formed in ten states, by 1920 the momentum for compulsory health insurance had stalled.[14] Not coincidentally, that was also the year the AMA, influenced by a revolt from conservative segments of its membership against the national leadership, formally declared its opposition (which would last for over half a century) "to the institution of any plan embodying the system of compulsory [medical] insurance . . . controlled or regulated by any state or the federal government."[15] Changing medical opinion also reflected concerns that compulsory health insurance would threaten the growing incomes and social status American physicians were achieving, fears fed by exaggerated accounts of the plight of European doctors under national health systems. A political chasm had been exposed between the medical profession's urban, academic-medicine-oriented national leadership, such as AMA president Dr. Alexander Lambert, and county and state medical societies led by rural and private practice physicians.[16] Enraged over the leadership's initially favorable stance on compulsory insurance, the 1920 meeting of the AMA's House of Delegates "periodically broke into the chant 'Get Lambert!'"[17]

In addition to the turnaround by organized medicine, national health insurance fell victim to a wide array of interests whose hostility to compulsory health insurance the AALL seriously underestimated, including the insurance industry, pharmaceutical companies, employers, and American Federation of Labor leader Samuel Gompers.[18] The American entry into World War I sealed the fate of health reform. Opponents exploited the association of health insurance with the enemy, Germany. Fredrick Hoffman, vice president of Prudential Insurance and a prominent spokesman for opponents of health reform, declared national health insurance a "German plot."[19] The AALL did not effectively counter this opposition, "naively assuming that a reform which they thought should be deemed good by everyone would triumph on its own merits."[20] The AALL's "coolheaded language of expertise was no match for the fiery rhetoric of its detractors."[21]

The chances for enactment of compulsory health insurance were even more remote in the 1920s. Conservative Republicans consolidated their hold on national politics, while Progressivism gave way to a public philosophy critical of government activism and content with the prevailing social order. The identification of compulsory health insurance with Bolshevikism following the 1917 Russian Revolution, which triggered fears of a socialist takeover in the United States, further hindered reformers. "The methods of rational argument and statistical persuasion that the AALL preferred," the historian Beatrix Hoffman notes, "were impotent against the rhetorical frenzy of the Red Scare."[22] The activists of the AALL were branded traitors, and national health insurance "un-American."[23] Before World War I, American reformers looked to Europe for policy models and argued that the United States had fallen behind its European counterparts in social policymaking, necessitating emulation of foreign-born solutions. Now, that strategy had backfired. "The very explicitness of the American borrowings," Daniel Rodgers explains, "the theme of backwardness that social insurance proponents favored, their arguments from preexisting European experience, all became potential liabilities after 1917."[24] In the United States, national commissions continued to study issues pertaining to the costs and distribution of medical care, but in the absence of favorable political circumstances, health insurance remained a topic for intellectual inquiry rather than government action.[25]

The second wave of the campaign for national health insurance arrived with the 1932 election of Franklin Roosevelt and the coming of the New Deal. Though unemployment and old-age insurance were clearly priorities in the midst of the depression, the political climate of federal activism appeared favorable for enactment of health reform.[26] The mandate of the Committee on Economic Security, created by FDR in 1934 to draft a program of social insurance legislation, included health insurance. Nevertheless, the ensuing Social Security legislation of 1935, which encompassed old-age pensions, unemployment insurance, and aid for dependent children, omitted any program of national health insurance. The original Social Security bill had contained a single line authorizing a study of health insurance, prompting a concerted campaign of AMA opposition. Edwin Witte, executive director of the Committee on Economic Security, famously remarked "that little line was responsible for so many telegrams to the members of Congress that the entire social security program seemed endangered until the Ways and Means committee unanimously struck it out of the bill."[27] The Roosevelt administration, fearing the controversy would jeopardize the enactment of the Social Security bill, refrained from pushing health insurance and ordered the line removed from the legislation. National health insurance became "the lost reform," politically abandoned by reformers and consequently separated from the creation of the modern American welfare state.[28]

The failure of the Roosevelt administration to sponsor national health insurance legislation in 1935 did not, however, spell the end of New Deal health insurance proposals. In 1939, Senator Robert Wagner of New York introduced a national health bill, and beginning in 1943, the introduction of national heath insurance legislation in Congress, cosponsored by Senator James Murray of Montana and Representative John Dingell, Sr., of Michigan, both Democrats, became an annual event. The Wagner-Murray-Dingell legislation was significantly broader than Progressive Era proposals, providing for comprehensive health insurance for all residents of the United States, not just industrial workers.[29] Yet FDR remained reluctant to endorse the proposals, though there were indications he intended to push anew for health insurance legislation following his reelection to a fourth presidential term in 1944.[30]

The third campaign for national health insurance coincided with the ascension of Harry Truman to the presidency following Roosevelt's death. Truman supported the Wagner-Murray-Dingell bill and thus became the first American president to formally endorse national health insurance legislation, though his commitment to health reform also served a strategic purpose. He pressed for its enactment in 1948, aware that it had no chance of passing the Republican Congress—infamously labeled the "do-nothing Congress"—but knowing its obstruction could be a valuable issue in that year's presidential contest.[31] After winning the 1948 election, Truman again pressed for the enactment of his health insurance program. However, despite favorable public opinion and presidential sponsorship, national health insurance failed to pass the Congress.[32] The medical profession launched an intense political effort against the legislation, taking advantage of emergent Cold War fears to redefine the health debate as an issue of socialized medicine. The AMA declared that supporters of the Truman plan included "all who seriously believe in a Socialistic State. Every left-wing organization in America . . . [and] the Communist Party."[33] The AMA, though, went far beyond crude red-bashing in its offensive against the Truman administration: in 1949 it launched the most expensive lobbying campaign in American history to raise public anxieties about national health insurance; warned that government insurance would inevitably erode the quality of medical care by giving the government control over medical services, overcrowding hospitals, and reducing the incentive for physicians to provide quality care;[34] forged political alliances with hundreds of pressure groups, such as the Chamber of Commerce, which found common cause in its distrust of big government; and, in conjunction with the insurance company Blue Cross, pushed the alternative of private ("voluntary") insurance as the "American way."[35]

The reputed political power of the AMA had reached its zenith. The organization was widely regarded as the most powerful interest group in America, combining vast financial resources, the willingness to engage in hardball tactics, and the social prestige as well as ubiquitous presence of physicians across the country.[36] In 1950, AMA efforts were credited for defeating at least three congressmen who had been prominent supporters of the Truman plan.[37] Yet the attention lavished on the AMA obscured another principal barrier to enactment of national health insurance: the political strength of the conservative coalition of southern Democrats and Republicans that, in effect, ruled Congress. Indeed, even though Democrats held a majority in both the House and Senate after the 1948 elections, the conservative coalition constituted the de facto majority. The coalition rejected not just health insurance, but much of President Truman's Fair Deal domestic agenda.[38]

THE ORIGINS OF THE MEDICARE STRATEGY

By 1950, then, national health insurance was already "three times denied."[39] The failure of Progressive, New Deal, and Fair Deal health insurance proposals persuaded advocates to reconsider their strategy. Those advocates included two officials in the Truman administration, Wilbur Cohen and I. S. Falk, who had been involved in developing health insurance proposals since the 1930s. Cohen and Falk, advisers to Federal Security Agency administrator Oscar Ewing, sought to reverse reformers' losing fortunes by "resurrect[ing] health insurance in a dramatically new and narrower form."[40] They developed a plan to provide federal health insurance to beneficiaries of Social Security payments for Old Age and Survivors Insurance (OASI). In June 1951, Ewing publicly announced a proposal for sixty days of hospital insurance a year for the seven million elderly retirees receiving Social Security, saying "it is difficult for me to see how anyone with a heart can oppose this."[41]

The Medicare strategy rested on three crucial decisions. The first involved restricting the beneficiaries of government health insurance to the aged. In contrast, the Truman proposals had sought to provide health insurance to the entire population. By restricting the scope of eligible beneficiaries, the architects of Medicare intended to capitalize on the political appeal of the elderly, who were demonstrably "sicker, poorer, and less insured than other adult groups."[42] Private health insurance had spread to American workers in the 1940s and 1950s as a result of union gains and federal tax policies. But most of the aged lacked adequate medical insurance. The elderly had medical expenses twice as high as those under sixty-five and were twice as likely to have a chronic illness, and their hospital stays were on average twice as long as those of younger Americans.[43] Yet fewer than half of retirees had any form of health insurance, because they commonly lost their employment-based group coverage and affordable individual policies were rarely available.[44] For commercial insurers, the expensive medical needs of the elderly simply made them a bad risk not worth insuring. And by the late 1950s, Blue Cross and Blue Shield had raised premiums substantially for retirees, in response to intense competition from commercial insurers who attracted younger, employed groups by offering them lower premiums.[45] The elderly confronted an obvious dilemma: "Among the groups least well covered by the rapid postwar expansion of private health insurance were retired people. They were generally ineligible for group plans designed for employed persons; if they had belonged to group plans during their working years, their participation was often terminated upon retirement; [and] to obtain coverage on an individual basis, they had to pay high rates that were often prohibitive to those living on retirement incomes."[46] It was little wonder, then, that "the need for a means of paying the high cost of medical care echoed throughout . . . [1950s congressional] hearings as the single greatest problem of America's retired generation."[47]

The substantive case for a public health insurance program for the aged was buttressed by an equally compelling political logic: namely, the opportunity to attach federal health insurance to the favorable public reputation of the elderly. Unlike other groups, such as able-bodied working-age adults, the elderly "could be presumed to be both needy and deserving . . . through no fault of their own."[48] Consequently, a health insurance program for the elderly would command public sympathy and thereby circumvent traditional American skepticism toward government-provided social welfare assistance.[49] It would also take advantage of building national attention to the "problems of aging" that surfaced during the 1950s at both the state and federal level. Wilbur Cohen later observed that federal health insurance for the aged drew on middle-class anxieties about having sufficient resources to care for their parents while paying for their children's college education.[50] The architects of the Medicare strategy were tired of losing battles over health care reform. From their perspective, focusing on the elderly offered the best opportunity to enact federal health insurance; Cohen called the proposal for the aged "America's form of national health insurance."[51]

The second decision was to build on the existing Social Security system. Social Security provided Medicare's architects with their formative administrative and political experiences.[52] They attributed the widespread public support the program enjoyed by the late 1950s to its social insurance design and concluded that health insurance could be enacted and successfully operated if built on the same model.[53] Social Security paid out benefits as an earned right to workers who had contributed payroll taxes to the program, giving old-age pensions the appearance of private insurance. Beneficiaries believed they deserved benefits because they had paid for them, just as individuals purchased private insurance coverage through payment of premiums.[54] In a country traditionally skeptical of public assistance to "undeserving" recipients, the notion that social welfare benefits had been earned was politically crucial. Medicare advocates also favored the social insurance approach in order to avoid establishing a means-tested program, which they regarded as demeaning to those forced to demonstrate eligibility. A Florida retiree, appearing before the Senate Special Committee on Aging, dramatically echoed their concerns about means-testing federal health insurance, testifying: "I live with my wife and my income is $1500 a year. Well, we are old people and we don't require much. . . . We don't eat much so we get by in a manner. But I want to ask you . . . what do we do if something happens and we need medical care on $1500 a year? . . . I will have to seek some charity institution and submit to the humiliation of what they call a necessity, and pronounce to the

Old Age and Survivors Ins.

whole world that I am only a pauper, a beggar. Now if I alone were involved in this personally, I might suffer it. I would take it and swallow it. But if my children are brought into that, then I say, 'No, never.' I would rather die than submit to that humiliation and that degradation."[55]

The legitimacy of Social Security made it possible to provide health insurance without the usual stigma associated with welfare programs. Proponents were eager to wrap Medicare in the popularity of old-age insurance, promoting the slogan "health insurance through Social Security."[56] Both the eligibility and financing of Medicare were linked to the OASI program, which paid pensions to retirees and their survivors. As with OASI, Medicare would be financed from employer and employee payroll taxes paid into an earmarked trust fund. Retirees who qualified for OASI benefits would automatically be eligible for hospital insurance. However, the political benefits of relying on Social Security carried a substantial cost. Only seven million elderly, out of a total population of twelve and one-half million aged, would have been eligible for Medicare in 1952, since only those seven million were then receiving Social Security benefits. Federal health insurance, already restricted to those over sixty-five, would not reach almost half of the elderly population.[57]

The third decision of Medicare strategists was to restrict the scope of benefits. The Truman national health program provided for comprehensive coverage of hospital, medical, dental, and nursing home costs. In contrast, the first Medicare proposal offered only sixty days of hospitalization coverage a year. By limiting Medicare benefits, advocates hoped to weaken opposition from the medical profession (physicians' services were not covered) and fiscal conservatives who objected to the expense and tax burden of federal health insurance. Given political constraints, the goal was to protect the elderly from financial catastrophes resulting from medical care, and hospitalization represented the largest threat of such a catastrophe. Medicare's designers understood the limitations of their proposal but believed such limits were the political price that had to be paid to win enactment of federal health insurance.[58] Yet the name "Medicare" connoted, incorrectly, government insurance coverage for a broad range of medical care services. "Hospicare" would have been a more appropriate name for the proposed program.[59]

In sum, the narrowing of the Truman national health insurance proposal into Medicare reflected an incrementalist strategy of "consensus-mongering."[60] The aim was to identify less controversial problems and more politically feasible solutions than had previous health insurance proposals. However, despite their carefully crafted strategy, there would be no easy consensus on Medicare.

The Legislative Contest: Medicare, 1957–65

The 1952 elections foreclosed any immediate possibility of Medicare's enactment. The Republican Party gained majorities in both the Senate and the House of Representatives, and the national political mood moved in a conservative direction. Dwight Eisenhower came to the presidency on a Republican Party platform that condemned federal health insurance proposals for their "crushing cost, wasteful inefficiency, bureaucratic dead weight, and debased standards of medical care."[61] In 1954, the Democrats regained control of both houses of Congress. Still, the prospects for Medicare were not favorable. The Democratic majority in Congress did not produce a liberal programmatic majority capable of enacting federal health insurance for the aged. The House Ways and Means and the Senate Finance committees, the two committees with primary jurisdiction over Social Security legislation, offered substantial resistance. Lacking presidential sponsorship, a committed programmatic majority, and the endorsement of key committees, Medicare had no chance of becoming law during the Eisenhower administration.[62]

Congressional consideration of Medicare began in 1957 with the proposal of a bill by Representative Aime Forand (Democrat, Rhode Island). In 1958, Ways and Means began hearings on Medicare, but the Forand bill, opposed by Arkansas Democrat Wilbur Mills, the new committee chair, did not make it out of committee and was again rejected the following year.[63] Yet the Forand hearings made health insurance for the aged a public issue. As a consequence, the same political cleavages that had characterized the Truman insurance proposals re-formed. The AMA had ignored Medicare at the start, believing that with the defeat of the Truman plan it had once and for all defeated national health insurance.[64] By 1958, the AMA had taken notice. David Allman, AMA president, declared the Forand bill "at least nine points evil and one part sincerity."[65] The medical profession, seeing a threat to its professional and financial sovereignty, as well as an opening wedge to a national health insurance system, denounced Medicare as an unwarranted intrusion of the government into private medical practice. The AMA argued rather dubiously that "the aged as a group are substantially better off on average than younger Americans" and cited an equally dubious study by the Health Insurance Association of America that predicted without government action, 90% of the elderly would be covered by private insurance by 1970.[66] In order to attract the support of conservative interest groups, the AMA framed its opposition in ideological terms, warning in the midst of the Cold War that health insurance for the aged represented the first step to national socialism.[67]

The Medicare strategy of liberal reformers therefore did little to calm the ideological tenor of the medical profession's exaggerated rhetoric. Under the Medicare proposals, the existing organization of medical care in the United States would be maintained and physicians would remain private entrepreneurs. However, to the AMA, federal health insurance for the aged still constituted "socialized medicine" and, above all, a dangerous first step toward national health insurance. The magnitude of the threat ascribed to Medicare by the medical profession was illustrated in a 1962 speech recorded for the AMA by Ronald Reagan, as part of a home lobbying campaign known as Operation Coffee Cup. Reagan urged Americans to voice their opposition to health insurance for the aged: "Write those programs now; call your friends and tell them to write them. If you don't, this program, I promise you, will pass just as surely as the sun will come up tomorrow. And behind it will come other federal programs that will invade every area of freedom as we have known it in this country. Until one day . . . we will awake to find that we have socialism. And If you don't do this, one of these days you and I are going to spend our sunset years telling our children and our children's children what it once was like in America when men were free."[68]

The AMA mobilized against Medicare in the late 1950s and 1960s as it had earlier organized against the Truman proposals, lobbying Congress, attempting to influence public opinion, and courting allies of its past struggles against national health insurance, including the American Hospital Association and various business organizations. On the other side, labor rallied to Medicare's cause, with the AFL-CIO the most prominent proponent (forming the National Council of Senior Citizens to lobby for the program).[69] With the two sides of the dispute over national health insurance reconfigured, the debate over the appropriate role of the federal government in health insurance reopened. The narrowing of national health insurance failed to prevent controversy from surrounding federal health insurance for the aged. However, the Medicare strategy succeeded in shifting the terms of the debate. "It was," as Theodore Marmor argues, "one thing to write off socialism, but the risks of writing off the aged would give the wise politician second thoughts."[70]

The AMA's political attacks actually raised the public profile of Medicare. Moreover, a series of public meetings in thirty-eight cities between 1959 and 1961 by the newly formed Special Senate Subcommittee on Aging, chaired by Pat Macnamara (Democrat, Michigan) and including Senator John F. Kennedy, generated substantial publicity across the country.[71] The Eisenhower administration remained staunchly opposed to the Forand bill, echoing the AMA's argument that it needlessly abandoned voluntary insurance.[72] But the administration came under increasing pressure from Vice President Richard Nixon, who feared the impact that doing nothing would have on his 1960 presidential bid, to announce its own proposal, which it put forward in February of 1960.[73]

By that point, the pressure for federal health insurance for the aged was also sufficiently strong to prompt a counterproposal from congressional conservatives. It came in the form of a bill, sponsored by Senator Robert Kerr of Oklahoma and Wilbur Mills, proposing expanded federal aid to states providing medical care assistance to the elderly poor.[74] The Kerr-Mills bill, consistent with the Eisenhower administration's plan, provided for federal matching grants of 50%–80% of the costs to participating states and promised broader benefits than the Medicare proposals.[75] The dynamics of the 1960 presidential election campaign drove congressional action. Influenced by the public opinion polling of Louis Harris, the Kennedy campaign identified medical care for the aged as an ideal issue to distinguish its candidate from Richard Nixon. John F. Kennedy accordingly made Medicare one of the major themes of his campaign, pushing for a plank favoring the legislation at the Democratic convention and at a special session of Congress held in August of 1960.[76] Kennedy's emphasis on the issue enhanced Medicare's position on the national agenda, which in turn generated the pressures that helped lead to the passage of Kerr-Mills.

The AMA, after initial reluctance to endorse any bill at all, reconsidered and supported Kerr-Mills as a preferable alternative to Medicare. Wilbur Cohen, one of Medicare's architects, actually helped draft the legislation at Senator Kerr's request, arguing that it represented "a step up the ladder" on the way to a Social Security—style health program for the aged.[77] However, for members of Congress opposed to such a program, Kerr-Mills was not to be a first step, but a final step to avoid passage of Medicare. Kerr-Mills won out over Medicare in 1960, as it passed both houses of Congress and Eisenhower signed the legislation. Vice President and presidential aspirant Richard Nixon hailed the apparent defeat of Medicare, arguing "The American people . . . do not want, they must not have, a compulsory health insurance plan forced down their throats . . ."[78] But Kerr-Mills failed dismally in practice, as many states did not participate in the program; by 1965 only five states accounted for 90% of Kerr-Mills funds.[79]

Kennedy's victory over Nixon in the 1960 presidential elections gave

Medicare the presidential sponsorship it had lacked during the Eisenhower years. In his first state of the union address, on January 30, 1961, President Kennedy called for enactment of "measures to provide health care for the elderly . . . this year."[80] The administration's Medicare bill, sponsored by Senator Clinton Anderson of New Mexico and Representative Cecil King of California, provided for 90 days of hospitalization coverage, 240 days of home health services, 180 days of nursing home care, and outpatient diagnostic services. The administration launched a public campaign in favor of Medicare, culminating in a series of rallies and a nationally televised appeal in 1962.[81]

Kennedy's efforts, however, failed to secure Medicare's enactment. Program advocates considered the president's public relations campaign for Medicare a disappointment. And as during the Truman years, presidential sponsorship again proved to be an insufficient condition for the adoption of federal health insurance. Kennedy, like Truman before him, lacked a firm programmatic majority in Congress. The conservative coalition of southern Democrats and Republicans in Congress remained strong enough to frustrate much of the liberal domestic agenda. Moreover, Medicare still lacked the approval of Ways and Means chairman Wilbur Mills, who feared the fiscal consequences the program would have on Social Security solvency, as well as a majority on the full committee—derided by program advocates as the "In No Way and by No Means Committee"—without whose support the legislation could not reach the floor.[82]

The landslide victory of Lyndon Johnson over Republican Barry Goldwater in the 1964 presidential election guaranteed Medicare's passage. Medicare now had not only presidential sponsorship but also a clear programmatic majority in both houses of Congress. The wide margins of Democratic control (295-140 in the House, 68-32 in the Senate) brought enough liberals into Congress to break the grip the conservative coalition had held on federal health insurance since the New Deal. Yet the circumstances of the Johnson victory caught Medicare advocates unprepared. For over a decade, they had pursued a strategy of securing passage of an incremental program of federal health insurance limited to hospitalization coverage for the elderly. Now, when the stunning electoral outcome permitted a broader vision, Medicare advocates stuck to their original proposal, which had been conceived at a time when the political constraints on Medicare were far stronger than they were in 1965. The Johnson administration proposal thus maintained the Medicare strategy of securing maximizing consensus on minimum benefits as a prelude to future expansion. In the 1965 version of the King-Anderson bill, Medicare coverage remained restricted to sixty days of hospitalization benefits and sixty days of nursing home care.[83]

Whereas supporters of Medicare did not alter their strategy, Republicans perceived that Medicare's passage was now inevitable and rushed to avoid being seen as obstructionists. They criticized Medicare for offering inadequate benefits. John Byrnes, ranking Republican on Ways and Means, offered his own bill for a voluntary program of federal payments to subsidize the purchase of private insurance by the elderly. The program's benefits were much broader than Medicare, covering physician and pharmaceutical expenses in addition to hospital costs.[84] Byrne's proposal, supported by the House Republican leadership, would be financed from general revenues (two-thirds of the funding) and beneficiary premiums.[85] The AMA was slower to grasp the new political landscape that made Medicare's passage inevitable. They offered Eldercare, a state-administered program to subsidize the purchase of private health insurance for the elderly poor. It essentially maintained the failed Kerr-Mills approach, and apart from the AMA and its two congressional sponsors, "no one in Congress took . . . [Eldercare] . . . very seriously."[86]

The final Medicare legislation embodied an ingenious combination of all three proposals. Wilbur Mills, knowing he could no longer stop Medicare, decided to shape its passage. Mills used his position as chair of Ways and Means to create a legislative package that had not been previously considered by any of the major actors. Mills combined what were seen as mutually exclusive alternatives, the Johnson administration, AMA, and Republican bills, together into a "three-layer cake" of hospital insurance for the aged (Medicare part A), a voluntary program of physicians' insurance for the elderly (Medicare part B), and an expanded Kerr-Mills program of federal assistance for state medical services payments for the poor (Medicaid). By shifting from "opponent to manager," Mills defused criticisms that Medicare's benefits were too limited and "forestalled subsequent demands for liberalization."[87] Under the expanded legislation, insurance for physicians' services was funded by general revenues and beneficiary premiums, preempting its expansion through the Social Security system (which Mills opposed), and Medicaid coverage of the nonaged poor removed a potential source of pressure for national health insurance.[88] The move stunned both Medicare opponents and proponents. Wilbur Cohen, then assistant secretary for legislation in the Department of Health, Education, and Welfare, perhaps the most influential individual shaping Medicare since its beginnings in 1951 and a skilled political operator in his own right, believed that: "It was the most brilliant legislative move I'd seen in 30 years. The doctors couldn't complain because they had been carping about Medicare's shortcomings and about it's being compulsory. And the Republicans couldn't complain, because it was their own idea. In effect, Mills had taken the AMA's ammunition, put it in the Republicans' gun, and blown both of them off the map."[89]

The contest over Medicare thus ended with a broader government role in health insurance than anyone had anticipated. Not only would the federal government provide hospitalization coverage to the elderly, but it would also operate a program of physicians' insurance and subsidize state medical assistance to the poor. Moreover, the final bill extended Medicare coverage initially to the nearly three million seniors who were not eligible for Social Security.[90] The final outcome was significantly less than the Truman administration's proposals for national health insurance, but substantially more than Medicare strategists had believed possible. Recognizing its origins in the campaign for national health insurance, Lyndon Johnson signed the legislation on July 30, 1965, in the presence of Harry Truman in Independence, Missouri, declaring that the enactment of Medicare meant that "no longer will older Americans be denied the healing miracle of modern medicine. No longer will illness crush and destroy the savings that they have so carefully put away over a lifetime so that they might enjoy dignity in their latter years. No longer will young families see their own incomes, and their own hopes, eaten away simply because they are carrying out their deep moral obligations"[91]

MEDICARE AS LAW: PROGRAMMATIC FOUNDATIONS AND ASSUMPTIONS

Tables 2.1 and 2.2 summarize Medicare benefits and other programmatic arrangements as enacted in 1965. It is worth unpacking the assumptions behind these arrangements, since they have proven to be both a crucial source of stability and, since 1995, conflict in program politics. The first assumption was that a central goal of Medicare should be to bring the elderly into the mainstream of American medicine. Medicare's benefits, reimbursement mechanisms, administration, and structure of insurance all reflected prevailing practices in the American private sector. In concrete terms, this meant that Medicare followed the Blue Cross–Blue Shield model of health insurance; emphasized coverage for acute-care services; contracted out program administration to private insurers; and paid physicians and hospitals generously, retrospectively, and with little oversight. In all of these features, Medicare adopted the norms of the private insurance industry. The embrace of mainstream medicine served the dual purpose of assuring the elderly access to high-quality medical care and re-

Table 2.1 Medicare Program Benefits and Eligibility, 1965

Part A, hospitalization insurance
    60 days of inpatient hospital services during any spell of illness, after $40
        deductible (deductible scheduled to rise over time to reflect increases in
        average cost of hospital day)
    30 days of hospitalization coverage subject to daily coinsurance set at 25% of
        the deductible
    Posthospital extended care (nursing home) services up to 100 days
    Posthospital home health visits up to 100 days
    Outpatient hospital diagnostic services, with 20% coinsurance
    Lifetime maximum of 190 days of inpatient hospital psychiatric services
Part B, supplementary medical insurance
    Payment for 80% of "reasonable charges" for physicians' services for office
        visits, surgery, and consultation, after $50 deductible; 20% coinsurance
        required
    Home health services up to a 100 days a year; 20% coinsurance required.
    Outpatient psychiatric and mental health treatment (with 50% copayment
        required)
    X-ray tests and diagnostic laboratory tests
    Ambulance service
Eligibility
    Eligibility for hospitalization insurance initially open to all persons age 65 and
        above; after 1968, eligibility restricted to individuals 65 and older who were
        entitled to Social Security benefits; part B was a voluntary program, open to
        anyone eligible for Medicare part A who paid the required premium

Note: "Spell of illness" was defined as beginning the first day of hospitalization and ending with the
close of the first period of 60 consecutive days during which the patient was not hospitalized or enrolled
in an extended care facility.

assuring the medical profession that the federal government would not disrupt the existing order in the health system.[92] The latter goal proved particularly critical given growing sentiment within the medical community in 1965 for a physicians' strike against Medicare.

The second assumption was that Medicare should provide all elderly with the same health insurance coverage. Regardless of their income before or after retirement, all beneficiaries would participate in the same program with the same benefits, premiums, and cost-sharing requirements. Higher-income elders, for example, would not be charged any additional fee for Medicare coverage. This principle of universalism reflected the thinking of Medicare proponents, who embraced social insurance and disliked means-tested programs. But it also reflected the public impression of the elderly as, on average, a substantially poor and dependent group (a largely accurate impression in 1965) that deserved sympathy and warranted government assistance. Because the elderly were generally assumed

Table 2.2 Medicare Financing and Provider Payment Arrangements, 1965

Financing
    Medicare part A funded through an earmarked payroll tax on workers and
        their employers; the payroll tax was initially set at .35% on an earnings base
        of $7,800 and was scheduled to rise in five increments to .80% in 1987
    Medicare part B funded through equal contributions from general revenues
        and monthly premiums (initially 3$) paid by beneficiaries; the premium was
        to increase over time so that the sum of beneficiary contributions would be
        maintained at a level of 50% of the total costs of part B
Provider payments
    Hospitals reimbursed retrospectively for their "reasonable costs"
    Physicians reimbursed retrospectively for "reasonable charges"
Program administration
    Claims processing and bill auditing contracted out by the Bureau of Health
        Insurance of the Social Security Administration to private fiscal
        intermediaries and carriers (mostly Blue Cross and Blue Shield plans)

to be poor, only limited public support existed for differentiating among income groups within the retired population.

The third assumption, held strongly, though silently, by the architects of the Medicare strategy, was that Medicare represented a beginning, not an end. As Robert Ball, former commissioner of the Social Security Administration and an important participant in crafting the Medicare strategy, later explained: "we all saw insurance for the elderly as a fallback position, which we advocated solely because it seemed to have the best chance politically . . . we expected Medicare to be the first sep toward universal national health insurance, perhaps with 'Kiddicare' [federal insurance for children] as the next step."[93] On this score, at least, the AMA had been right. Despite their repeated denials during the Medicare debate, advocates envisioned the program as an opening wedge to secure a universal health system for the whole population. It should be remembered that the political world of Medicare advocates was that of New Deal and Great Society liberalism. Given this background, and the politics of the time, from their perspective it was reasonable to assume that liberal predominance would continue and provide opportunities in the not-so-distant future for reformers to expand on Medicare to achieve their ultimate goal, national health insurance.[94]

The final assumption reflected in the 1965 legislation was that Medicare should be a system of public health insurance guided by the federal government. In the parlance of contemporary health policy, Medicare was created as a single-payer program, similar in structure and philosophy to

Medicare
could have
went another
way. So
why this
way?

the health systems employed in Canada and in parts of Western Europe.[95] This was not, however, the only programmatic form that Medicare could have taken. One alternative would have been to provide elderly retirees with federal subsidies or vouchers to purchase insurance policies from private, commercial insurers. In fact, conservative and medical profession critics of Medicare legislation favored this approach.[96] Why, then, did Medicare emerge in 1965 as a public insurance program, rather than as a system of subsidized private insurance? The most important reason is that the shape of Medicare was largely determined by the preferences of the social insurance advocates who designed it. And they assumed public insurance offered the appropriate, efficient, and just model of medical care delivery. The glaring inability of the private insurance market to cover retirees at the time of the Medicare debate reinforced that view. The most compelling argument that the medical care needs of the elderly could be met only though public insurance was simply that the market had already had its opportunity and had failed. - market failed

Finally, in the aftermath of the 1964 elections, the programmatic structure of Medicare mirrored the dominant political current of liberalism. The structure of a public program carries with it a corresponding set of values, social commitments, and political dynamics. In 1965, the properties of public health insurance matched the values and social commitments favored by the liberal majority of policymakers: universalism, government responsibility for social welfare provision, and public accountability. At a different time, under different ideological and electoral circumstances, Medicare might well have been a very different program.

In subsequent years, the idea that federal health insurance for the elderly should be organized as a public, single-payer program was institutionalized in American politics and policy. That idea became what I term here the "Medicare consensus." During the next three decades, that consensus and the assumptions underlying it were not seriously challenged. In fact, the choices made in 1965 became so deeply embedded in American political thinking that the Medicare consensus was rarely openly acknowledged. Yet political quiescence should not be mistaken for lack of influence. Indeed, I argue here that the consensus is the key to understanding contemporary conflicts over Medicare, as well as emergent directions in program development.

The next three chapters explore Medicare's development from 1966 to 1994 in three major areas of program policy: benefits, regulation, and financing. Although there were conflicts in all three areas, often driven by tensions in Medicare's original structure, those conflicts were largely contained within broad agreement that Medicare should remain a public insurance program. The politics of Medicare as single-payer insurance—with more limited benefits and weaker cost controls than health systems in other countries, and with an inherently unstable financing system—is the first part of my story.

THREE

Going Nowhere

THE POLITICS OF BENEFITS

For many Americans, Medicare represents a promise to the nation's elderly of protection against the potentially devastating costs of medical care. Medicare, though, has never fully delivered on that promise. The program has greatly increased the access of the elderly to medical services and shielded many aged and disabled persons, as well as their families, from the economic insecurities of illness.[1] Yet persistent gaps in Medicare benefits have left beneficiaries vulnerable to the rising costs of American medical care. Medicare pays for less than half of all health expenses incurred by the elderly, a burden that falls heavily on the elderly poor.[2] And despite frequent assertions that the United States cannot afford to maintain the level of coverage the program now provides, Medicare benefits are hardly generous compared to the international standard. Senior citizens in other industrial democracies, who generally receive coverage in universal health insurance systems rather than separate programs for the aged, are exposed to substantially less financial risk from seeking medical care than their American counterparts.[3]

This chapter explores two puzzles in the politics of Medicare benefits policy. The first is why Medicare benefits remained stable for so long despite obvious limitations and the wide gap between the program's promise to the elderly and its performance in delivering on that promise. Medicare benefits in 1995 were almost identical to those first offered in 1965. The stability of Medicare benefits during the era of program consensus is particularly puzzling given political and social forces, such as the reputed political power of the elderly, that presumably created pressures for program expansion. Yet Medicare politics was governed by a "negative consensus" that emphasized cost containment over benefits improvement despite public opinion that favored expanding Medicare benefits. The politics of consensus in Medicare benefits policy, then, reflected elite rather public attitudes. I examine the origins of that consensus and the political influences on benefits stability in Medicare.

The second puzzle concerns the one substantial reform of Medicare benefits that took place during the program's first three decades, the 1988 addition of catastrophic health insurance. Catastrophic health insurance redressed gaps in Medicare coverage that left beneficiaries susceptible to the unlimited costs of prolonged hospital stays and out-of-pocket spending on medical services. However, only sixteen months after its passage, catastrophic coverage was repealed following intense protests from segments of the elderly population. In retrospect, it is difficult to decide what is more perplexing about the catastrophic insurance case: that when significant Medicare expansion finally arrived, it came during a period of fiscal deficits and welfare state retrenchment, or that a program hailed as a major improvement in health coverage for the elderly was overturned because of opposition from the elderly. I examine the anomalous rise of catastrophic insurance as an issue in Medicare policy and argue that the same political forces that contained program expansion for two decades ultimately led as well to its demise.

THE DEVELOPMENT OF MEDICARE BENEFITS

Medicare Benefits, 1965

Medicare in 1965 was designed to cover a substantial portion of the expenses of the elderly for acute medical care. Modeled after Blue Cross and Aetna insurance plans, the core of program benefits provided protection against the costs of hospital stays and physician services.[4] Medicare did not, however, aim to pay the entire medical care bill of the elderly. Indeed, in the 1960s Medicare advocates rebutted the AMA's charges that enacting the program would eliminate the private insurance market by pointing out that "the proposed health insurance benefits would not cover . . . all the health care costs of the aged. Many aged persons will want to buy [supplemental private] insurance protection."[5] Medicare consequently had a number of significant coverage limitations (see tables 3.1, 3.2). There was no cap on the medical care expenses paid by beneficiaries ("out-of-pocket costs") and physicians were free to bill patients extra for amounts well beyond what the government paid doctors ("balance

Table 3.1 Medicare Cost Sharing for Hospitalization Insurance

YEAR	DEDUCTIBLE ($)	DAILY COINSURANCE, DAYS 61–90 ($)	DAILY COINSURANCE, DAYS 91–150 (LIFETIME RESERVE) ($)
1966	40	10	—
1970	52	13	26
1980	180	45	90
1985	400	100	200
1986	492	123	246
1987	520	130	260
1988	540	135	270
1989	560	0[a]	0[a]
1990	592	148	296
1991	628	157	314
1992	652	163	326
1993	676	169	338
1994	696	174	348
1995	716	179	358
1996	736	184	368
1997	760	190	380
1998	764	191	382
1999	768	192	384
2000	776	194	388
2001	792	198	396
2002	812	203	406

Source: Health Care Financing Administration.
Note: The deductible is for each benefit period, which starts when the beneficiary first enters a hospital and ends when there has been a break of at least 60 consecutive days since inpatient hospital or skilled nursing care was provided. There is no limit to the number of benefit periods covered by hospitalization insurance during a beneficiary's lifetime; however, inpatient hospital care is normally limited to 90 days during a benefit period, and copayment requirements apply for days 61–90. If a beneficiary exhausts the 90 days of inpatient care available in a benefit period, he or she can elect to use days of Medicare coverage from a nonrenewable "lifetime reserve" of up to 60 (total) additional days of inpatient hospital care. Copayments are also required for such additional days.
[a]The 1989 deductible for hospital insurance was applied on an annual rather than benefit period basis. Once the beneficiary paid the deductible, Medicare paid the balance of covered hospital services, regardless of the number of days of hospitalization.

billing"). After ninety days, hospitalization coverage ran out. Mental health services required a sizable 50% copayment with limits on inpatient stays in psychiatric hospitals and a $250 cap on annual outpatient services. Outpatient prescription drugs, medical physicals, hearing aids, eyeglasses, and dental care were not covered at all. And for services that were covered, beneficiaries were responsible for considerable amounts of cost sharing, including deductibles and coinsurance for both hospital and physician services that rose substantially over time.[6]

Nor did Medicare provide broad protection against the costs of chronic

Table 3.2 Medicare Cost Sharing and Premium Amounts for Supplementary
Medical Insurance (Including Physicians' Services), Medicare Part B

YEAR	ANNUAL DEDUCTIBLE ($)	COINSURANCE (%)	MONTHLY PREMIUMS ($)
1966	50	20	3.00
1967	50	20	3.00
1970	50	20	5.30
1975	50	20	5.30
1980	50	20	9.60
1981	50	20	11.00
1982	75	20	12.20
1983	75	20	12.20
1984	75	20	14.60
1985	75	20	15.50
1986	75	20	15.50
1987	75	20	17.90
1988	75	20	24.80
1989	75	20	31.90
1990	75	20	28.60
1991	100	20	29.90
1992	100	20	29.90
1993	100	20	36.60
1994	100	20	41.10
1995	100	20	46.10
1996	100	20	42.50
1997	100	20	43.80
1998	100	20	43.80
1999	100	20	45.50
2000	100	20	45.50
2001	100	20	50.00
2002	100	20	54.00

Source: Health Care Financing Administration.

illness. Home health and nursing home care were restricted to short-term posthospital rehabilitation, with no coverage for long-term care. Nursing home policy received little attention in the Medicare debate, despite the fact that by 1965 under Kerr-Mills, the joint state-federal health insurance program for low-income elderly people enacted in 1960, some three hundred thousand beneficiaries were receiving payments for nursing home care.[7] Bruce Vladeck notes that Medicare's architects, including Wilbur Cohen, feared that inclusion of nursing home benefits "would open a bottomless budgetary pit that would destroy the politically delicate budget for health insurance."[8] The reason that Medicare contained any coverage at all for nursing home services was that Cohen and others were concerned about rising hospital costs. They believed that transferring patients from hospitals to long-term care facilities in the latter stages of illness would save money—an expectation that would not be borne out.[9]

The limitations in Medicare benefits reflected both political constraints and prevailing practices in the health insurance market. Opposition from the medical profession and fiscal conservatives worried about Medicare's expense led program architects to restrict the scope of benefits. They abandoned the comprehensive medical care benefits envisioned by the Truman national health insurance proposals for Medicare's limited benefits package in the name of political feasibility. Yet in its adoption of extensive cost-sharing measures to deter unnecessary utilization of medical services and control program costs, and in its omission of coverage for a broader range of services, Medicare actually followed the standard benefits package offered by private insurers at the time.[10] The core assumption behind Medicare was that the elderly should be brought into the mainstream of American medicine, and in 1965 the mainstream of American medicine focused on acute care. There was no discussion of the possibility that the elderly had different health needs, such as a higher prevalence of chronic illness, than younger, employed populations and therefore required different health coverage.[11]

Medicare Benefits, 1966–86

The two decades following Medicare's enactment witnessed few significant changes in program benefits. A 1967 statute added a sixty-day lifetime reserve for hospitalization (along with a 50% coinsurance rate), and coverage of hospice care for terminal illness was incorporated in 1983.[12] Otherwise, benefits under Medicare part A remained unchanged. Physician service benefits were similarly stable, though over time Medicare expanded to cover a few specialty services such as podiatry.[13] There was more movement in home health care. Coinsurance requirements were removed in 1972, and the deductible, one-hundred-day limit, and prior hospitalization requirements were eliminated in 1980, though the benefit remained restricted by other means.[14]

The Addition of End-Stage Renal Disease and Disabled Patients to Medicare

Eligibility for Medicare extended beyond the aged in 1972 to encompass two new categories of beneficiaries: the disabled and end-stage renal disease (ESRD) patients. Extension of Medicare coverage to Social Security beneficiaries on disability insurance was viewed as a natural, almost automatic step by program architects, though they gave little forethought to its future costs and the different medical needs of persons with disabilities. Extending Medicare to disabled persons had been recommended by the 1965 Advisory Council on Social Security, proposed by the Johnson administration in 1967, and passed by both the Senate and House in 1970 only to be held up as part of negotiations over broader Medicare legislation in conference committee.[15] In contrast, the enactment of ERSD coverage was not anticipated at all during the Medicare debate. Instead, its addition to Medicare in 1972 was a product of "serendipity . . . [rather] than the result of a grand design."[16] And the passage of ESRD coverage was more than a little peculiar, since it represented the first and only extension of Medicare to a specific disease category.[17]

The medical procedure for dialysis had been invented in 1960, and by 1965 the Veterans Administration as well as the Public Health Service had initiated efforts to fund dialysis for patients with kidney disease.[18] In 1967 the Gottschalk committee, convened by the Bureau of Budget in response to growing awareness of the financial implications of federal involvement in dialysis, released a report that declared transplantation and dialysis effective therapies for treating ESRD. The commission recommended adding an ESRD benefit to Medicare, though it had little impact on a Congress concerned with more pressing issues in Medicare implementation.[19] The National Kidney Foundation and a small "high command" of physician kidney specialists continued to lobby Congress for federal action to increase access to dialysis for ESRD patients.[20] The group, however, emphasized adding coverage for dialysis by expanding existing federal programs (such as opening the Veterans Administration to non- veteran ESRD patients), rather than creating a new program.[21]

After 1965, introduction of legislation in Congress to increase federal funding for dialysis became an annual event, and in November 1971, the House Ways and Means Committee heard testimony about the emergent ESRD issue as part of hearings on national health insurance. The testimony of Shep Glazer, vice president of the National Association of Patients on Hemodialysis (NAPH), underscored the extent to which ESRD differed from other diseases; access to dialysis made a clearly demonstrable, dramatic, and immediate difference between life and death. Glazer implored the committee to provide government assistance: "I am 43 years old, married for 20 years, with two children ages 14 and 10. I was a salesman until a couple of months ago until it became necessary for me to supplement my income to pay for the dialysis supplies. I tried to sell a non-competitive line, was found out, and was fired. Gentleman, what should I do? End it all and die? Sell my house for which I worked so hard, and go on welfare? Should I go into the hospital under my hospitalization policy, then I cannot work? Please tell me. If your kidneys failed tomorrow, wouldn't you want the opportunity to live? Wouldn't you want to see your children grow up?"[22] In a controversial move opposed by many kidney disease advocates who worried both about the appearance of sensationalism and the consequences of failure, Glazer was then dialyzed before the committee—a move that came close to backfiring when he encountered, unbeknownst to the committee, medical complications during the procedure.[23] While the dialysis episode attracted substantial media attention and subsequently entered American political lore, there is little evidence that it was ultimately decisive in congressional adoption of ESRD.[24]

Congressional interest in ESRD continued to grow. Wilbur Mills, chair of the House Ways and Means Committee, sponsored legislation in December 1971 to provide federal financing for dialysis through a budgeted program. And in early 1972, Senator Vance Hartke (Democrat, Indiana) introduced a bill to expand access to dialysis for patients unable to pay through the Public Health Service.[25] At the same time, members of the National Kidney Foundation focused their lobbying efforts on Ways and Means and the Senate Finance Committee. The provisions of the 1972 Social Security amendments that created the Medicare ESRD program owed their existence to the prior agreement on adding the disabled to the Medicare population, thus enabling kidney disease to be seen as a disability fitting program eligibility criterion, and to horse trading between Ways and Means and Senate Finance conference committee members.[26] The Finance Committee, chaired by Russell Long, had passed a provision adding some outpatient prescription drug coverage to Medicare. However, he failed to persuade the conference committee, in the context of concerns over costs and opposition from the Nixon administration, to accept drug coverage and instead received Ways and Means's assent on ESRD, "so that the Senate came away with something."[27] Long, a supporter of catastrophic health insurance as an alternative to comprehensive national health insurance proposals that were then en vogue, viewed Medicare ESRD coverage as a demonstration of a universal health insurance system based on catastrophic insurance. "Ironically," as Senate staffer James Mongan later commented, "rather than serving as a demonstration or pilot, the ESRD legislation proved to be the last train out of the station for national health insurance. No other group has had a chance to get on board."[28] Coverage for ESRD, though, was overshadowed by the welfare as well as Medicare and Medicaid provisions of the Social Security amendments and drew little public attention until after its enactment.

The Medicare eligibility expansions to the disabled and ESRD patients significantly broadened Medicare's reach across American society and diversified its clientele to populations under age 65. By 1987, there were three million nonelderly disabled Americans on Medicare (including over one hundred thousand dialysis patients), constituting 10% of all program enrollees.[29] But while these eligibility changes brought new populations into Medicare, they were not intended to expand benefits for aged Medicare enrollees.[30] For the elderly, still the primary and most politically influential constituency in Medicare, program benefits did not increase. The most striking development in Medicare benefits for the elderly during the program's first two decades was surely the extent to which they did not develop.

Why Medicare Benefits Did Not Expand

Writing in 1973, the political scientist James Q. Wilson predicted "in time, Medicare benefits may also experience more or less automatic increases," repeating the expansionary record of Social Security.[31] According to Wilson, Medicare provided benefits to a relatively large constituency and spread program financing broadly across the population, giving legislators strong incentives to expand benefits, since they could receive political credit for such policies without fear of creating any political losers.[32] Yet expectations of automatic increases in Medicare benefits were not borne out. The failure of Medicare benefits to expand substantially in the two decades following the program's enactment was an extraordinary outcome considering the political influences favoring expansion. There were four potential sources of pressure for Medicare expansion: the popular appeal of the aged and public opinion favoring increased program benefits; the political power of organizations representing the elderly; the limited scope of program coverage; and the political strength of Medicare's programmatic structure.

The enactment of Medicare drew on the popular appeal of the elderly. Medicare advocates counted on public sympathy for the elderly to weaken the political obstacles that had previously frustrated advocates of national health insurance. The same dynamics that helped secure Medicare's enactment—the reputation of the aged for deservingness and the consequent political appeal of enacting government benefits for them—should have produced expansions of Medicare. The popular appeal of legislating benefits for the aged presumably did not end in 1965. As an existing public program, Medicare provided a high-profile, politically attractive, and administratively convenient opportunity for lawmakers to do something for the elderly. Indeed, public opinion data showed strong public support for increasing program benefits. For example, in a 1986 poll, over 80% of the public favored or strongly favored expanding Medicare, including adding

Table 3.3 Public Willingness to Pay Additional Taxes to Create a Federal
Long-Term Care Program for the Elderly

YEAR	WILLING TO PAY MORE TAXES FOR LONG-TERM CARE (%)	NOT WILLING TO PAY MORE TAXES FOR LONG-TERM CARE (%)	NOT SURE (%)
1981	49	31	20
1982	53	27	20
1983	43	32	24
1985	58	25	17
1988	71	24	5
1989	58	39	3
1990	72	25	4
1991	74	24	2
1992	73	21	3
1993	69	28	3

Source: Roper Center Public Opinion Database; surveys from Cambridge Reports Research
International, Louis Harris and Associates, EBRI, and Gallup.
Note: The 1989 survey asked specifically about raising the FICA payroll tax, and the 1990–93 surveys
asked about increasing income taxes. All other surveys asked about willingness to pay more taxes
without specifying income or payroll taxes. No data were available for 1986 and 1987.

coverage for nursing home care. And a 1991 survey found that 68% favored increasing Medicare benefits.[33] Throughout the 1980s and early 1990s, public support for establishing a federal long-term care program for the elderly remained strong, increasing as the issue gained public prominence in the late 1980s, with majorities often willing to pay additional taxes to fund the new program (see table 3.3).[34] If public policy had followed the dictates of public preferences, Medicare benefits would have expanded.[35]

The second potential influence favoring expansion was the reputed political power of the aged. While interest groups representing the aged exerted little influence on the enactment of Medicare, political organizations representing the elderly grew substantially in the years following the introduction of the program. The so-called gray lobby came to comprise a wide range of organizations, including the National Council of Senior Citizens, the Gray Panthers, the American Association for Retired Persons (AARP), the National Committee to Preserve Social Security and Medicare, and the National Alliance of Senior Citizens.[36] These groups focused largely on federal benefits for the aged offered through Social Security and Medicare.

The AARP, in particular, gained a reputation for political muscle, flexed on behalf of the twenty-eight million members it enjoyed at the close of the 1980s.[37] Founded in 1947 as a retired teachers association, the AARP in 1959 had a membership under one million but then opened itself to all occupations and maintained an important business component as a large seller of both health (underwritten by Colonial Penn) and life insurance policies to seniors. In the 1970s, the AARP was criticized for too cozy a relationship with Colonial Penn, and the group broke its exclusive ties to the insurer, leading to greater AARP involvement in Washington politics, a more liberal political stance on policy issues, and, perhaps most crucially, more legitimacy as an advocacy group.[38] By the late 1980s, the AARP had emerged as the most visible and influential interest group representing the elderly and had created an organizational structure capable of mobilizing large numbers of seniors, as well as a research department that could provide policymakers with valuable data on issues relating to senior well-being as well as Medicare and Social Security.[39] Henry Pratt, a leading scholar of old-age political groups, labeled the AARP "the largest, and probably the wealthiest," voluntary organization in the world; it had thirty-seven hundred local chapters, a paid staff of thirteen hundred, and a budget of nearly $250 million, published the largest-circulation magazine in the country (*Modern Maturity*), and offered popular product discounts and travel plans.[40] By 1990 the AARP had arguably replaced the AMA as the most prominent interest group engaged in Medicare politics.

There was good reason to believe that the AARP and other groups representing the elderly would win Medicare benefits expansions. Public policymaking in the United States frequently takes the form of "servicing of the organized."[41] Interest groups that possess the resources to monitor the policy process and influence the electoral circumstances of politicians (through campaign contributions, organizational assistance, and publicity), command a degree of deference. Aged groups, to the extent they represent a broadly based and geographically diffuse constituency, are well positioned in the American political system.[42] That position, and political deference to their influence, should have generated pressures to expand Medicare and public policies that responded to those pressures.

In addition, the elderly vote in American elections at higher rates than younger citizens. Their share of the voting electorate expanded in the years following Medicare's enactment (table 3.4). They are, as table 3.5 shows, the only age group whose voting rate in the 1990s was higher than it was in the 1960s. And those approaching Medicare eligibility, the age cohort 45–64, had the second highest voting rate in the 1990s. If politicians make policy decisions based not simply on the preferences of the general public, but on who votes, then the ballot power of the elderly should produce political pressures for benefits expansion. Indeed, interest groups for the elderly have effectively used the "electoral bluff" of the vot-

Table 3.4 Votes Cast by Persons Aged Sixty-five and Older,
as Percentage of All Votres Cast in Presidential
Elections

YEAR	PERSONS AGE 65+ AS PERCENTAGE OF ALL PERSONS OF VOTING AGE	PERCENTAGE OF VOTES CAST BY PERSONS AGED 65+
1996	16.5%	20.3
1992	16.6	19.0
1988	16.2	19.4
1984	15.7	17.7
1980	15.3	16.8
1976	15.0	16.0
1972	14.7	14.9
1968	15.8	15.4

Source: Robert Binstock, "Older People and Voting Participation: Past and Future," *Gerontologist* 40, no. 1 (2000): 18–31; and U.S. Census Bureau, Current Population Surveys.

ing power of the aged to convince "many elected officials and journalists that they ignore the interests of older people at their own peril."[43] That threat ignored the diversity of political attitudes among seniors: like that of younger Americans, individual seniors' voting behavior varies significantly along partisan, ideological, and class and income lines.[44] But the perception of the elderly as a bloc vote carried political weight among policymakers regardless of its validity. The electoral bluff of the elderly may have been a myth, but for interest groups representing the elderly, it proved a useful myth.

Third, Medicare benefits policy could have followed an expansionary course simply because of the limited scope of the original benefits package. Since Medicare coverage was severely restricted in the range of services it covered, as well as the cost-sharing requirements it imposed on beneficiaries, there was certainly ample room for improvement. As already noted, Medicare paid less than half of all the medical expenses of the aged, and for some critical services, such as outpatient prescription drugs, it paid nothing at all.[45] Furthermore, the gap between Medicare and the standard for workers in the private insurance market widened over time as the program failed to keep pace with benefits such as prescription drug and dental care coverage that became commonplace in the commercial market. In 1965, fewer than 5% of Americans with private insurance had dental coverage. By 1981, over 50% carried such coverage and over 25% had insurance for prescription drugs, a rare benefit in the private sector in 1965.[46] And the Medicare population aged considerably over the program's first twenty years, increasing the prevalence of chronic illness among enrollees and strengthening the need for more comprehensive cov-

Table 3.5 Reported Voting Rates by Age in U.S. Presidential Elections

AGE (YEARS)	1964	1968	1972	1976	1980	1984	1988	1992	1996	2000
18–24	50.9	50.4	49.6	42.4	39.9	40.8	36.2	42.8	32.4	32.3
25–44	69	66.6	62.7	58.7	58.7	58.4	54	58.3	49.2	49.8
45–64	75.9	74.9	70.8	68.7	69.3	69.8	67.9	70.0	64.4	64.1
65 and over	66.3	65.8	63.5	62.2	65.1	67.7	68.8	70.1	67	67.6

Source: U.S. Census Bureau, Current Population Survey, November 2000 and earlier years.
Note: The figures are the percentages of people in the age groups who reported that they voted in the years shown.

erage.[47] If either the popular appeal of the aged or the political power of interest groups representing the elderly had been operative forces, recognition of Medicare's limitations could have catalyzed support for expansion.

Finally, Medicare benefits might have been anticipated to expand over time because of the experience of Social Security. The two programs share several key features. In both Social Security and Medicare, the elderly are the primary constituency, eligibility is universal and irrespective of income, and the primary financing mechanism is payroll taxes.[48] In the case of Social Security, these features coincided historically with a consistent pattern of benefits expansion. During its first four decades, policymaking for Social Security yielded increasing levels of benefits, new categories of benefits as well as beneficiaries, and political consensus on program growth.[49] Insofar as Medicare's financing and eligibility structure resembled that of Social Security, its benefits pattern could have been expected to follow a similar course of expansion.

Yet during Medicare's first two decades, this expansion never came, and despite programmatic similarities, Medicare did not follow the path of Social Security. Why did Medicare benefits fail to expand? There are three main explanations: the dominance of fiscal concerns in program policy, the development of private supplemental insurance, and confusion of beneficiaries regarding Medicare coverage.

Fiscal Concerns

Fiscal issues cast a shadow on Medicare politics from the start. Medicare quickly acquired a reputation in Congress and the executive branch as an uncontrollable burden on the federal budget. In its first years, Medicare costs far outpaced the actuarial projections that had been made at the time of its enactment. In 1968 and 1969, program costs rose at an average annual rate of 40.2%, and by that latter year, Russell Long, chairman of the Senate Finance Committee, warned that Medicare had become a "runaway program."[50] Early experience with cost overruns in the kidney dial-

Issue become controlling
cost over enhancing
Programs
benefits.

ysis benefit added to Medicare in 1972 reinforced the stigma of fiscal reck-lessness.[51] As a consequence of Medicare's inflationary beginnings, fiscal issues came to dominate the policy agenda. The key issue in Medicare pol-icy became how to restrain costs through regulatory and financing re-forms, rather than how to enhance the program's limited benefits.

The predominance of fiscal issues over Medicare policy was partly due to the program's primary legislative location in congressional financing committees, the House Committee on Ways and Means and the Senate Fi-nance Committee. These committees have traditionally conceived of their roles in Congress in terms of a norm of financial responsibility.[52] And Congress traditionally recognized their importance in protecting the U.S. national legislature from itself by serving as a restraint on overspending, establishing that no amendments would be allowed before the commit-tees' legislation reached a vote on the floor of the House of Representa-tives. Given the norm of responsibility and Medicare's perceived financial problems, increasing the scope of program benefits would have been re-garded as irresponsible. To use Senator Long's metaphor, expanding Medi-care coverage would have been equivalent to speeding up a runaway train. Rather than expansion, benefits policy came to be governed by a negative consensus that left Medicare coverage unchanged, despite persistent doubts about its adequacy and public opinion favoring expansion.

The fiscal pressures driving Medicare policymakers may also have de-terred interest groups for the elderly from pushing an expansionary agenda. In a political environment inhospitable to Medicare expansion, groups representing the elderly had organizational incentives to em-phasize protecting current benefits, rather than pushing for large-scale ex-pansions. Unsuccessful campaigns for Medicare expansion could have weakened their political clout among policymakers and eroded support among constituents disillusioned with legislative defeats. Protecting the status quo was a safer, if less imaginative, alternative.

Supplemental Insurance

The growth of supplemental health insurance for the aged created the sec-ond source of stability in Medicare benefits. Supplemental Medicare in-surance, often called Medigap, encompasses private health insurance policies carried by program beneficiaries to cover gaps in services and cost sharing left by Medicare coverage. The development of supplemental in-surance was driven by the limited scope of Medicare benefits, the con-comitant creation of a market niche for private insurers, and the desire of beneficiaries for first-dollar insurance coverage.[53]

As Medicare benefits failed to expand, the proportion of the aged carrying supplemental insurance increased. In 1967, 46% of elderly Medicare beneficiaries had private supplemental insurance; by 1984 that figure had risen to 72%.[54] Supplemental policies typically covered cost-sharing liabilities for Medicare-covered services. Virtually all plans covered the deductible and coinsurance payments for Medicare hospitalization benefits, as well as the 20% copayments for physician services.[55] However, there was significantly less private insurance available for services not covered by Medicare. Over 25 years after Medicare's enactment, fewer than one-half of such policies covered prescription drugs or any physician bills in excess of what Medicare paid as "reasonable charges."[56] Additional hospital days were usually covered, but additional nursing home days and coverage of nursing home stays not certified by Medicare were usually not. Coverage of dental care, eyeglasses, and hearing aids was rare. In addition, some elderly beneficiaries carried other types of supplemental insurance, including coverage for specific illnesses.[57]

Medicare beneficiaries acquired supplemental coverage in two ways: as a benefit of current or previous employment, or through individual purchase of so-called Medigap policies.[58] In 1984, 30% of the elderly received supplemental coverage as a benefit of present or past employment, where employers paid the majority of the supplemental premiums.[59] The remainder of Medicare beneficiaries who had supplemental coverage purchased Medigap policies individually from private insurance companies. On average, the elderly carried 1.25 supplemental policies per person, and private insurance policies paid for approximately 7% of medical care expenditures for the elderly in 1984.[60]

The development of the Medigap and supplemental insurance markets had an important political impact on Medicare, dampening pressures for program expansion. In this respect, the relation of supplemental policies to Medicare parallels that of private health insurance to public insurance in countries with national health systems. In these nations, health insurance is universally available and guaranteed by the government, but there often exists a small private market for citizens to purchase coverage in addition to that offered by the national system. Rudolf Klein, in his analysis of the British National Health Service (NHS), explains the political consequences of having a private-sector complement to a public health system. The existence of the private sector, he argues, contributes to the shortcomings of British public health services by encouraging government officials "to ignore consumer demands."[61] These demands for improvements in the NHS can be ignored on the assumption that they will be redirected to the purchase of private coverage. The private sector thus acts as a restraint on pressures for growth in the public health sector.

Klein contends that the existence of a private sector encourages patients to leave the NHS rather than fight for a particular service from within: "if the most articulate and demanding patients exit into the private sector, then the NHS is rid of its most troublesome customers. Conversely, if the most articulate and demanding patients were denied the exit option, they would be forced to use voice: to engage in the politics of protest." [62] This dynamic operates in Medicare as well. As with the NHS, exit weakened beneficiaries' voice in the politics of Medicare benefits, undercutting pressures for program expansion by siphoning off those beneficiaries most likely to generate pressure for reform.

There are substantial differences within the Medicare population both in terms of who owns supplemental insurance and who owns the best policies. Ownership of Medicare supplemental insurance is correlated with income, race, education, and health status. Whites are almost twice as likely as nonwhites to have supplemental coverage. The elderly below the poverty line are less than one-half as likely to have private insurance as the aged with incomes twice the poverty level. Medicare beneficiaries with thirteen years of education are almost twice as likely to be covered than those with fewer than eight years of education. And while 75% of the elderly who considered themselves to be in excellent health carried private insurance, only 45% of those self-described as in poor health did so.[63] There are also significant disparities among supplemental policies. Employer-sponsored plans generally provide better benefits, such as prescription drugs, than individually purchased Medigap policies.[64] In short, "the Medicare beneficiaries who are least able to afford the costs of major illnesses—and therefore are most in need of supplemental coverage—are the least likely to have it."[65]

The existence of income, race, and education differentials among supplemental Medicare ownership suggests that those beneficiaries most likely to generate political pressures on Medicare are precisely those most likely to benefit from private health coverage. Political activism in the United States is highly correlated with socioeconomic status.[66] It is the elderly of this higher socioeconomic status who have the best supplemental coverage. The politically active class of the elderly, in other words, is the class least dependent on public Medicare benefits. The voice of beneficiaries is consequently dulled by the exit of elder participants with higher incomes into private supplemental insurance, eroding the ability of political organizations of the elderly to mobilize for Medicare expansion.

*medilend five [69]
Basic services for
the poor*

The Special Case of Long-Term Care

The failure to adopt long-term care coverage, however, had little to do with the existence of private coverage, for the simple reason that there was none. There are a number of barriers to purchasing private long-term care insurance, including prohibitive costs for seniors, inadequate coverage that often does not adjust for medical care inflation, and the difficulty of selling future policies to younger, employed populations with more immediate concerns.[67] In 1992, fewer than 5% of the elderly had private long-term care insurance.[68] There was, however, another source of nursing home coverage for the elderly: Medicaid. Enacted as a legislative comple- /
ment to Medicare in 1965, Medicaid mandated state coverage of five basic services for the poor, including care in "skilled nursing homes."[69] Although it was not widely acknowledged or understood at the time because the program's constituency was believed to be the nonelderly poor, Medicaid continued the precedent of Kerr-Mills payments for long-term care. The guarantee of nursing home coverage and its implications for the future of Medicaid were not seriously contemplated: "first nursing home coverage under Medicare was limited; then Medicaid was added to Medicare; then nursing homes were included under Medicaid—and then the process stopped."[70] In 1992, payment for long-term care services represented over one-third of all Medicaid expenditures, and although the aged made up less than 10% of the Medicaid population, 30% of program spending went to services for the elderly.[71]

To the extent that Medicare beneficiaries qualified as poor or medically indigent, they could receive Medicaid nursing home benefits.[72] In long-term care, then, the availability of public supplemental coverage for the elderly through Medicaid reduced pressures for Medicare expansion. However, the stigma, emotional pain, and administrative burdens that seniors endured in applying for welfare coverage after they had spent so much of their financial resources that they qualified for Medicaid made this an unpopular benefit. Medicaid's payment policies also encouraged institutionalization in nursing homes rather than home or community care.[73] To many elders, Medicaid long-term care was unacceptable; a 1985 AARP poll found that 40% of seniors remained reluctant to establish their eligibility for Medicaid.[74] As a result, organizations representing the elderly continued to push for a national long-term care program, a demand that went unmet. Since 1965, federal policymakers had consistently regarded long-term nursing home care as a costly, highly unpredictable commitment that Medicare could not afford to make, and ultimately, not as critical as coverage for acute medical care.

Medicaid reduced pressure for Medicare expansion

-74

Confusion about Benefits

The final source of stability in Medicare benefits was confusion among the elderly about the scope of Medicare and lack of knowledge about their health coverage. Studies have consistently demonstrated low levels of understanding among the elderly of Medicare and supplemental insurance benefits.[75] Quite simply, many of the elderly do not understand the limitations of Medicare coverage, especially with regard to long-term care. A 1984 study found that less than 40% of seniors understood Medicare's limited benefits for nursing home care, and only 13% and 22%, respectively, gave correct answers about Medicare coverage for prescription drugs and mental health services.[76] In another study of Medicare beneficiaries in six states in 1982, between 31%–45% of seniors in all the states did not know that Medicare failed to cover outpatient prescription drugs, while 53%–75% of beneficiaries across the states overestimated Medicare coverage for long-term nursing home care.[77] Medicare beneficiaries also tend to overestimate the coverage provided by their privately purchased Medigap policies. And the complex relationship between Medicare part A, Medicare part B, and Medigap policies leaves many beneficiaries and their families unsure of what services are covered by which insurer. This confusion is exacerbated by the reliance of the program on Blue Cross and Blue Shield plans as administrative intermediaries. Some beneficiaries mistakenly assume that their Medicare benefits come from the "Blues," rather than the federal government, because of their role in claims processing.

Confusion among the elderly regarding Medicare and the scope of its benefits has undercut the efforts of advocacy groups for the elderly to mobilize for benefits expansion. As Mark Schlesinger and Terrie Wetle argue, "with such widespread misunderstanding, mobilizing political support for changes in coverage is difficult."[78] If the elderly had better understood the limitations of Medicare coverage, they might have generated more pressure to expand benefits. The confusion of elderly beneficiaries regarding Medicare coverage is mirrored in the working population, with a similar effect on program politics. A 1995 poll, taken in the midst of a Medicare reform debate that should have raised public awareness about the program, found that fewer than half of all Americans knew that Medicare did not cover long-term care in nursing homes and only 41% knew Medicare did not cover outpatient prescription drugs.[79] If younger employees properly understood the burden that Medicare's coverage limits would place on their grandparents, parents, and eventually, themselves, more intense public desire for expansion might have materialized.

In sum, the predominance of fiscal concerns, the development of private supplemental insurance, and confusion among the elderly regarding health coverage helped to sustain a negative consensus on Medicare benefits during the program's first two decades. These forces both weakened the demand for expansion from the elderly and their political organizations and reduced the appetite of policymakers to extend program benefits. As a result, Medicare benefits remained stable, even as the costs of medical care to program enrollees grew.

REVERSAL OF FORTUNE: CATASTROPHIC HEALTH INSURANCE, 1986–89

The pattern of stability in Medicare benefits broke off sharply in 1988 with the enactment of the Medicare Catastrophic Coverage Act.[80] The emergence of catastrophic insurance onto the government agenda in the mid-1980s was strikingly anomalous. In addition to the constraints on benefits reform previously described, the largest expansion of Medicare benefits in program history came during the tenure of a conservative Republican administration committed to downsizing the welfare state, in the midst of ascendant deficit politics that constrained the domestic policy agenda, and during the same period in which federal officials were enacting substantial cuts in Medicare spending.[81] David Stockman, the president's controversial director of the Office of Management and Budget, candidly summarized the administration's ambitious mission to remake American social policy: "The Reagan revolution . . . required a formal assault on the welfare state. . . . Accordingly, forty years' worth of promises, subventions, entitlements, and safety nets issued by the federal government to every component and stratum of American society would have to be scrapped or dramatically modified."[82] Yet the initial impetus for catastrophic insurance came from the Reagan administration. While the previous two decades had witnessed occasional efforts by members of Congress to sponsor legislation expanding Medicare benefits, the Reagan administration surprisingly established itself as the first presidential administration since the program's enactment to make Medicare expansion a top priority.

How did catastrophic insurance rise to the top of the federal agenda despite such seemingly unfavorable political conditions? Much of the answer lies with the political entrepreneurship of Reagan's secretary of health and human services, Otis Bowen. Reagan appointed Bowen, a former family physician and governor of Indiana, secretary of health and human services in 1985 to succeed Margaret Heckler. From 1982 to 1984, Bowen had chaired the federal Advisory Council on Social Security, which was also charged with reviewing Medicare. As part of its 1984 report, the Advisory Council recommended expanding Medicare's hospitalization benefit to an unlimited number of days and eliminating coinsurance payments for hospital and skilled nursing facility care.[83] In addition, the Advistory Council, or Bowen commission, recommended a voluntary benefit that would cap out-of-pocket expenses for Medicare part B (physician) services.[84]

Bowen proposed a Medicare catastrophic insurance plan that followed the design recommended by the Advisory Council during his December 1985 confirmation hearing.[85] There is no evidence, though, that President Reagan nominated Bowen knowing that the new secretary would begin a campaign for Medicare expansion. Bowen's emphasis on catastrophic coverage represented his own initiative and commitment, not a broader decision by the administration on Medicare policy.[86] President Reagan did not, however, discourage Bowen's efforts. As governor of California, Reagan had proposed a catastrophic insurance program of his own and looked upon Bowen's proposal favorably.[87] The political appeal of doing something for the elderly may also have influenced Reagan's thinking. The administration had proposed highly unpopular Social Security cuts in 1981, and some Reagan advisers saw catastrophic insurance as a way for the president, as well as the Republican Party, to improve its standing with seniors.[88] In his 1986 state of the union address, Reagan authorized Bowen to conduct a study and formulate a proposal addressing the problem of catastrophic costs.[89]

Yet the president's initial permissiveness did not guarantee the administration's endorsement of catastrophic insurance. "The hardest thing about passing catastrophic," observed Tom Burke, Bowen's chief aide at Health and Human Services, "was getting it through the White House."[90] Domestic policymaking was concentrated under the authority of the Domestic Policy Council (DPC), which had been created at the start of Reagan's second term. Chaired by Ed Meese, then attorney general, the DPC comprised cabinet members whose departments were involved with domestic issues and it had authority to review domestic initiatives and make recommendations to the President.[91] In order for catastrophic insurance to emerge from the White House with Reagan's sponsorship, it first had to run "the gauntlet" of the DPC.[92]

A core group of administration conservatives—led by Meese, Office of Management and Budget director James Miller, chair of the Council of Economic Advisers Beryl Sprinkel, and Secretary of Interior Donald Hodell—opposed catastrophic insurance on ideological grounds. They argued that catastrophic insurance represented an unwarranted expansion of the federal government. Meanwhile, private insurers involved in selling supplemental policies to Medicare beneficiaries lobbied the White House against catastrophic coverage, fearing a reduction in their market. Their demands found a sympathetic audience among Meese and other administration conservatives.[93]

Bowen ultimately triumphed over the conservative faction by courting other cabinet members and by convincing Reagan that his plan was administratively simpler than conservative alternatives that preserved a broader role for the Medigap industry.[94] The considerable opposition within the administration to Bowen's plan underscored the degree to which his political entrepreneurship drove the emergence of catastrophic insurance. Without Bowen, there would have been no advocate in the administration willing to push catastrophic health insurance, and without such an advocate, Medicare expansion would not have received presidential sponsorship.

The idea of adding catastrophic coverage to Medicare found a much more receptive audience in Congress. Ironically, congressional enthusiasm for Medicare expansion was generated in part by recent congressional cuts in the program. There was a growing sense that previous federal policies had eroded Medicare coverage. Between 1980 and 1985, Medicare beneficiaries' out-of-pocket costs for hospital services covered by the program increased by 49%, and for physician and outpatient services, by 31%.[95] And by 1984, the elderly paid as much in out-of-pocket health costs as a percentage of their income (15%) as they had in 1965, when Medicare was enacted.[96] These cost increases were not solely the result of intentional increases in cost-sharing measures. By adopting changes in hospital payment policies that encouraged hospitals to shorten the hospital stays of Medicare patients, Congress inadvertently drove up the deductible that Medicare beneficiaries pay for hospital coverage, which was linked to the average cost of a hospital day. As hospital days shortened and costly procedures were crammed into a shorter stay, that average increased significantly. The deductible rose almost one hundred dollars between 1985 and 1986, the largest one-year increase in Medicare history. Congressional Democrats, as well as some Republicans, had come to believe that after all the increased costs imposed on Medicare beneficiaries, the time had arrived to do something for the elderly.[97]

Congressional concern over limitations in Medicare coverage overlapped with political motivations. In November 1986, immediately before the release of the Bowen report on catastrophic insurance, the Democrats captured the Senate for the first time since 1980, gaining majority control of both houses. Bowen's proposal provided a convenient vehicle for Democrats to pursue liberal social policy aims that had eluded them during the Reagan years. It also enabled, and forced, members of Congress to take positions on improving health care for the elderly, an issue certain to be popular with both aged and nonaged constituents.[98] The negative consensus on Medicare benefits had been sustained largely because of the low visibility of the issue in the public domain. In the absence of presidential support, and given the predominance of fiscal concerns among both parties in Congress, expanding Medicare was not a prominent public issue during the program's first two decades. That obscurity proved critical, since the public supported expanding program benefits at much higher levels than policymakers. By keeping the issue off the agenda, the negative consensus limited the influence of the public for program expansion. At the same time, for the most part both political parties abandoned their ideological dreams: Republicans accommodated to living with Medicare as a federal insurance program and Democrats gave up on expanding the program. Instead, a bipartisan consensus on rationalizing the program through controlling costs and enhancing efficiency dominated the agenda.[99] Political pragmatism, defined as reining in Medicare spending, ruled benefits expansion out.

The Bowen proposal fundamentally changed that dynamic. What was easy to do away from the public eye—namely, avoid expanding Medicare benefits—was much harder to maintain once the issue emerged on the national political agenda. Public opinion, which favored program expansion, had been activated. Not only were the potential political benefits of expanding Medicare now increased, but so too were the political costs of inaction. For the first time since 1965, politicians would be judged by their responsiveness to pressures for expanding health care benefits for the elderly. As a result, Secretary Bowen's proposal for catastrophic health insurance broke the hold of the negative consensus that had governed Medicare politics for its first two decades.

Legislating Catastrophic Insurance

In view of the subsequent backlash among the elderly against the Medicare Catastrophic Coverage Act, the key provisions of the legislation now seem curious. The programmatic form adopted for catastrophic insurance in 1988 raises two questions. First, what explains the choice of benefits proposed by the Reagan administration and legislated by Congress? And second, what explains the bipartisan decision to rely on self-financing and income-related premiums to finance catastrophic coverage?

Benefits

The 1982 Advisory Council on Social Security, chaired by Otis Bowen, recommended expanding Medicare hospitalization coverage to an unlimited number of days, eliminating hospital and skilled nursing facility coinsurance requirements, and offering an optional benefit for part B (physician services) that would establish a cap on out-of-pocket expenses by beneficiaries.[100] These benefits became the basis for the catastrophic insurance plan Bowen proposed as secretary of health and human services. The Bowen report, released in November 1986 after President Reagan's authorization of a study on catastrophic costs, proposed to make Medicare coverage of hospitalization days unlimited and to limit beneficiaries' annual out-of-pocket expenses to two thousand dollars.[101] But the Medicare Catastrophic Coverage Act enacted by Congress in 1988 expanded substantially on Bowen's proposal. Table 3.6 lists its benefits.[102]

There was, then, a large discrepancy between the administration's initial proposal and the final legislation. Bowen's proposal reflected his perception of what was both desirable and achievable, given political and fiscal constraints. The problem he saw in Medicare was the threat of beneficiaries' losing a lifetime's savings to the costs of catastrophic illness.[103] From his perspective, expanding Medicare hospitalization coverage and limiting liability for out-of- pocket costs solved this problem. Of course, it did not address all or even the most important dimensions of the problem. There were other sources of catastrophic costs for Medicare beneficiaries, including prescription drugs and long-term care, that were far more consequential than limited hospitalization coverage. Crucially, however, the 1982 Advisory Council chaired by Bowen did not endorse coverage of these items, regarding both as too expensive to add to Medicare.[104]

The limited benefits proposed by Bowen also embodied political constraints. In order to secure approval from the Reagan administration, Bowen produced a benefits package that did not add to the deficit and that was funded solely from beneficiary contributions. These assumptions of budgetary neutrality (new policies could not increase the federal deficit) and self-financing (Medicare beneficiaries should finance benefits expansions) are discussed in detail later in this chapter. Their impact here was to restrict the scope of benefits that Bowen could propose, since higher levels of benefits would have had to be funded by beneficiaries, creating an unaffordable burden for many Medicare enrollees. Finally, Bowen and his staff proposed limited benefits, understanding that Congress was likely to expand catastrophic insurance, though they did not anticipate just how large that expansion would become.[105]

Table 3.6 Provisions of the 1988 Medicare Catastrophic Coverage Act

---

Expansion of Medicare hospitalization coverage to an unlimited number of days
and limitation of the deductible to only once a year

Elimination of coinsurance requirements for inpatient hospitalization

Reduction in coinsurance requirements for care in skilled nursing facilities;
previously, there was no coinsurance for the first 20 days, but coinsurance was
required for days 21–100; the new law required coinsurance for only the first
8 days of a stay in a skilled nursing facility and extended coverage from 100 to
150 days

Elimination of 3-day prior hospitalization requirement for skilled nursing facility
benefits

Extension of hospice care benefits for the terminally ill

Limitation on out-of-pocket expenses for Medicare part B to $1,370; this cap
was to be indexed thereafter to inflation; the cap included part B deductible
and 20% part B coinsurance

Expansion of covered home health services to 38 consecutive days

Coverage of mammography screening

Coverage of outpatient prescription drugs, implemented in stages until requiring
20% coinsurance and payment of a deductible ($652 for 1992)

Requirement for states, under Medicaid buy-ins, to pay for Medicare premiums,
deductibles, and cost sharing of all beneficiaries below the federal poverty line

Requirement for states to extend Medicaid coverage to pregnant women and
infants up to age one with incomes at or below 100% of the federal poverty
level

Protection against spousal impoverishment for institutionalized beneficiaries
with Medicaid coverage; provision for beneficiaries to keep more income and
still qualify for Medicaid coverage of nursing home care

Note: Previously, beneficiaries could pay more than one deductible a year, since Medicare benefits were based on "spell of illness," defined as beginning when a beneficiary entered the hospital and ending 60 days after the patient was discharged. If beneficiaries experienced more than one spell of illness during a year, they had to pay the deductible for hospitalization services again.

The Bowen plan envisioned a limited and simple expansion of Medicare. By the time Congress enacted the Medicare Catastrophic Coverage Act in 1988, catastrophic insurance had become considerably less limited and considerably more complicated. The enhanced scope of the legislation reflected congressional political dynamics. The Democratic Party's capture of the Senate in 1986 bolstered their desire to move forward on domestic policy goals, and catastrophic insurance provided that opportunity. It also presented a challenge. Since the Reagan administration had initially sponsored catastrophic insurance, the Democrats found themselves in the unusual position of risking ceding credit for Medicare expansion to the Republicans. As a consequence, the Democratic leadership in Congress had an incentive to add benefits in order to put the party's stamp on the catastrophic insurance legislation. This partisan incentive played a role in the financially most significant expansion of catastrophic coverage: the addition of prescription drugs. In meetings with congressional party leaders, Jim Wright, the new Speaker of the House of Representatives, emphasized the importance of prescription drug benefits to making catastrophic coverage a Democratic program.[106] Wright urged both Ways and Means and Energy and Commerce to add the drug benefit.[107]

Beyond partisan incentives, there were members of Congress, especially those on committees with health care jurisdictions, such as California Democrats Pete Stark and Henry Waxman, who believed that the Bowen plan did not go far enough in addressing Medicare's limitations.[108] The administration's proposal for catastrophic insurance provided the instrument through which previously desired but deferred Medicare reforms could be realized. Expansion of hospital coverage and limitation of out-of-pocket expenses grew "into a legislative vehicle for a wide variety of Medicare changes long sought by many Congressional health policymakers."[109] Expanded coverage of home health services, hospice services, care in skilled nursing facilities, and mandates on state coverage of cost sharing for poor Medicare beneficiaries were the result.[110] And the reforms went well beyond Medicare. Driven by the work of Henry Waxman, chair of the House Energy and Commerce Subcommittee on Health, the Medicare Catastrophic Coverage Act also substantially expanded Medicaid coverage of low-income pregnant women and children.

Yet this expanded package was not sufficiently comprehensive for Rules Committee chair Claude Pepper (Democrat, Florida), the preeminent congressional voice for the elderly. When the Bowen plan had been released, Pepper sardonically remarked: "The President calls this a giant step forward. This isn't a step taken by a giant, it's one taken by a pigmy."[111] Speaker Wright had hoped that adding drug coverage would mollify Pepper, whose opposition as the congressman most associated with the causes of the elderly could prove damaging to the legislation's chances for passage. Still, the law did not go far enough for Pepper, who, seeking to leverage the political capital he had earned by mobilizing elderly voters for Democrats in the 1982 congressional elections, threatened to introduce an amendment to the legislation for long-term home care, only to be persuaded by Speaker Wright to hold off any floor vote on the expensive program.[112]

Finally, the expanded benefits package incorporated political calculations. Increasing the scope of federal health insurance for the aged was undoubtedly politically popular. But organizations representing the elderly were not pleased with the limited benefits in Bowen's proposal. As the

Bowen plan was announced, the AARP and the Villers Foundation (later Families USA) were preparing to launch "Long Term Care '88," a campaign to generate publicity and pressure for enactment of a national long-term care program during the 1988 election.[113] The campaign was supported by more than one hundred national organizations. In 1987, interest groups representing the elderly wanted above all else long-term care; there was no clamor in their memberships for unlimited hospitalization insurance.[114] After all, only a small percentage of the elderly exhausted Medicare's hospital benefits. Only .5% of Medicare beneficiaries would be affected by the elimination of hospital coinsurance and limits on covered hospital days.[115] That hardly represented a mass political constituency. Moreover, the changes made in hospital payment policies during the 1980s were inducing hospitals to shorten the stays of Medicare patients. The already small problem of exhausting hospitalization benefits was apparently becoming even smaller.

In addition to the limited benefits, groups representing the elderly disliked catastrophic insurance's financing arrangements. Congressional leaders consequently were concerned with securing the support of the elderly for catastrophic insurance. While the addition of prescription drugs put a Democratic stamp on the legislation, it also had the advantage of offering political organizations representing the elderly one of their legislative priorities. They could take prescription drug coverage to memberships disappointed by catastrophic insurance's financing arrangements and its failure to cover long-term care. In this context, there were discussions between the Committee on Ways and Means and groups representing the elderly, most notably the American Association for Retired Persons (AARP), regarding prescription drug coverage. From the perspective of the committee, the addition of prescription drugs to the catastrophic insurance package represented a deal in exchange for the AARP's support of the legislation.[116] Prescription drug coverage was the price for securing the political support of groups representing the elderly on Medicare reform. And the political value Congress placed on prescription drugs was evident in its adoption despite strenuous opposition from the pharmaceutical industry, which feared that federal coverage would inevitably lead to price controls.[117] *Opposition from Pharmaceutical industry.*

Financing

The Bowen catastrophic insurance plan introduced a major change in Medicare financing. Since the program's enactment, Medicare hospitalization insurance had been funded exclusively from payroll taxes on employers and their workers. This financing system followed the logic of social insurance, which spreads financing (in the form of payroll taxes) across one's own lifetime and different age groups in order to insure against the risks of lost income inherent in not working, such as retirement and disability. All people contribute to social insurance funds when they can, while working, to create a pool that will provide benefits to those who need them when they experience the loss of income.[118] Beneficiaries contributed premiums for physician services, but by the 1980s, the premiums covered only 25% of part B costs. In contrast, Bowen's plan assumed that Medicare beneficiaries alone would fund the new benefits. Catastrophic insurance would be financed entirely by a $4.92 increase in the monthly premiums that beneficiaries paid for physician services.[119]

Bowen's proposal relied on the principle of self-financing for two reasons. First, the Advisory Council on Social Security had rejected general tax increases for Medicare, including sin and payroll taxes. Because of strong antitax sentiment in American politics at the time, proposals that avoided general taxes were more politically attractive. Moreover, as a result of the 1983 Social Security reforms, payroll taxes had been raised, and raising them again so soon was not considered an option. Second, Bowen's catastrophic coverage plan assumed budget neutrality. The new program could not add to the deficit, a condition of President Reagan's support.[120] Since general taxes had been ruled out, budgetary neutrality required Medicare beneficiaries to finance benefits expansion. Fiscal politics in the 1980s led inexorably to the unprecedented step of having beneficiaries finance their own benefits.

Despite objections from interest groups for the elderly, Congress never seriously challenged self-financing as the funding mechanism for new benefits. Indeed, a bipartisan consensus existed for self-financing. The Democratic-controlled House Ways and Means Committee operated on the assumption of budget neutrality, and members of Congress were reluctant to raise general taxes for fear of electoral retribution. And there was widespread agreement that the 1983 Social Security reforms had brought payroll taxes to their political limit—not the first time this limit had, in the opinion of Congress, been reached.[121] Self-financing was widely seen as the only feasible way to expand Medicare, given the fiscal and political constraints of the federal deficit. It may not have been many Democratic members' preferred option, but if it enabled a benefits expansion, it would have to do.

The Rise of Intergenerational Equity Concerns

The justification of self-financing on fiscal grounds obscured changing conceptions of the deservingness of the elderly and the influence of these conceptions on catastrophic insurance. Congressional acquiescence to self-financing represented a transformation in political thinking about the aged. Medicare advocates had chosen the elderly for introduction of federal health insurance because they commanded public sympathy. But by the time catastrophic insurance emerged as in issue in the mid-1980s, this sympathetic stereotype had been substantially revised.[122] Many policymakers now regarded the elderly as relatively privileged, not disadvantaged. And instead of being seen as deserving of government aid, the elderly were increasingly charged with receiving too much government money. As one member of Congress remarked, "demographic data show that the elderly are in better shape than the non-elderly. This is particularly true with respect to the affluent elderly. In light of this, it wasn't right to ask the non-elderly to finance their benefits [i.e., the benefits of the elderly] in the case of catastrophic care."[123]

There were four elements in what amounted to a new politics of intergenerational equity that emerged in the 1980s. First, the elderly were said to consume too great a proportion of the federal budget. In 1985, 25.9% of all federal outlays went to the aged.[124] Proponents of intergenerational politics frequently linked this spending on the elderly to low levels of public spending on children; while the poverty rate of the elderly had fallen from 28.5% in 1966 to 12.2% in 1990, poverty rates among children had risen from 17.6% to 20.6%.[125] It was a short step from there to attributing the high numbers of children in poverty in the United States to federal spending on the aged.[126] Second, Social Security and Medicare were identified as prime causes of the federal deficit. To the extent that the deficit was believed to be the source of national economic troubles, the elderly become the culprit. Critics complained that public programs for the elderly were "off limits" due to the political power of the aged.[127] Third, these same programs were said to be unsustainable because of long-term demographic changes that were producing a graying of the population. In 1980, the elderly (those sixty-five and older) were 11% of the population. The share of the population that was over sixty-five was projected to rise to around 20% in 2025, with especially large growth in the "very old" population over eighty-five. At this rate, the future burden of Social Security and Medicare was portrayed as unaffordable. Fourth and finally, critics claimed that too many well-off elderly Americans received government benefits although they did not need them, at the same time that these benefits were financed by younger populations that could not afford the taxes and would not receive as generous benefits in the future.[128] By 1982, the poverty rate among the elderly had dropped below the overall national poverty rate, and the 1960s public image of the poor elder dependent on

Social Security had been replaced by the 1980s image of the affluent retiree playing golf and enjoying lavish vacations.[129]

These intergenerational equity concerns were reinforced by conservative interest groups whose ideological hostility to big government and concern for deficit reduction often matched the financial self-interest of business constituents in lowering federal taxes and shrinking the size of government.[130] The most influential of these groups, the Concord Coalition, was founded in 1992 by Peter Peterson, an investment banker and former secretary of commerce, and former senators Paul Tsongas and Warren Rudman. The group found a receptive audience on Capitol Hill for its message that fiscal responsibility, and ultimately America's national economic future, required cuts in entitlements for the elderly that had created an unsustainable burden.

To be sure, much of the logic of intergenerational equity was specious.[131] Data showing lower poverty rates among the elderly than other age groups obscured the large number of seniors living with modest means just above the federal poverty line.[132] There was no established causal connection between federal spending on the elderly and spending on children. And there was no guarantee that money not spent on the elderly would go to children, rather than to defense, tax cuts, or any other national priority. Indeed, public spending on the elderly in the United States was not out of line with that in other Western democracies. Instead, elders' share of the welfare state appeared lopsided because the share of the welfare state for the nonaged was small compared to the share in other countries, as exemplified by the lack of a universal health care program. And warnings about the declining number of workers per retiree neglected to mention that the overall dependence ratio—the number of nonworkers per worker—would actually decline even as the country aged. Yet, whatever its flaws, the intergenerational argument gained political momentum.

The new, less favorable picture of the elderly and the emergent politics of intergenerational equity were significantly stronger at elite than at mass levels. The public continued to support Medicare and Social Security at high levels and continued to have a favorable impression of the elderly. Many policymakers, however, saw the aged in a less benign light, perhaps because their knowledge of program costs and proximity to the federal budgetary process raised concerns that the elderly were consuming too many public resources, as well as resentment over perceived heavy-handed political tactics by groups such as the AARP. In a 1986 survey of attitudes on social welfare programs, Fay Lomax Cook and Edith Barrett found wide disparities between public and congressional views on Medicare. As table 3.7 demonstrates, the public showed substantially more support for increasing benefits of programs for the elderly than members of Congress. The public was twice as likely as congressional representatives to support expansion of Medicare benefits and five times as likely to support increases in Social Security benefits. And whereas the public ranked the elderly as the group most deserving group of federal assistance, members of Congress ranked children first.[133] As one member of the House of Representatives told the researchers, "We have successfully, to a degree, eradicated the problem of poverty among the elderly. . . . And so . . . here we are making tremendous strides against povertization of our elderly, nobody is paying attention to the children."[134] As catastrophic insurance rose to the top of the agenda in 1986, then, it did so at a time when concern had grown over international equity among federal policymakers.

The idea that the elderly should fund their own benefits expansion thus meshed squarely with policymakers' emergent fiscal, demographic, and generational equity concerns. The erosion of the reputation of the elderly for deservingness made the already strong fiscal-political appeal of self-financing all the more attractive. Self-financing did not add to the deficit and did not increase younger generations' financial responsibility for the aged, instead putting the burden of rising program costs on the elderly themselves. Changing views of the elderly, specifically, recognition of the financial heterogeneity of the aged population, also reinforced support for

Table 3.7 Comparison between Public and Congressional Support for Increasing, Maintaining, or Decreasing Benefits for Social Welfare Programs

PROGRAM	PUBLIC SUPPORT (%)	CONGRESSIONAL SUPPORT (%)
Medicare:		
Increase	67.6	32.4
Maintain	29.9	55.6
Decrease	2.5	10.9
SSI:		
Increase	57.3	23.8
Maintain	40.0	68.0
Decrease	2.7	8.2
Social Security:		
Increase	56.7	11.7
Maintain	40.0	85.5
Decrease	3.3	—

Source: Fay Lomax Cook and Edith J. Barrett, *Support For the American Welfare State: The Views of Congress and the Public* (New York: Columbia University Press, 1992), 86.
Note: Supplemental Security Income (SSI) is a federal program that provides cash assistance to low-income elderly, disabled, and blind Americans.

another provision of the catastrophic insurance legislation: income-related premiums.

Income-Related Premiums

Otis Bowen's 1986 proposal funded catastrophic insurance through flat increases in beneficiary premiums. However, the Medicare Catastrophic Coverage Act of 1988 also incorporated income-related premiums. For the first time in program history, Medicare premiums were formally related to income. Under the new law, all beneficiaries would pay an additional amount on their monthly part B premiums (four dollars in 1989). In addition, higher-income beneficiaries were required to pay a "supplemental premium" for catastrophic insurance benefits, capped at a maximum of eight hundred dollars for 1989.[135]

In large measure, congressional·expansion of the benefits in the catastrophic insurance legislation necessitated a new financing mechanism.[136] In order to remain deficit-neutral, the expanded benefits package required additional financing. Since self-financing had been assumed as a constraint, having all beneficiaries pay equal amounts for the new benefits would have imposed a considerable burden on lower-income beneficiaries. Yet the introduction of income-related premiums represented more than a straightforward response to the financing demands of expanded benefits. For several years, the idea of income-relating Medicare premiums had been gaining adherents in Congress among both Democrats and Republicans. Democrat Pete Stark, chair of the House Ways and Means Subcommittee on Health, had proposed linking Medicare premiums to beneficiaries' ability to pay in 1985. Stark's plan did not pass, but he continued to push income-related reform of Medicare financing.[137]

The idea of differential Medicare premiums appealed during this period to an unusual alliance of liberals and conservatives. Liberal Democrats such as Stark were concerned that continued increases in the part B premium would price poorer beneficiaries out of the program. Since part B was voluntary, liberals feared that further increases in costs would force low-income beneficiaries to withdraw from program coverage of physician services. Income-related premiums provided a means of increasing Medicare's revenues without increasing the financial burden on poorer beneficiaries.[138] Income-related premiums also enhanced the progressivity of Medicare financing, along the lines of Social Security. Social Security provides for redistribution toward lower-income beneficiaries in both its benefits and financing. Lower-income retirees receive a higher rate of return on their contributions than wealthier Social Security contributors. And, as a result of the 1983 Social Security reforms, higher-income retirees had to pay federal taxes on their Social Security benefits. In contrast, Medicare benefits were the same irrespective of income and the program had no visible progressive financing mechanism focused on beneficiaries, though the fact that general revenues from progressive income taxation funded part B was frequently neglected. Income-related premiums offered liberals an opportunity to make Medicare financing more progressive and to follow the redistributive direction that had been set for Social Security. The 1983 introduction of income-related benefits into Social Security without any significant political furor set a precedent for extending progressive financing to Medicare.

While liberals were concerned about the fate of the elderly poor, some conservative lawmakers worried about the program's coverage of the more affluent aged. They disliked Medicare's universalism, objecting to Medicare's coverage of those of the elderly who they believed could afford to purchase private health insurance on their own; this constituted, in their view, an unnecessary and expensive form of government largesse.[139] Indeed, the opposition of contemporary conservatives to federal health insurance for all the elderly regardless of income echoed that of conservatives during the Medicare debate in the 1950s and 1960s.[140] From the conservative perspective, income-related premiums were favored as a means to redress the inefficient government subsidy to wealthy individuals promoted by universal eligibility.

By 1986, then, an emergent compatibility had developed between liberal and conservative thinking regarding the adoption of progressive financing for Medicare. The House Ways and Means Committee had worked out an income-related design for financing Medicare *before* catastrophic insurance was proposed.[141] The introduction of income-related premiums was a case of a solution searching for a problem.[142] Catastrophic insurance did not provide only the vehicle for benefits reforms sought by congressional health policymakers. It also provided the opportunity to enact financing reforms that were considered vital to Medicare, as well as to potential subsequent expansions of the welfare state during an era of fiscal restraint. Congress deemed income-related premiums and self-financing as critical to the enactment of catastrophic insurance and the future of Medicare. Ironically, these same provisions proved critical to the legislation's demise.

The Collapse of Catastrophic Insurance

Sixteen months after catastrophic insurance was enacted, Congress voted overwhelmingly for its repeal. The scope of the reversal was striking. The Medicare Catastrophic Coverage Act had passed in the Senate 86-11, and in the House, 328-72. Now, the House voted for repeal 360-66, and the Senate voted 73-26 to strip much of the program away (in conference committee, it went along with the House version).[143] Although there had been some opposition to catastrophic coverage during its enactment, lawmakers assumed that once enacted, the issue was closed.[144] The rapidity with which repeal came, and the extent to which almost all of the new law's benefits were canceled, shocked those involved in the passage of catastrophic insurance.[145] What made the repeal of catastrophic insurance even more unusual was that its impetus came from the intended beneficiaries of the program. The only substantial expansion in program history was rolled back because of opposition from segments of the elderly population.

Why did catastrophic insurance collapse? The most important factor in its demise was opposition among the elderly to its financing provisions. The new benefits were to be financed entirely by Medicare beneficiaries. All beneficiaries would pay at least a flat increase on their premiums for physician service. In addition, 40% of the more affluent elderly would pay a supplemental premium varying with their income, up to a maximum annual cost of eight hundred dollars. Only 5% of beneficiaries initially would be liable for the maximum, though the percentage of the elderly paying the maximum supplemental premium and the amount of the premium would rise over time. It was precisely these upper-income beneficiaries, however, who carried the most extensive supplemental insurance policies. The 30% of the elderly who received supplemental insurance from former employers already carried coverage more generous than that offered by the Medicare Catastrophic Coverage Act.[146] The costs of catastrophic insurance, in other words, were imposed disproportionately on those who needed the benefits the least. This was an invitation to political trouble, and the rhetorical transformation of "new taxes" into "supplemental premium" did little to ameliorate the sense of increased burden.

"A mere five months after passage of the Medicare Catastrophic Coverage Act," Richard Himmelfarb observes, "senior citizens were in open revolt against the program."[147] A national campaign for repeal of the legislation began, led by the National Committee to Preserve Social Security and Medicare, associations representing federal retirees and former military personnel, and organizations founded specifically to oppose the legislation, such as the Seniors Coalition against the Catastrophic Act. By 1989, the National Association of Retired Federal Employees and the Retired Officers Association had put together a formidable coalition for repeal of organizations with large senior memberships, comprising forty-four groups with nineteen million members.[148] The coalition generated intense pressure on Congress through mailings, rallies, and angry appearances at meetings in members' home districts.

Catastrophic insurance relied on a transparently redistributive financing mechanism, taxing the higher-income elderly to pay for coverage that would most benefit lower-income Medicare enrollees. Forty percent of Medicare beneficiaries would pay 82% of the costs of catastrophic coverage: "for the first time in the history of American social insurance the most affluent participants would, on average, get back less then they contributed (in terms of the Medicare Catastrophic Coverage Act alone)."[149] Yet though opposition to catastrophic insurance was led by more affluent beneficiaries, it was by no means limited to them. After all, over 60% of Medicare enrollees would receive benefits from the legislation greater than their costs, creating a potentially formidable constituency to back the legislation.[150]

However, as table 3.8 shows, after enactment in July 1988, support for the Medicare Catastrophic Coverage Act eroded precipitously among seniors of all income groups—even those who stood to gain the most from the legislation. In particular, the level of support among less wealthy beneficiaries was substantially lower than AARP leaders expected.[151] This was largely attributable to widespread misunderstanding about the program. Surveys found that only 39% of the elderly knew that the Medicare Catastrophic Coverage Act covered outpatient prescription drugs, and fewer than 50% understood that not all beneficiaries would pay the sup-

Table 3.8 Support for and Opposition to the Medicare Catastrophic Coverage Act among Elderly Americans Age Sixty-five and Over

POSITION OF RESPONDENTS	NUMBER HOLDING POSITION (%)		
	DECEMBER 1988	FEBRUARY–MARCH 1989	AUGUST 1989
Low income:			
Support	70	52	47
Oppose	13	23	27
Difference	+57	+29	+20
Moderate income:			
Support	62	49	38
Oppose	23	33	45
Difference	+39	+16	−7
High income:			
Support	63	47	38
Oppose	31	43	57
Difference	+32	+4	−19

Source: Richard Himmelfarb, *Catastrophic Politics: The Rise and Fall of the Medicare Catastrophic Coverage Act of 1988* (University Park: Pennsylvania State University Press), 63, using AARP survey data.

plemental premium (fewer than 6% of beneficiaries actually would pay the maximum).[152] The perception that all the elderly would pay the supplemental premium, or "seniors tax," as opponents derisively called it, was particularly damaging. This confusion was fostered by some interest groups, most prominently the National Committee to Preserve Social Security, whose misleading mailings gave the false impression that all the elderly were subject to the extra premium.[153] Proponents of the program failed to counteract this confusion or to explain the scope of the new benefits. And any congressional urge to stand up to the growing campaign for repeal was weakened by Congressional Budget Office estimates that showed the prescription drug benefit would be five times as high as initially forecast when Congress enacted the legislation.[154]

Assessing Blame

It is easy to conclude that the collapse of catastrophic insurance was caused by the political folly of its congressional advocates. After all, Congress enacted catastrophic insurance with no sense of the controversy that it would produce, apparently heedless of the dynamics of Medicare politics and social insurance. In retrospect, this political miscalculation is hard to justify. Clearly, congressional policymakers underestimated the significance of the existing Medigap and supplemental insurance market. Many elderly people were attached to their already privately acquired supplemental coverage and were not enthusiastic about replacing it with government benefits. Contemporary politics and policy options were constrained by the historical development of private insurance to an extent that those involved in planning catastrophic insurance failed to appreciate. Congress, as well as the Reagan administration, also overestimated the value to the elderly of the benefits that were actually enacted. As health economist Marilyn Moon noted, "the term *catastrophic* evoked images of long-term care benefits . . ."[155] As a result of the defeat of Claude Pepper's legislation to enact a long-term care program, widely viewed as too expensive, the Medicare Catastrophic Coverage Act did not cover the most catastrophic expense of the elderly, nursing home care, which then accounted for 42% of the out-of-pocket costs of the elderly.[156] The absence of long-term care coverage prevented Congress from offering the affluent elderly a benefit that their private insurance plans did not include, a benefit that may have prevented the backlash against the legislation.

Finally, Congress also miscalculated the impact of the program's financing provisions. Only 40% of the elderly may have been scheduled to pay the supplemental premiums, but for those paying the premium at higher rates, the costs were considerable. The eight-hundred-dollar maximum supplemental premium for 1989 was almost three times as much as beneficiaries were paying in premiums for part B coverage of physician services.[157] For seniors subject to the higher rates of the supplemental premium, catastrophic insurance appeared to be an enormous tax for marginal benefits. Congress similarly failed to anticipate the reaction against self-financing and differential premiums or to understand how far the legislation had deviated from established principles of social insurance. Instead of spreading risk and financing across the life span and whole population, catastrophic insurance broke new ground by concentrating financial responsibility on Medicare beneficiaries alone and then further concentrated that cost on higher-income beneficiaries. The catastrophic insurance legislation contradicted the core element of social insurance: pooling risk. It replaced the communtiarian idea that we all pay into social insurance funds to protect everyone with the radically different, and anticommunitarian, concept that those using the benefit must finance the benefit themselves. There was predictable (and yet unanticipated) resentment that the elderly alone would finance the benefits, and fear that the introduction of income-related charges meant that Medicare was becoming a means-tested program.

The failure to anticipate this response was due in part to misrepresentations by the AARP of opinion among the elderly that misled congressional supporters of the legislation. Based on its own internal surveys, the AARP showed overwhelming support for the legislation among the elderly, rising from 78% in April 1987 to 91% in May 1988. But the AARP surveys did not focus on the potentially controversial financing mechanisms and thus provided the organization and policymakers an exaggerated view of the degree of support among the elderly for catastrophic insurance.[158] The leaders of the AARP realized the potential for opposition from more affluent seniors whose costs would far exceed benefits from the new program, but "they reasoned that this group was small in number, representing no more than 10 to 15 percent of seniors, and therefore could be easily withstood."[159] The group ignored evidence from its own surveys that there was little support among the elderly for self-financing or income-related premiums and saw no need to mobilize a grass-roots effort in favor of the legislation.[160]

In all of this, Congress and other program advocates badly miscalculated, and, even with the knowledge that policy science rarely offers the tools necessary to predict the political future, it is reasonable to believe that program advocates could have better forecast the consequences of their decisions. However, the "stupidity thesis" that catastrophic insurance collapsed because of lawmakers' miscalculations neglects the role of

American political institutions in shaping this outcome. The key question is, *Why* did Congress miscalculate? In fact, members of Congress involved in designing the catastrophic insurance legislation were not ignorant of strategic calculations. They were sufficiently concerned about potential opposition by the elderly to the program to add prescription drugs as a means of securing the support of political organizations representing the elderly. By offering a benefit of primary importance to the aged, congressional policymakers believed they had struck a deal for support among the elderly for catastrophic insurance.

In a corporatist political system such as exists in much of western Europe, this negotiated deal probably would have held.[161] In these systems, policymaking often takes the form of centralized negotiations between the government and "peak associations" that represent various categories of private interests, such as employers, labor unions, and medical professionals. But the relationship between interest groups and government in the United States is not as structured as it is in a corporatist system. There are no clearly defined peak associations officially representing societal interests in the United States. The AARP could not, as subsequent events vividly demonstrated, force a deal with the federal government on other groups representing the elderly. In fact, the AARP was not able, as both Congress and the AARP erroneously assumed it would be, to make a deal for its own members, let alone for others. In this sense, politicians and the AARP itself mistakenly accepted the myth of the AARP as the most powerful interest group in the country, a peerless political force that spoke for the elderly. The catastrophic insurance episode shattered that myth. After all, substantial opposition to catastrophic insurance existed within the AARP. The failure of the organization's leadership to anticipate or quell this opposition raised questions about the AARP's ability to act as an effective political force and about the linkages between the national leadership and membership, given the group's vast size and diverse composition. The experience with catastrophic insurance consequently had a restraining influence on the AARP's involvement in the 1993–94 debate over the Clinton health plan.

Ultimately, the looser, pluralistic character of interest group organization in the United States injects higher degrees of uncertainty and instability into political negotiation than exist in other democratic systems. The critical miscalculation in catastrophic insurance was that the support of the elderly could be guaranteed through corporatist-style policymaking that brokered a deal between government and social interests. Such deals are harder to reach in the United States due to fragmented organization of both social interests and the government, and even if struck, as the case of catastrophic insurance demonstrated, they are inherently volatile. In this sense, the failure of catastrophic insurance was a product of American political institutions, not merely individual error.

CONCLUSION

The expansion of Medicare benefits was restrained for two decades by a negative consensus supported by both political parties that privileged cost control over improvements in program coverage. Notably, that consensus prevailed in Medicare politics despite substantial public support for expanding benefits. The same forces that sustained that consensus ultimately contributed to the downfall of catastrophic health insurance. Fiscal concerns over the worsening federal deficit and reluctance to raise taxes led policymakers, with bipartisan support, to rely on financing arrangements (self-financing and income-related premiums) that precipitated the backlash against the program. The development of supplemental insurance reduced the support of the elderly for the expansion to catastrophic coverage by creating a constituency within Medicare that valued its private health benefits more than the prospect of new government benefits. And confusion among the elderly over Medicare's limitations and the benefits of catastrophic insurance enabled opponents of the legislation to persuade many beneficiaries that it was not in their interest. In the end, the politics of benefits expansion converged with that of benefits stability.

The failure of catastrophic insurance left several key legacies for Medicare. The generational equity concerns that played a role in structuring the catastrophic insurance proposal were deepened considerably by its repeal. The lasting public image of catastrophic insurance politics was that of senior citizens in Chicago pounding on the car of Ways and Means chair Dan Rostenkowski, upset by his continued support for the legislation after the drive to repeal catastrophic coverage had built momentum. The image provided a perfect advertisement for critics of "excessive" public spending on the elderly.[162] It suggested the elderly were political powerful, willing to resort to any means necessary, and greedy in rejecting a program that would have helped the less fortunate among them. This stereotype ignored the complexity of the case of catastrophic insurance, but as far as the media were concerned, the verdict was clear: *Newsweek* warned that "hell hath no fury like a senior scorned."[163] Catastrophic insurance helped, for a time, to make "greedy geezers" a new buzzword in American politics and fueled the resentment of some policymakers against political organizations representing the elderly.

Yet the repeal of catastrophic insurance left many Medicare beneficiaries vulnerable to soaring health costs. For all its faults, the catastrophic insurance legislation contained a number of important benefits, particularly the cap on out-of-pocket expenditures and the addition of prescription drug coverage. Without these benefits, the performance of Medicare in living up to its promise of protecting beneficiaries against the costs of medical care continued to fall short, and the gap between Medicare and private insurance widened in the years that followed.

Finally, the demise of catastrophic insurance also left the program politically vulnerable. As Medicare entered the 1990s, it did so with a seriously deficient benefits package. Medicare may have been single-payer insurance, but it was not, at least for beneficiaries and by international standards, generous single-payer insurance. As a consequence, the political constituency for Medicare was in some respects weaker than the constituencies that developed around national health insurance plans in other countries. That weakness would later be exposed when advocates of market-based reforms sought to restructure Medicare to carve out a broader role for private health plans.

There is one remaining puzzle in the case of catastrophic coverage. Income-related premiums proved to be the downfall of Medicare expansion. Yet only five years earlier, income-related taxes had been imposed on Social Security without any serious political backlash. And while in Medicare the new financing scheme was introduced at the same time as benefits were expanded, in Social Security income-related taxes accompanied benefits cuts. Why, then, did Medicare financing reform fail while Social Security succeeded? The different outcomes are largely attributable to the relative positions of the two programs' trust funds during the attempted reforms. How trust funds came to occupy an important position in Medicare, and their influence on program politics, is the subject of the next chapter.

Going Broke

THE POLITICS OF FINANCING

During the 1990s, the notion that Medicare was a program in crisis became a staple of American politics. Policymakers, journalists, and health
policy analysts all popularized the idea that Medicare was "going bankrupt," simultaneously feeding public fears about the program's future and
building political support for policy changes that would radically transform Medicare. Fears about Medicare's bankruptcy came to the fore in
1995, when congressional Republican leaders presented their reform
package as a necessary response to the projected insolvency of Medicare
in 2002. During the course of the ensuing Medicare reform debate, conventional wisdom over Medicare's financial condition was broadened and
redefined: the Republican leadership argued that Medicare not only faced
a short-term financial crisis, but in the absence of decisive action, it would
certainly go bankrupt as the baby boomers retired into the program beginning in 2010, doubling the number of Medicare beneficiaries in the
span of only two decades. Coupled with the same demographic challenge
confronting Social Security, many commentators wondered if America
could afford to grow old.[1]

The 1995 debate over the program's financial condition represented a
milestone in Medicare politics. Although fears that public programs for
the aged would go bankrupt were not new in U.S. politics—Social Security went through a similar dynamic in the late 1970s and early 1980s—it
marked the first time Medicare had experienced a trust fund crisis that
captured widespread public attention. Yet 1995 was not the first time that

Medicare's trust fund had run into trouble, nor was it the first time that policymakers had "discovered" a financial crisis that required programmatic changes. Indeed, the 1995 crisis was only the latest episode in a recurrent, and largely overlooked, pattern of crisis and reform that has driven Medicare politics since the program's enactment. While most analysts have concluded that Medicare's social insurance system of funding has helped to ensure the stability of the program, they have overlooked the role that same system has played in creating temporary funding crises in Medicare, and its decisive influence on program reform.[2]

This chapter analyzes the politics of Medicare financing, with a focus on three key questions. What explains the structure of Medicare financing arrangements? How have these arrangements—including payroll taxes, trust fund financing, and reliance on long-term actuarial forecasts—shaped Medicare financing politics? And what consequences have these same arrangements had on the timing and substance of Medicare reform? In answering these questions, I first trace the historical origins of Medicare's financing policies and their relationship to Social Security. This history is particularly important because, as I argue, decisions that were made about how to finance Medicare in the 1960s, based on the prior experience of Social Security, still exert tremendous influence over program politics four decades later. Next, I focus on the intermittent appearance of trust fund shortfalls in Medicare and explain their causes, as well as the politics of redressing funding shortfalls.

Finally, the chapter shows how policymakers have controlled the definition of both problems and solutions to financial crises in Medicare. I argue that across three decades of program history, political explanations for Medicare's financial problems focused on different problems, identified different solutions, and resulted in the adoption of different policy responses. Yet from 1965 to 1994, Democrats and Republicans generally agreed on policy responses to funding shortfalls, even as those responses changed course; in this era of consensus politics, potentially divisive trust fund crises were bipartisan events. As a result, financing shortfalls were not intensely public affairs, handled instead by Medicare policymakers often operating far from public view.

Changing understandings of the causes of financing shortfalls and "required" solutions underscore a critical point. Medicare trust fund crises are not merely objective events of fiscal duress that command automatic responses. Rather, trust fund crises are political events whose solutions reflect contemporary partisan alignments, ideological commitments, and policy analysts' thinking about what represents the solution du jour in the health system. Indeed, it is arguable that the cycle of crisis and reform in

Medicare financing is the single most important pattern in program politics, since it has, more than any other factor, driven the direction and timing of program reform. In other words, much of Medicare's political history can be understood through the lens of its financing arrangements. It is that lens that this chapter seeks to put in focus.

THE ORIGINS AND STRUCTURE
OF MEDICARE FINANCING

As enacted in 1965, Medicare contained two different financing systems. Medicare hospitalization insurance (part A) was funded through matching payroll taxes from current workers and their employers. In contrast, Medicare insurance for physician services (part B) was financed by beneficiary premiums and matching general revenues from the federal government.[3] Medicare's reliance on payroll taxes to fund hospitalization benefits differed from the logic of Social Security contributions. In Social Security, beneficiaries receive pension payments that vary according to the taxes they pay into the program during their working years. The higher the taxes paid into the system, the higher the pension benefits, though the benefits formula favors low-wage workers.[4] Medicare, however, does not operate on this principle of earnings-related benefits.[5] The amount of benefits received depends not on the amount of payroll taxes an individual pays into the Medicare trust fund as a worker, but on how much medical care a beneficiary receives as a retiree. The more medical care a Medicare beneficiary requires, the higher the program benefit to the individual. One of the main justifications for payroll tax financing of Social Security—that benefits are closely related to prior earnings—therefore cannot be applied to Medicare. However, Medicare's financing arrangements did resemble those in countries with social health insurance programs. In those systems, like Medicare, health insurance benefits are not proportional to earnings or taxes, a redistributive policy that ensures low-income workers the same access to government-sponsored health insurance as affluent employees.

Payroll tax financing of Medicare was a peculiar choice for a second reason. Because they are applied at an equal rate to all workers regardless of income, exclude income earned from interest, rents, and profits, and often tax only up to an established limit on earnings, payroll taxes are, in strict economic terms, a regressive form of financing.[6] Yet the architects of Medicare, who were New Deal liberals with close ties to the labor movement, advocated payroll taxation, instead of more progressive income or corporate tax schemes according to which the tax rate rose with income.[7] The reliance of Medicare on payroll taxes despite their regressive character is explained by the political commitment of Medicare's designers to an ideology of social insurance and in their related programmatic experience with Social Security. Understanding the historical roots of this commitment helps to explain Medicare's embrace of payroll taxes.

THE INFLUENCE OF SOCIAL INSURANCE

In the early twentieth century, American Progressives were drawn to a new wave of welfare state programs in European countries commonly known as "social insurance" or "workingman's insurance."[8] Social insurance sought to adapt the logic of private insurance to public programs.[9] The idea, as in private insurance plans, was to insure against identifiable risks by creating an insurance pool large enough to guarantee benefits payments to those who needed them when they experienced the covered risk. In the case of social insurance, the risks to be insured against were conditions, such as old age, disability, and sickness, that prevented people from working and therefore left them to the uncertainties of the market economy without stable income. Due to a number of sources of market failure, social insurance advocates argued that private insurance could never be universally available or affordable to protect all workers against these risks, which necessitated government programs to guarantee "true security."[10] And despite the allusion to private insurance, social insurance differed from private insurance in two crucial respects: it advanced societal purposes (such as income redistribution) and it represented a social rather than individual contract.[11]

In contrast to the American ideology of voluntarism that prevailed in the ninetennth and early twentieth centuries, social insurance advocates rejected the idea that private charity could provide adequate economic assistance to those in need. Social problems required government-organized action and programs.[12] But in contrast to existing public welfare programs that offered assistance only to those poor enough to qualify through a means test, social insurance aimed to keep workers out of poverty. By providing financial assistance to those unable to work, social insurance programs sought "to prevent and finally eradicate poverty . . . by meeting the problem at the origin, rather than waiting until the effects of destitution have begun to be felt."[13] And social insurance appealed to individual as well as communitarian logics: it presumed that it was "in everyone's interest to agree to the collective provision of affordable . . . insurance in order that they all have reasonable protection against foreseeable risks."[14]

Social insurance was an earned right of workers and, as such, rested on the principle of compulsory participation. Workers earned their right to benefits through mandatory payment of taxes on their wages, frequently termed contributions or premiums, into social insurance funds. These contributions were typically matched by employers. The notion of earned benefits maintained the analogy to private insurance, whose subscribers received benefits as a right of purchasing private policies.[15] Just as subscribers to private insurance qualified for benefits by paying premiums, so too would workers qualify for government benefits by making their own contributions. Advocates viewed compulsion as necessary to assure working-class and higher-income earners' participation in social insurance programs. Without compulsion, higher-wage workers might not join the insurance pools, leaving only lower-wage workers who lacked the financial resources to support a large-scale program. I. M. Rubinow, the preeminent American advocate of social insurance, summarized the dilemma in a 1916 study: "The class which needs social insurance cannot afford it, and the class that can afford it does not need it."[16] To solve this problem, social insurance required workers to participate in its financing.

Progressives launched a campaign to enact social insurance legislation in the United States in the first decade of the twentieth century. Chapter 2 discussed the role of the American Association for Labor Legislation (AALL), a group of academic and professional reformers founded in 1906, in advocating health insurance legislation.[17] The AALL also pressed states to enact industrial accident and unemployment insurance. However, the American social insurance movement generally enjoyed less success than its European counterparts. Most states enacted industrial accident insurance in the second decade of the twentieth century, but proposals during 1906–20 for medical, old-age, and unemployment insurance were either stalled or defeated.[18]

THE SOCIAL SECURITY CONNECTION

When the United States finally enacted national old-age insurance (Social Security) during the New Deal, it followed the social insurance model.[19] In 1934, Franklin Roosevelt created the Committee on Economic Security (CES), chaired by Secretary of Labor Frances Perkins, to make recommendations that addressed, in the president's words, "misfortunes which cannot be wholly eliminated in this man-made world of ours."[20] In 1935, the CES reported its findings and formally endorsed a compulsory system of old-age insurance. Workers, as well as their employers, would be required to contribute to retirement pensions during their working years. Their payroll taxes would go into a separate budgetary account, an old-age insurance trust fund, managed by the federal government. The trust fund would then pay out pension benefits to retirees who had contributed to the system.[21]

The reliance on payroll tax and trust fund financing had several key political advantages. First, since workers were compelled to pay taxes into an insurance fund, they established a moral claim on future benefits. As Martha Derthick has observed, "The whole philosophy of the [Social Security] program and the psychology of its public relations rested on the proposition that benefits were earned through the 'contributions' of individual workers."[22] The trust fund was seen, in effect, as the public property of the individuals who had paid into it, not simply as another government program that went to help "others."[23] Contributors to social insurance believed they were entitled to benefits. This sense of entitlement gave Social Security a strong public mandate. *Sense of entitlement*

Second, social insurance created an intergenerational political alliance. Both workers who were currently paying payroll taxes and retirees who had already paid payroll taxes regarded benefits as a right conferred by virtue of their own contributions. Since all Americans expected to receive Social Security when they retired, young and old found common cause in supporting benefits expansions and opposing program cuts. The program constituency, then, was numerically impressive and politically potent; it comprised not merely retirees but future retirees—in other words, the whole population.

Third, the notion of Social Security as earned benefits proved especially valuable within the conservative confines of American political culture. The designers of old-age insurance were sensitive to widespread opposition in the United States to government assistance for the "undeserving poor," who were regarded as personally responsible for their poverty— and for getting out of it.[24] In contrast, old-age insurance created a class of "deserving" beneficiaries who earned government payments through their work, enhancing its political acceptability. The association of pensions with work also enabled Americans "to accept government aid [for themselves] without feeling guilty."[25] Social Security (and later Medicare) enrollees were commonly referred to as beneficiaries, rather than recipients, a label restricted to Americans on welfare. The vocabulary of social insurance connoted images of deserving citizens rather than needy objects of government largesse.

Fourth, since payroll tax financing was compulsory, and since it was not limited to low-wage workers, old-age insurance produced a cross-class constituency. Unlike means-tested programs, whose recipients were restricted to those deemed poor enough to qualify for eligibility, Social Security included middle-class and higher-income workers. Compulsory financing created a politically stronger program by giving a stake in its operation and maintenance to politically active upper-income, as well as to low- wage, workers. Politically active beneficiaries could be expected to assure that the program remained in good financial and administrative standing, lest their own benefits suffer. In contrast, they would have no such incentive to maintain a program for the poor alone.

The 1935 CES proposal for old-age insurance embodied the principles of social insurance, with matching worker and employer contributions and compulsory participation regardless of income. However, the CES envisioned a time when the exclusive reliance on payroll taxes would end.[26] They argued that once Social Security taxes reached a rate of 2.5%, in an estimated three decades, general revenues should be introduced.[27] Beyond that point, the CES feared additional payroll taxes would impair workers' standard of living and employers would pass on the costs of additional taxes to their employees. Franklin Roosevelt, however, rejected the CES's recommendation for eventual use of general revenues. Roosevelt believed that payroll tax financing guaranteed the payment of pensions to future beneficiaries. He later justified the exclusive reliance of Social Security financing on payroll taxes by explaining that "We put those payroll contributions there so as to give the contributors a legal, moral, and political right to collect their pensions. . . . With those taxes in there, no damn politician can ever scrap my social security program."[28]

At Roosevelt's insistence, Social Security was enacted in 1935 with exclusive reliance on payroll taxes for its funding. The program would be "self-supporting," meaning that its financing came entirely from payroll taxes dedicated to Social Security, without any subsidy from general revenues.[29] That decision left an enduring historical legacy for Medicare.

MEDICARE AND PAYROLL TAX FINANCING

The federal officials who planned Medicare, including Wilbur Cohen and I. S. Falk, brought their administrative experience with Social Security, along with a political ideology of social insurance, to federal health insurance.[30] In designing Medicare, they simply extended Social Security financing.[31] Medicare would be financed as a self-supporting program, through an increase in the Social Security payroll tax on workers and their employers to fund federal health insurance, and benefits would be open to beneficiaries of Social Security pensions.[32] Like old-age insurance, payroll taxes collected for Medicare would be placed in a separate trust fund account from which the government would pay out benefits.

From the first proposals for federal hospitalization insurance for the aged in the 1950s, Medicare was based on the social insurance model of financing. Hospitalization benefits were to be financed exclusively from payroll taxes on current workers and their employers. The strategists who planned Medicare had presided over the substantial expansion of Social Security benefits and eligibility during the 1940s and 1950s. By encoding Social Security's financing arrangements and social insurance principles into Medicare, they intended to reproduce the political popularity and financial stability of old-age insurance in federal health insurance. The anticipated political advantages of payroll tax financing for Medicare were the same as those for Social Security. Health insurance benefits funded by payroll contributions would be widely viewed as an earned right. Since beneficiaries would contribute to the federal hospitalization insurance trust fund through taxes on their employment, they would be seen—and they would see themselves—as deserving claimants of Medicare benefits, not as recipients of government welfare. Medicare's political constituency, like Social Security's, would be cross-generational and cross-class. Since workers paid taxes into the program, they could be expected to support its maintenance in anticipation of their retirement. And since participation in Medicare financing was compulsory, the range of beneficiaries encompassed middle-class and upper-income, as well as low-income, seniors. All of these dynamics were expected to ensure the program's popularity and political success.

Yet payroll tax and trust fund financing appealed to fiscal conservatives as well as to advocates of social insurance. Because Medicare was self-supporting, increases in benefits had to be accompanied by increases in the Medicare payroll tax. Conservatives believed the reluctance of the public to accept increases in their payroll taxes would constrain the growth of the program in a way that reliance on general revenues would not.[33] In a 1965 congressional hearing on Medicare, Wilbur Mills, a leading fiscal conservative, explained the logic: "whenever you have a program financed by a specific tax, the willingness of people to pay that tax, that specific tax, limits the benefits of that specific program. . . . if you put a program, then, into the general fund of the Treasury, there is less likelihood that you control the package of benefits initially enacted than there is if you put it in a trust fund. . . . I can't help but reach the conclusion that a specific fund, supported by a payroll tax, is a more conservative method of financing something than to do it out of the general fund of the Treasury."[34] Payroll taxes consequently enjoyed broad political appeal from both liberals and conservatives as an instrument of public financing.

INSURANCE FOR PHYSICIANS' SERVICES

As chapter 2 detailed, insurance for physician services was added to Medicare only at the last stage of its enactment, and the origins of its financing were very different from the social insurance model of Medicare hospitalization insurance. The decisive influence on funding for physician services—what came to be known as Medicare part B—was Wilbur Mills, chairman of the House Ways and Means Committee. That committee had Social Security under its jurisdiction, and Mills strongly opposed further expansion of payroll taxes. Mills feared the impact that the high and uncertain costs of medical care would have on the Social Security trust fund, potentially forcing the payroll tax beyond acceptable limits, leading to "constituent and corporate revolt against Social Security."[35] Mills and others strongly believed (falsely, as it turned out) that the combined Social Security tax on employers and employees could not exceed 10%, a psychological barrier they presumed the American public would not cross.[36] Mills also worried that Medicare weakened the connection between payroll taxes and benefits that Social Security had established by using "wage related revenue to pay for non-wage related service benefits."[37] Finally, Mills was aware of the criticism that Medicare offered inadequate health insurance protection to the elderly because, in its initial legislative form, it covered only the costs of hospital services. Such perceptions of inadequate coverage could generate future demands for Medicare's expansion, leading to what he viewed as unaffordable increases in payroll taxes that would threaten both the solvency of Social Security and the vitality of the economy.

In order to assuage Mills, Medicare designers emphasized that the Medicare trust fund for hospitalization insurance would, for accounting purposes, be separate from Social Security's trust fund for old-age insurance.[38] In fact, this arrangement followed the precedent of disability insurance. When disability insurance was enacted in 1956 as an addition to Social Security, congressional critics such as Oklahoma senator Robert Kerr argued that due to the ambiguous nature of eligibility determinations for disability, program enrollment was unpredictable and could overwhelm the Social Security trust fund, hurting retirees and survivors.[39] As a result, disabiltiy insurance was placed in a separate trust fund account to assure Kerr and others that it would not harm the finances of old-age insurance. Now, a decade later, the creation of a separate Medicare trust fund served to reassure Mills about the impact of a new program with uncertain costs on the financial security of Social Security. However, in order to assuage Mills's concerns, Medicare's designers took a step beyond what they had done for disabiltiy insurance. Instead of funding Medicare hospitalization insurance through an increase in the existing Social Security tax, as they initially wanted, they changed their proposal to incorporate a separate Medicare payroll tax that would be earmarked for the Medicare trust fund.[40] Medicare hospitalization insurance would be supported strictly from the revenues collected from its own payroll tax.

However, Mills's fiscal concerns regarding Medicare still were not satisfied. He added physicians' insurance to the final Medicare legislation in 1965, funded in equal parts by general revenues and beneficiary premiums rather than another increase in payroll taxes. By extending Medicare coverage to physician services through general revenue financing, Mills assured that payroll taxes would be confined to Medicare part A, hospitalization insurance. As Medicare began operation in 1966, it consequently contained two sets of financing mechanisms with strikingly different historical roots and political philosophies. Incongruously, one part of Medicare was designed to expand social insurance, while the other attempted to restrain it.

THE POLITICAL CONSEQUENCES OF MEDICARE FINANCING

Since its enactment, Medicare has been one of the nation's most popular social programs. That popularity can be attributed, in part, to its financing design. The Medicare payroll tax has created the sense of public entitlement that its architects anticipated. It has also served to reinforce the notion that Medicare beneficiaries are deserving claimants on the public purse rather than the recipients of government welfare. These developments would seem to confirm the political power of the program's financing arrangements. However, it is worth noting that there is no evidence of differentiation in public attitudes toward Medicare part A, funded through payroll taxes, and Medicare part B, which is funded primarily by general revenues. That there is no distinction in public support for the two parts of Medicare may simply indicate the extent to which, in the public mind, the payroll tax is associated with the entire program, not simply with part A. And since part A accounts for the majority of program expenditures, the payroll tax is arguably the most important financing mechanism in the program. But it may also indicate that the influence of payroll tax funding on Medicare's popularity has been exaggerated at the expense of emphasizing the importance of the program's universal coverage to its success. After all, programs that cover an entire population or population category regardless of income need not be financed through payroll taxes or even earmarked taxes. And universal health insurance programs in nations such as Canada that are funded through general revenues rather than payroll taxes enjoy strong public support.

Regardless of the source of Medicare's political strength, though, analysts have often overlooked the impact of the program's financing arrangements on its politics. That impact has been profound, and, contrary to conventional wisdom, it has not always promoted Medicare's political stability. Indeed, the influence of Medicare's financing system on program politics has in important respects been the opposite of what the program's architects expected. In particular, during its first three decades Medicare experienced a series of intermittent funding shortfalls that fueled fears the program was going bankrupt.

There have been three periods of financial crisis in Medicare's history: 1969–72, 1982–84, and 1995–97. All three periods were marked by organized attention from policymakers to Medicare crises. Congressional hearings on Medicare financial crises were held by the Senate Finance and House Ways and Means Committees during 1969–70, 1984, and 1995.[41] The 1982–84 crisis was also addressed by a presidential advisory commission on Medicare.[42] In two of the three periods, organized attention by policymakers to Medicare trust fund shortfalls was matched by substantial attention from the national media, in 1983–84 and again in 1995.[43] This is not to suggest that these are the only periods when Medicare's financial condition has been a political issue. On the contrary, concern with Medicare's growing rate of spending has been present virtually from the start of program operations; fiscal duress has been a persistent feature of program politics. But what distinguished these three acute periods from chronic scrutiny of financing was the sharp focus on the threat to Medicare's ability to fund benefits, as exemplified by warnings that the program was "going bankrupt" and that the trust fund faced immediate "insolvency" and "exhaustion."

INSTITUTIONAL SOURCES OF BANKRUPTCY CRISES

As viewed from the perspective of most other government programs, the character of Medicare financing politics is unusual. We do not talk of the military "going bankrupt" or becoming "insolvent." Nor do other federal programs, such as foreign aid, poverty assistance, loans for education, or funding for the arts experience bankruptcy crises. Such programs may be the targets of criticism that they are spending too much money, or that their spending is not accomplishing stated goals. They may be said to be in financial trouble. But they are not subject to bankruptcy rhetoric.[44]

Why is Medicare different? The distinctive form of Medicare financing politics can be explained by analyzing the one prominent federal program other than Medicare that has been subject to a bankruptcy crisis: Social Security. In 1977, unexpected sharp increases in program costs precipitated a financial crisis in Social Security, prompting the passage of "rescue" legislation by the Carter administration and Congress. However, the rescue proved short lived, and by 1982 the Social Security trust fund was again "going broke." The crisis had all the elements, including high-profile political attention, media coverage, and warnings of impending bankruptcy, that are by now familiar to Medicare politics.[45] Paul Pierson locates the cause of the Social Security bankruptcy crises within the program's own financing arrangements. He argues that Social Security politics is "trust-fund driven" and that it is consequently prone to crisis.[46] Financing for Social Security is self-supporting; that is, it is funded exclusively from payroll taxes that go into an earmarked federal trust fund. Social Security benefits are paid out of the trust fund, not out of general revenues collected by the federal government. This arrangement is crucial, because it means that Social Security funds are treated as an account that is separate from the rest of the federal government's finances. When the revenues in this trust fund account appear low, a financial crisis is claimed to ensue.[47] In other words, the potential for bankruptcy crises is inherent in Social Security's design.

The trust-fund-driven logic of Social Security politics can be extended to Medicare as well. The hospitalization insurance portion of Medicare is similarly funded from payroll taxes on current workers and their employers. And like Social Security, for accounting purposes these funds are dedicated to a trust fund specific to Medicare hospitalization insurance. If the revenues in this trust fund appear to be low or insufficient to pay program costs, then Medicare too appears in danger of bankruptcy. If Medicare hospitalization insurance were instead financed out of the general revenues that fund other government programs, and if it did not have an independent trust fund, there would not be bankruptcy crises in Medicare, because there would not be a separate account to go bankrupt.

The primary cause of Medicare financing crises is thus the structure of Medicare financing itself. By relying on a system of payroll tax and trust fund financing that is self-supporting, Medicare has created a system that is inherently vulnerable to cycles of bankruptcy. The irony is that the structural arrangements of Medicare financing that cause its bankruptcy crises are precisely the mechanisms that Medicare's architects favored as essential to its political stability. Payroll taxes and trust fund financing were to be the cornerstones of Medicare's political popularity and financial stability. Instead, they became sources of periodic program instability, albeit instability that has led to policy innovation.

Physician Insurance and Financing Politics

The institutional basis of Medicare financial crises is underscored by the contrast between financing arrangements in hospitalization and physician insurance. Medicare part B, physicians' insurance, is not a self-supporting financing system. It too has a trust fund, but since its annual costs are funded from beneficiary premiums and general revenues, the supplementary medical insurance trust fund cannot be exhausted in the same sense that the hospitalization insurance trust fund can. Figure 4.1 compares the annual rate of increase in Medicare outlays for hospitalization and physicians' insurance. In fourteen of Medicare's first twenty-seven fiscal years for which data exist, the annual rate of growth in Medicare for physician outlays exceeded that for hospitals. Nevertheless, Medicare part B has never experienced a bankruptcy crisis, nor has a shortfall in the trust fund for physicians' insurance ever sparked a broader program crisis. Bankruptcy crises are not, then, only the result of high rates of increase in program costs. Rather, they are the function of a distinctive set of financing arrangements, namely a self-supporting system of payroll taxes and a trust fund. The absence of this system in physician insurance has given its politics a different character than that of hospitalization insurance, one that is not driven by bankruptcy crises.

Timing

How do we explain the timing of Medicare financial crises in 1969, 1982, and 1995? Is there a pattern to when these crises occur? Does the timing of crises reveal anything about their causes? Table 4.1, utilizing data from the board of trustees of the federal hospitalization insurance trust fund, compares the date of onset of Medicare crises with two measures of the program's financial condition: the number of years until the Medicare hospitalization insurance trust fund is predicted to be exhausted and the size of the long-term deficit in the hospitalization insurance trust fund. These projections are computed by actuaries within the Health Care Fi-

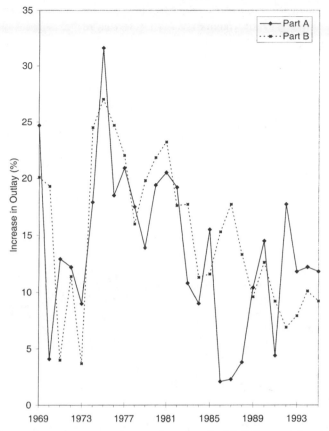

Fig. 4.1. Annual percentage increase in outlays for Medicare parts A and B.

nancing Administration (now the Center for Medicare and Medicaid Services, or CMS), the federal agency that administers Medicare, and presented to Congress, in compliance with federal law, in annual reports by the board of trustees.[48]

Two trends are evident. First, Medicare's long-range actuarial balance has been negative—that is, its revenues have been projected as insufficient to cover costs for the next twenty-five years—for almost all of the program's history. In twenty-six of the first thirty years of Medicare's operation, federal actuaries forecast a long-range trust fund deficit, and there was no positive actuarial balance from 1974 to 1994. Second, there is no consistent relationship between the size of the long-range deficit and the onset of Medicare financial crises. The three Medicare funding crises—

Table 4.1 Financial Status of the Medicare Hospitalization Insurance Trust Fund

YEAR OF REPORT	ESTIMATED DATE OF EXHAUSTION	YEARS TO EXHAUSTION	ACTUARIAL BALANCE
1966	1990	24	0
1967	1991	24	0
1968	1992	24	.03
1969	1976	7	−.29
1970	1973	3	−.48
1971	1974	3	−.62
1972	1976	4	−.61
1973	1997	24	−.04
1974	1998	24	.02
1975	1998	23	−.16
1976	1992	16	−.64
1977	1988	11	−1.16
1978	1990	12	−1.12
1979	1992	13	−1.04
1980	1994	14	−.99
1981	1992	11	−1.31
1982	1988	6	−1.85
1983	1990	7	−1.17
1984	1991	7	−1.30
1985	1999	14	−.60
1986	1997	11	−.41
1987	2004	17	−.38
1988	2007	19	−.41
1989[a]	—	—	—
1990	2004	14	−.70
1991	2005	14	−.70
1992	2002	10	−1.00
1993	1999	6	−2.11
1994	2001	7	−1.65
1995	2002	7	−1.33

Source: *Annual Reports of the board of trustees of the Federal Hospital Insurance Trust Fund*, 1966–95.
Note: "Year of Report" lists the year the actuarial report was issued. "Estimated Date of Exhaustion" gives the estimated date of trust fund exhaustion as predicted by each report. The estimated date of trust fund exhaustion represents the year in which the money in the trust fund is projected to be insufficient to pay all of Medicare's costs. "Years to Exhaustion" lists the number of years from the issuing of each report until the trust fund is predicted to run out. "Actuarial Balance" lists the trust fund's long-range actuarial balance expressed as a percentage of taxable payroll, the measure used by Medicare actuaries. The long-range actuarial balance is defined as the difference between Medicare's projected income and projected costs during the next twenty-five years. Taxable payroll is the amount of workers' income subject to Medicare payroll taxes. If projected revenues exceed costs over a twenty-five-year period, Medicare is said to have a "favorable actuarial balance." If the number is negative, it means that Medicare has a projected deficit in its finances over the next twenty-five yeaars, i.e., an "actuarial deficit."
[a]No long-range forecasts were made in 1989 because of uncertainty regarding the Medicare catastrophic health legislation.

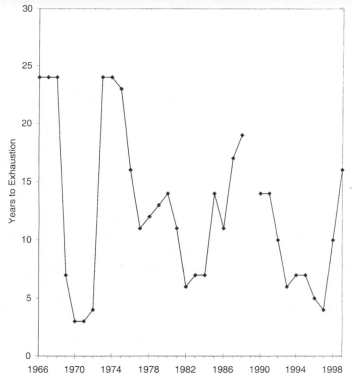

Fig. 4.2. Estimated time until hospitalization insurance trust fund exhaustion.

1969, 1983, and 1995—began at different levels of long-range deficit: −.29, −1.85, and −1.33. There is not, then, a "magic number" in the program's long-range actuarial balance that triggers Medicare crises.

Figure 4.2 displays the number of years, as estimated by program actuaries, to trust fund "exhaustion." Trust fund exhaustion represents the year Medicare actuaries predict that program revenues will not cover all program costs.[49] The results are striking, revealing a strong relationship between the number of years to trust fund exhaustion and the onset of Medicare crisis. There have been three periods in which the estimated time until trust fund exhaustion has been seven years or less: 1969–72, 1982–84, and 1993–95. Medicare financial crises have occurred in all three periods. In two cases, the onset of each crisis came in years when the actuaries predicted seven years to exhaustion, 1969 and 1995. In the other case, 1982, the crisis began at an estimated date to exhaustion of six years. There has been, then, a consistent pattern to the onset of Medicare financial crises. That pattern in turn reflects in large part the influence of actuaries on Medicare financing policy.

THE PRIVILEGED POSITION OF MEDICARE ACTUARIES

The dynamics of Medicare financing crises shed light on a crucial set of actors in program policy who have rarely been examined: actuaries. Medicare borrowed its practice of relying on actuarial estimates from Social Security. From its inception, Social Security employed federal actuaries who released annual reports with data on the program's finances and forecasts of its future prospects. Social Security financing emphasized the insurance principle of "actuarial soundness." An actuarially sound pension system was defined as "one which sets forth a plan of benefits and the contributions to provide these benefits, so related that the amount of the present and contingent liabilities of the plan as actuarially computed as of any date will at least be balanced by the amount of the present and contingent assets of the plan actuarially computed as of the same date."[50] As in private pension plans, then, forecasts were made to provide an annual accounting of program finances and to ensure that Social Security would have adequate assets in its trust fund to pay out future benefits obligations.[51] The inclusion of an actuarial system in Social Security maintained the analogy to private insurance by assuring that the program would follow the same financial standards that private pension plans used. It also served to legitimate the program in the eyes of the professional actuarial community, an important function for a new government program regarded at the time as economically unsound by much of the business community.

By focusing on the concept of actuarial soundness, Social Security financing guaranteed that the forecasts by government actuaries would occupy a privileged position in the program. Since Social Security financing was self-supporting, actuarial forecasts were essential to determining the payroll tax schedule necessary to meet program costs. If actual costs exceeded predicted costs by wide margins, the program trust fund could be threatened by insolvency. Forecasts provided an aura of certainty, permitting Congress to set payroll taxes at specified levels to meet expected costs. The financial stability of the Social Security system thus depended, in large measure, on the reliability of actuarial forecasts. And in practice, actuarial forecasts in Social Security were conducive to program expansion. During the program's first three decades of operation, conservative assumptions employed by actuaries in their forecasts helped assure that Social Security's revenues usually exceeded expenditures, creating surpluses that were frequently spent on benefits expansions (though these expansions were also largely necessitated by inflation).[52]

Medicare adopted the same principle of actuarial soundness when it began operation. Whereas estimates of Social Security's financial condition were originally made into "perpetuity," and then adjusted to seventy-five-year projections,[53] long-range forecasts for Medicare initially covered only a twenty-five-year year period (they were subsequently expanded to seventy-five years in 1984). The reason, according to federal actuaries, was that there were greater uncertainties in predicting the costs of medical care than pension payments. Indeed, forecasting Social Security benefits, based predominantly on demographic trends and projections of benefits owed to contributing workers, is relatively straightforward compared to long-range forecasting of Medicare spending. Forecasts of Medicare expenditures, to be accurate, require estimates of numerous variables including utilization rates, medical practice patterns, technological changes in medical services, changes in the structure of the health care system, trends in health status and prevalence of disabilities and chronic conditions, and fluctuations in medical care inflation and prices—a daunting list. In fact, while it was common practice for private insurers to make long-term forecasts about the financial condition or "actuarial soundness" of pension plans, at the time of Medicare's enactment private health insurers typically made only annual projections of outlays in order to adjust their premiums and did not rely on long-term forecasting.[54] The unpredictability of these measures led the 1971 presidential Advisory Council on Social Security to recommend that Medicare forecasts be restricted to ten-year periods.[55] In their efforts to reproduce Social Security's political success in Medicare, then, program architects borrowed a practice from pensions that was not as suitable for health insurance. However, whatever the technical limitations of long-term Medicare forecasts, once made, they were politically potent.

The adoption of actuarial soundness as a standard for the Medicare trust fund gave the annual actuarial forecasts a critical role in defining the parameters of program financing policy. The power of federal actuaries to predict the date of trust fund exhaustion and to define the balance of Medicare finances enables them to substantially influence perceptions both of Medicare's present state and its future course. These forecasts assume so much influence because Medicare financing is self-supporting.[56] If Medicare were funded from general revenues and its assets were not maintained in a separate account, actuarial estimates would not exert as much influence, since the program's finances could not be "exhausted" in the same sense that they are under current financing arrangements.

In Social Security, actuarial estimates historically served as a stabilizing influence on program politics.[57] Government actuaries such as Robert Myers enjoyed high levels of respect among the congressional financing committees that oversaw Social Security and both the Democratic and Republican parties. The office of the actuary within the Social Security Administration had a large degree of independence in making its forecasts.[58] And the presumed reliability of actuarial estimates gave congressional policymakers the confidence that program costs would not exceed revenues, enabling frequent increases in benefits.

In Medicare, though, the system of actuarial estimates has had an unanticipated, less stabilizing influence. Forecasting medical costs has proven a far more difficult task than predicting pension benefits. Federal actuaries have frequently underestimated Medicare costs, leading to recurrent trust fund shortfalls. While Social Security had not experienced any funding crises prior to Medicare's enactment, and did not endure its first until four decades after the program's introduction, Medicare's first financial crisis came in 1969, only four years after it started. Still, actuaries in Medicare enjoyed a privileged position in the program, one that has been relatively unchallenged, despite the growth of other organizations, such as the Congressional Budget Office, that possess similar expertise.[59]

ARE MEDICARE CRISES POLITICAL CONSTRUCTIONS?

Crises offer an extraordinary opportunity to remake existing public policies.[60] The rhetoric of crisis is a powerful stimulus to action, suggesting that something must be done quickly to avert or end the crisis situation. Trust fund crises, which are typically accompanied by claims that action must be taken to save programs from bankruptcy, have particular resonance.[61] In such circumstances, it may be easier to overcome program-based interests that resist changes in current policies, as their political influence may be weakened by the presumed urgency of the situation. In some cases, crises become public events, bringing the force of mass opinion and other heretofore latent political forces into normally less visible political contests, thereby changing the balance of power over a policy struggle, perhaps to the disadvantage of vested interests. The need for action that crises evoke may also induce acceptance of policy ideas that were previously regarded as too risky or unnecessary. As Carroll Estes argues, crises may be purposefully created by policymakers who already have a solution in mind and seek to arouse public anxiety in order to gain "expanded authority . . . [for] the adoption of formerly unthinkable solutions."[62]

There is a large literature in political science and sociology that argues political crises are socially constructed. In other words, crises are said not to reflect any changes in objective conditions that indicate a worsening problem. Rather, crises are generated by the subjective assessments of political actors who want to create a crisis to serve political purposes. The Medicare experience provides only partial support for this perspective. As discussed in the next section, Medicare policymakers have certainly exploited hospitalization insurance trust fund shortfalls to promote their own solutions and policy ideas. And there have been attempts to generate a mood of crisis surrounding Medicare. For example, in 1969, Senator Russell Long, chairman of the Senate Finance Committee, and John Williams, the ranking Republican on the committee, *wanted* to create the perception that a crisis existed in Medicare.[63] They did so by holding hearings and issuing reports critical of Medicare policies and administration that warned of impending funding problems.

Medicare financing crises, however, are not merely political constructions. There is an undeniable relationship between objective financial conditions and the onset of Medicare financing crises. As figure 4.2 shows, the three periods of crisis have all come when trust fund reserves were declining and the forecast date of trust fund exhaustion was less than a decade away. Admittedly, the relationship is not perfect. In 1995, for instance, both the predicted year of exhaustion (2002) and the long-range actuarial balance (-1.33) were actually more favorable than they had been in the previous two years. In other words, Medicare was in better financial shape in 1995 than in previous years. Yet there was no Medicare crisis in 1993 or 1994.

Indeed, there is no clearly demarcated actuarial border of years to exhaustion or long-term deficit that, if Medicare crosses it, constitutes a program crisis.[64] That makes the consistent relationship between actuarially predicted years to exhaustion and the onset of crisis puzzling. In all three periods of Medicare history when government actuaries have forecast trust fund exhaustion as imminent in seven years or less, there have been financial crises. And there have been no financial crises in years where the forecast time to trust fund exhaustion is eight years or more. Yet there is no special actuarial significance to this number. There is no more actuarial basis for saying that seven years is a crisis in Medicare than eleven years or three years.

Why, then, have Medicare crises occurred at similar points in actuarial forecasts? One explanation for this pattern may lie in the psychology of perception. Congressional policymakers may attach particular significance to estimates of Medicare exhaustion that are under a decade. When the forecasts reach this point, the date of exhaustion in program financing may appear so close as to constitute a crisis, or so close as to be sufficient to convince *others* that a funding crisis exists. When the trust fund's balance falls below a decade, entrepreneurs with Medicare reform plans already in hand can seize the opportunity to create a crisis environment that allows them to adopt these plans. The political meaning attached to estimates of trust fund exhaustion that are seven years or less may consequently reflect the political uses of psychological biases in how policymakers perceive the proximity of Medicare bankruptcy according to various estimates.[65]

Still, the relationship between objective changes in the trust fund and the advent of crises is clear. Here the crucial point is that the Medicare hospitalization insurance trust fund acts as a sort of internal alarm; when projected program finances are low, it sounds. How loud it sounds and for how long, as well as what steps are taken to shut it off, depend on the actions of politicians.

MANAGING TRUST FUND SHORTFALLS: FINANCING AS POLITICAL CHOICE

Program actuaries set the parameters of Medicare financing policy. They define how much additional funding Medicare needs, and how soon it needs it, if the program is to remain solvent. But it is Congress and the president who determine how that additional funding is to be obtained. There is no single, predetermined response required by trust fund exhaustion, though policymakers often talk and act as if there were. Rather, trust fund shortfalls in Medicare present a political choice between four potential responses: introducing general revenues, increasing revenues from payroll taxes, increasing the costs to beneficiaries, and decreasing program costs through regulation of payments to medical providers.

GENERAL REVENUES

One response to shortfalls in Medicare financing would be to augment program revenues from payroll taxes with general revenues from federal income, excise, and corporate taxation. General revenues could be introduced whenever there was a shortfall in the Medicare trust fund, or as a permanent financing mechanism for hospitalization insurance, as they are already a part of physician insurance. Alternatively, the program's existing financing system could be replaced by financing Medicare entirely out of general revenues.

There have been periodic calls to restructure Medicare financing, especially from the Federal Advisory Councils on Social Security.[66] The advisory councils began in 1937 as an instrument of Social Security policy-making, and when Medicare was enacted in 1965, federal health insurance was added to their responsibilities.[67] During Medicare's first fifteen years, the Social Security advisory councils consistently advocated changing the structure of Medicare financing. The 1971 council recommended combining Medicare hospitalization and physician insurance into one fund and financing it with equal, one-third contributions from employees, employers, and general revenues. The 1975 advisory council noted that Medicare benefits, unlike Social Security pensions, were not related to workers' payroll tax contributions, but to their health costs as retirees. "Under such circumstances," the council concluded, "there does not seem to be any real reason for funding such [Medicare] costs by a tax on wages."[68] Payroll tax financing, it said, should be replaced by a system of general revenue financing that would become the "sole source" of funding for hospitalization expenditures.[69] The 1979 council suggested that earmarked taxes be retained for Medicare, but that the taxes be collected from personal and corporate income, not wages.[70]

There is also some evidence that the public supported greater reliance on general revenue financing of Medicare. Surveys conducted from 1979 to 1982 consistently found either pluralities or majorities in favor of using more general revenues in Medicare.[71] Forty-three percent of respondents in a 1979 survey supported higher amounts of general revenue financing of Medicare (with 35% opposed), even if it required paying higher income taxes. And in 1982, a record 62% favored additional general revenue funding for Medicare.[72] Due to the limited polling data available, only a tentative conclusion is possible. But, at a minimum, it appears that there was public support during Medicare's 1982 funding crisis for enhancing the role of general revenues in the program, mirroring the position held by the Social Security advisory councils.

Yet Medicare financing for hospitalization insurance has remained exclusively reliant on payroll taxes. The introduction of general revenues, either as a supplement or replacement, has never attracted sufficient political support to win adoption. The major source of opposition has been fiscal. Policymakers have been concerned that if Medicare payroll tax financing were ended, so too would any financial discipline in the program, since benefits expansions would not have to be accompanied by specific tax increases.[73] From this perspective, general revenue financing of Medicare would, echoing the earlier fears of Wilbur Mills, "obscure the true cost [of the program]."[74] Congress has thus been reluctant to end Medicare part A's self-supporting financing structure.

More recently, the rise of antitax sentiment in national politics has strengthened opposition to introducing general revenues to Medicare hospitalization insurance. The 1982 Social Security advisory council, the first council to issue a separate report on Medicare, rejected any increases in general taxes to meet Medicare's projected fiscal problems. "In an era when the government is experiencing substantial annual deficits," the council wrote in its 1984 report, "reliance on general revenues would only serve to exacerbate the problem of increasing deficits."[75] In other words, there would be no new general revenues for Medicare. Medicare's exclusive reliance on payroll taxes to fund hospitalization insurance remained unchanged.

PAYROLL TAXES

A second potential response to Medicare financing shortfalls is to increase the program's income from payroll taxes. There are two ways to increase payroll tax income: raising the tax rate itself or raising the amount of income subject to Medicare taxes. Table 4.2 shows the historical experience of Medicare payroll taxes for hospitalization insurance (known as "contribution rates") and the maximum taxable amount of annual earnings.

How have policymakers altered payroll taxes in response to financial crises? In 1972, Congress raised the scheduled future rates for Medicare taxes, as well as the maximum amount of income subject to the tax. In 1982, no change was made in either the payroll tax rate or the maximum taxable earnings. And in 1995, there was no discussion of raising payroll taxes. Indeed, the Republican congressional leadership flatly rejected even considering the possibility of Medicare tax increases.

The pattern in Medicare, then, has been one of reluctance to raise payroll taxes in response to financing shortfalls. Only in the first Medicare trust fund crisis did widespread agreement exist between Congress and a presidential administration that payroll taxes should be increased to meet program funding problems.[76] Moreover, the current rate of 1.45% assessed on workers and their employers has remained unchanged since 1986, though the ceiling on maximum income subject to the payroll tax was removed in 1993. Policymakers, especially those on the congressional financing committees that oversee the program, have long justified their reluctance to raise payroll taxes by citing a "political limit" on the level of Medicare and Social Security taxes. This refers to an apparent limit on the willingness of the public to accept additional payroll taxes. With considerable public opposition, the argument goes, it is simply not feasible to raise the rate of payroll taxes for Medicare and Social Security.

Table 4.2 Medicare Payroll Tax Rates

YEAR	TAX RATE (%)	MAXIMUM TAXABLE EARNINGS ($)
1966	.35	6,600
1967	.50	6,600
1968–71	.60	7,800
1972	.60	9,000
1973	1.00	10,800
1974	.90	13,200
1975	.90	14,100
1976	.90	15,300
1977	.90	16,500
1978	1.00	17,700
1979	1.05	22,900
1980	1.05	25,900
1981	1.30	29,700
1982	1.30	32,400
1983	1.30	35,700
1984	1.30	37,800
1985	1.35	39,600
1986	1.45	42,000
1987	1.45	43,800
1988	1.45	45,000
1989	1.45	48,000
1990	1.45	51,300
1991	1.45	125,000
1992	1.45	130,200
1993	1.45	135,000
1994	1.45	no limit
1995	1.45	no limit
1996	1.45	no limit
1997	1.45	no limit
1998	1.45	no limit
1999	1.45	no limit
2000	1.45	no limit
Scheduled in present law:		
2001–	1.45	no limit

Source: *Annual Report of the board of trustees of the Hospital Insurance Trust Fund,* 1995.

Opinion polls on public attitudes toward Medicare payroll taxes have been conducted only sporadically. Nevertheless, two patterns emerge. First, when increasing payroll taxes is included as one option in a menu of choices to redress Medicare financing problems, the public does not choose it as a top option and it receives only minority support.[77] And second, when the public is asked about specific dollar amounts of proposed tax increases in Medicare, their opposition is often strong. For instance, in a 1984 survey, only 22% of respondents expressed willingness to increase their payroll taxes by $250 for Medicare, with 67% opposed; in 1983 opponents outnumbered supporters of a $750 increase 48%-30%.[78] This follows a more general trend in American polling on health care programs. Public support for national health insurance drops significantly when respondents are asked about their willingness to pay specific dollar amounts to fund it, as opposed to when they are queried more generally about support for a national health program.[79]

At first glance, then, the reluctance to raise payroll taxes can be interpreted as an example of the influence of public opinion over Medicare payroll taxes. Public resistance to tax increases appears to have constrained the range of policymakers' responses to Medicare funding crises. And politicians' claims that they have heard a strong cry of "no new taxes" from the public seem to ring true.

Yet this simple picture of public influence does not hold up to further scrutiny. It is, in fact, not at all clear that the public has decisively influenced Medicare financing policy, despite politicians' claims that they are responding to the public will, or in this case, lack of will to raise Medicare taxes. Crucially, the wording of questions has exerted substantial influence on polling results from surveys measuring the extent of public support for Medicare financing options. While the aforementioned surveys from 1983 and 1984 questioned respondents about higher "taxes," a series of surveys by the Employee Benefit Research Institute and Gallup from 1990 to 1993 asked instead about "willing[ness] to pay an increased Social Security *contribution* (italics added)."[80] This terminology followed that used by Social Security and Medicare administrators. The result: in 1992 and 1993, a majority of the public, 53% and 51%, respectively, were willing to pay higher Social Security contributions for Medicare, and in 1990, 48% favored higher contributions, with 47% opposed.[81] And a 1986 AMA poll that asked about support for raising payroll taxes given that "some observers have predicted that the Medicare system will go bankrupt without additional funding" found 70% of those surveyed were willing to pay additional taxes.[82]

These results do not merely reinforce the importance of question wording in shaping survey results and cautious interpretation of poll data derived from different questions (though due to these limitations, no conclusion can be reached about trends in public support for Medicare payroll tax increases over time).[83] More important, these polls suggest that policymakers can mobilize public support for raising Medicare taxes if they present a message that draws on core public support for Medicare, such as "contributing" to maintain benefits, or taps into concern about the program's future. Bipartisan appeals to raise the payroll tax out of a national obligation to maintain Medicare's social contract and protect the elderly would surely have been heeded by the public; they just were never made. For all the talk of an antitax popular mandate, in Medicare's first three decades there were no instances of mass public opposition to, or demonstrations against, rising program payroll taxes (nor for that matter were there any in Social Security). The American public has long abided payroll tax increases in Medicare and Social Security, and there is no reason to expect that they would not have abided tax increases to redress financial distress in a program that provides health insurance to their parents and grandparents. A public education campaign that explained the necessity of raising payroll taxes to save Medicare from bankruptcy would have elicited, at a minimum, a permissive consensus from the public to increase payroll taxes (especially given the already noted support for increasing general revenues devoted to Medicare).

The public, then, has not been the main obstacle to raising payroll taxes in Medicare. Instead, financing policy has been constrained primarily by political elites in Congress and the presidency. Recall that there is strong evidence of a gap between popular and elite support for Medicare, with the public favoring spending increases on Medicare at levels twice as high as that among members of Congress.[84] There has also been strong public support for benefits expansions in Medicare. There are two key implications. The first is that if public support for increasing Medicare spending and benefits exceeds that of policymakers, it is likely that the public would also look more kindly on payroll tax increases. While public antitax sentiment has grown in the United States since the 1970s, it cannot be assumed that this sentiment necessarily extends to Medicare. Medicare is a distinct case in financing politics. Its taxes are specifically directed at a popular program that serves a well-liked constituency—one that virtually all Americans living to age sixty-five will join—that is viewed as both deserving of government aid and entitled to earned benefits.

The second implication is that congressional policymakers are less likely to support payroll tax increases than the public because they believe Medicare costs are already excessive. Intergenerational equity concerns regarding the share of the elderly in public resources are more pronounced in Congress than in the public.[85] From the intergenerational perspective, payroll taxes take resources from younger, less well off workers and hand them over to seniors who already have too large a share of the public budget. There is, then, less to the publicly set political limit on raising Medicare payroll taxes than meets the eye. The public has been more willing to accept payroll tax increases than Medicare policymakers have acknowledged. And ultimately, the political limit on Medicare payroll taxes has been less a function of public opinion than of elite preferences.[86]

BENEFICIARY COSTS

A third response to financial crises in Medicare could be to increase the costs of hospitalization insurance to beneficiaries. These costs could be raised in three ways. First, existing cost-sharing amounts, including the deductible that beneficiaries pay for Medicare hospitalization coverage, could be raised. Second, new cost-sharing measures could be introduced. Beneficiaries could be charged a monthly premium for hospitalization coverage such as exists in Medicare physicians' insurance.[87] Or more affluent beneficiaries could be charged a higher premium for Medicare, as the Medicare Catastrophic Coverage Act imposed. Third, the retirement age for Medicare eligibility could be raised.

In general, however, increasing beneficiary costs has not been a prominent response to funding shortfalls in Medicare hospitalization insurance. The Medicare deductible has been, since the program's enactment in 1965, tied to the average daily cost of hospital stays, and increases in the deductible have been adjusted automatically to reflect changes in that cost. There was no legislated increase in hospitalization cost sharing in response to the 1969–72 crisis. During the second Medicare financial crisis in 1982, there was a 12% increase in the deductible as a consequence of a technical change in the formula through which it was calculated.[88] This change, however, paled in financial significance in comparison to savings from regulatory changes that were made in Medicare at the same time. And new cost-sharing requirements for hospitalization insurance, such as a premium, have not been introduced to the program.

The limited increase in beneficiary cost sharing as a response to financial crises reflected three main factors. First, the deductible for Medicare hospitalization insurance grew to be substantially higher than the deductible for most private health insurance plans.[89] Since the deductible was already viewed as a burden on beneficiaries, there has been little inclination to raise it further. Second, beneficiaries have been viewed, especially by the Democratic congressional majorities that were the norm from Medicare's passage in 1965 until 1994, in a more favorable light than hospitals and physicians (who also tend to be a more Republican constituency than the elderly). As a consequence, Congress sought to impose more costs on medical providers than on elderly and disabled Medicare patients. Finally, the financing system of hospitalization insurance confers a sense of earned benefits. This has diminished the political opportunities for introducing a new system of cost sharing, such as premiums for hospitalization insurance, since it would be widely regarded by retirees, as well as the public, as a violation of Medicare entitlement.[90]

[handwritten marginalia: charge wealthy more or cut benefits.]

However, there has been significant public support for charging wealthier Medicare beneficiaries more or cutting their benefits.[91] This support, though, did not translate from 1965 to 1994 into any congressional action to impose either more costs or benefits cuts on higher-income Medicare beneficiaries, other than the income-related premiums legislated in 1988 as part of the short-lived Medicare Catastrophic Coverage Act. The collapse of catastrophic insurance dramatically demonstrated why such a move had not been tried earlier: charging wealthier Medicare enrollees more concentrates costs on a politically active group that regards such a move as an abandonment of Medicare's social insurance contract. In addition, introducing higher costs for wealthier Medicare enrollees has always had more symbolic than financial significance. Quite simply, the financial savings of such measures are not substantial, since the large majority of seniors have incomes well below the usual threshold proposed for income-related premiums or taxes on Medicare benefits.[92] Given the likelihood of political opposition and the small financial payoff, it is no surprise that imposing more costs on higher-income seniors was not adopted during any of the periods of fiscal duress.

Nor has the Medicare eligibility age changed since the program's enactment in 1965. There have been some pressures do so. Advocates of raising the Medicare eligibility age often point to the example of Social Security, which began a process of increasing the age of eligibility for full benefits from sixty-five to sixty-seven in 1983 as a result of that year's Social Security reform legislation (sixty-seven will be fully phased in as the new age for Social Security benefits in 2022). The argument is that Medicare and Social Security should have a consistent standard for eligibility, perhaps as high as seventy. It is also argued that since the average life expectancy of Americans has increased significantly since 1965, it make sense to raise the age of eligibility for Medicare to reflect changing demographic realities. Such a move could save the program significant money by shifting the costs of medical care before the raised eligibility age to retirees, workers, and employers.

Despite the fiscal attraction, proposals to raise the Medicare eligibility age during 1965–94 did not come anywhere close to being enacted by Congress. Opponents have noted that such a change would be highly regressive. Lower-income workers die earlier than high-income workers, so an increase in the retirement age would effectively reduce their benefits. Lower-income workers are also more likely to work in more physically demanding jobs, meaning that maintaining employment to receive health insurance in lieu of Medicare is more difficult than for high-wage earners. The main explanation for the reluctance to raise the eligibility age,

[handwritten marginalia: supports not raising age.]

though, is that the specter of creating a new class of elderly uninsured is too much for most politicians to bear. And the political costs of creating new uninsured retirees have only increased since 1980 with national attention to the growing ranks of Americans without any health insurance.

REGULATION

The fourth potential response to Medicare financial crises is to lower program costs through regulation of program payments to medical providers. Chapter 5 addresses the substantive and political trajectory of Medicare regulation in depth, so here I only wish to note the correlation between Medicare funding shortfalls and the enactment of regulatory reforms. As figure 4.3 shows, there has been a strong relationship between Medicare financial crises and the introduction of such reforms. The 1969 shortfall was followed by the establishment of professional standard review organizations (PSROs), regulatory bodies that were to monitor the medical care Medicare patients received in hospitals. By reviewing care, PSROs were supposed to cut down on excessive utilization of medical services and thereby achieve substantial savings in Medicare payments for hospital services. The 1982 shortfall was followed by enactment of a new prospective payment system (PPS) for hospitals that replaced the existing retrospective reimbursement system for hospitals with an administered pricing system determined by the federal government.[93]

Medicare financial crises, then, have proven a powerful impetus to the adoption of regulatory reforms. The first two financial crises in Medicare were both accompanied by programmatic innovations. And the 1972 and 1983 reforms constituted the first two significant changes in Medicare regulation of medical providers. The 1995 crisis also led to the adoption of important regulatory changes—namely, the reform of payments for home health services and Medicare HMOs. The one significant regulatory reform in program history that did not occur during a period of acute financial stress, the enactment of the Medicare fee schedule in 1989, targeted Medicare part B. This was to be expected, since part B's programmatic dynamics are not necessarily driven by the logic of the part A trust fund.

That regulation of medial providers has been a central response to funding shortfalls in Medicare is not a political revelation. Of the choices presented above, this one has the least political fallout, since, in theory at least, it leaves the quality of care for beneficiaries as well as their cost-sharing bill for the program untouched.[94] When it comes to distributing the costs of policies designed to redress trust fund shortfalls, physicians

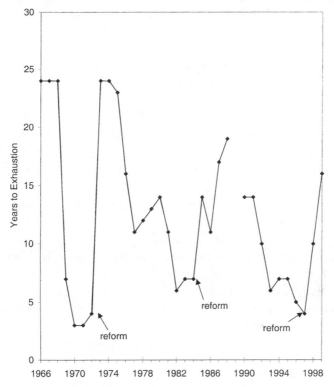

Fig. 4.3. Timing of Medicare reform and estimated time until
hospitalization insurance trust fund exhaustion.

and hospitals, rather than elderly and disabled program enrollees, have
been the primary targets.

CONCLUSION

In sum, the dominant issue in Medicare financing politics has been the
causes, timing, and consequences of the financial crises that have intermit-
tently beset the program. This chapter has located the primary cause of
these crises in the structure of Medicare financing itself, a structure copied
from Social Security in an effort to emulate its political success. But these
financing arrangements produced different political outcomes in Medicare from those experienced in Social Security's early years, highlighted by

recurrent alarms that Medicare was "going bankrupt." This has in turn generated a specific rhythm in program politics, a cycle of crisis and reform whereby Medicare reforms and innovations follow points at which a shortfall arrives. The structure of Medicare financing remained stable for the program's first three decades. Ironically, this stability generated an element of instability in program finances.

This is not to argue that if Medicare were funded through alternative arrangements, there would never be any Medicare crises or major reforms of program policies. The rate of growth in Medicare expenditures has been sufficiently high and its impact on the federal budget sufficiently strong that, regardless of its financing arrangements, reforms would have been adopted. After all, government efforts to contain the costs of health insurance programs are a common feature of public policy in all industrial democracies.[95] And in Medicaid, which is funded out of general revenues, governors periodically declare funding crises and then attempt to enact preferred policy changes. Has not Medicaid, then, gone through a similar cycle of crisis and reform without a payroll tax or trust fund? And if so, does this undercut the importance attributed here to Medicare's social insurance financing arrangements?

Medicare politics fundamentally differ from Medicaid politics. Medicaid has a political constituency comprised primarily of low-income women, children, and welfare recipients. There are few high-profile interest groups of Medicaid recipients organized around the program. Medicare has an entirely different clientele, one that has resources, is mobilized, is well liked by the public, and is represented by major interest groups. There has been no comparison on the federal level in terms of the pressure exerted on the Health Care Financing Administration in program administration; congressional interest in Medicare policy has dwarfed requests for help or information from administrators on Medicaid.[96] Moreover, changes in the status quo for the elderly in Medicare attract much more scrutiny from the public, media, and politicians than changes in the Medicaid status quo for the poor. And there is more potential political fallout with voters for the politician taking on Medicare reform than for the politician cutting Medicaid. In short, Medicare is harder to reform than Medicaid, and therefore the cycle of crisis and reform generated by its trust fund financing system is critical to generating opportunities for changing a program whose politics are biased toward the status quo.

Moreover, the crucial point is that the *timing* and consequently the *character* of Medicare reform would be altered by a different financing system. If there had not been a trust fund and payroll tax, Medicare reforms would not necessarily have come at the same points in the pro-

gram's history as those that were proposed when the hospitalization insurance trust fund was running low on reserves. Timing is a critical, and
too often overlooked, factor in public policy. As John Kingdon argues,
policy change is the product of three separate influences: how a policy
problem is understood, what solutions are preferred to address the problem, and what partisan alignment and ideology control the government.[97]
At two different times, for example, the same policy problem may be
viewed as requiring quite different solutions, perhaps because electoral
outcomes have changed the political environment or because policy specialists have adopted a new idea. The substance of policy change is contingent on the particular configuration of problems, solutions, and politics
that exists at any given time.

That contingency is illustrated by the changing character of the problems that have been defined and the solutions that have been proposed
during trust fund shortfalls in Medicare, as shown in table 4.3. In the first
crisis, the problem with Medicare was understood to be unnecessary utilization of medical services and fraud and abuse by medical providers. The
response was to create regulatory boards operated by physicians—
PSROs—that would monitor beneficiaries' care to ensure it was medically
necessary. In the second crisis, the problem was defined as the inflationary
nature of Medicare's retrospective reimbursement system for hospitals.
The response was to implement a new prospective payment system to
limit expenditures. In the 1995 crisis, the problem with Medicare was defined as the federal government's reliance on an "antiquated" fee-for-
service insurance model and its failure to keep up with innovations in the
private health care system. The reforms eventually adopted as part of the
1997 Balanced Budget Act consequently introduced an expanded market
of private insurance into Medicare (known as Medicare + Choice) and attempted to accelerate the growth of managed care in the program. Given
an alternative funding structure, program funding crises and reforms

Table 4.3 Changing Problems and Solutions Associated with Medicare Trust
Fund Shortfalls

YEARS	PROBLEM	SOLUTION	POLICY STRATEGY
1970–72	Over-utilization, fraud, and abuse	Professional self-regulation	Professional standard review organizations
1982–84	Retrospective reimbursement	Prospective payment	Diagnostic-related groups
1995–97	Fee-for-service system	Managed care, competition	Medicare + Choice

could have been triggered at different times, leading to the enactment of quite different solutions that reflected the prevailing thinking and political distribution of the day.

The reforms that have been adopted in Medicare, then, are products of the particular policy environment that existed when the program was in financial crisis. There are no objective problems or solutions produced by bankruptcy crises, only politically determined definitions and responses. Yet it is noteworthy that the first two Medicare trust fund shortfalls were characterized by the politics of consensus. In both 1969–72 and 1982–84, Democrats and Republicans broadly agreed on how to manage financing problems, even as federal management strategies radically changed course from the 1970s to the 1980s, a remarkable fact given subsequent political developments and the potential for making trust fund shortfalls into high-profile partisan affairs. Even when Medicare experienced states of crisis in financing politics the bipartisan consensus that governed Medicare politics from 1965 to 1994 remained intact. As a result, the 1972 and 1982 trust fund crises were not intensely public events, their resolution arrived at in relative quiescence and without much controversy.

The bipartisan responses to Medicare funding shortfalls are also noteworthy for what was not seriously contemplated: program restructuring. After all, another option other than raising revenues, beneficiary costs, or regulating payments to doctors and hospitals would have been to adopt a new structure for the program that would have promised, in theory at least, substantial savings. Certainly, some health policy researchers dreamed of such restructuring, often envisioning the transformation of Medicare into a voucher system or competitive market. But despite the appearance of funding shortfalls, those proposals fell on deaf ears in Washington until 1995. For three decades, the liberal Medicare consensus that favored maintaining federal health insurance for the elderly as a public, single-payer insurance program proved untouchable, even as the program veered in and out of financial trouble. Given the constraints of that consensus, bipartisan support emerged for a more incremental policy strategy: strengthening federal regulation of Medicare payments.

FIVE

The State Rises

THE POLITICS OF REGULATION

In many respects, Medicare regulatory policy has been the most prominent battleground in program politics. An enormous amount of money is on the line in regulatory decision making; not surprisingly, it has frequently drawn policymakers' attention. And for hospitals, physicians, and other medical care providers, influencing regulatory policy is their primary aim in program politics. After all, for health care providers Medicare spending is income, income that is central to their financial success given the high utilization rates of hospital and physician services by elderly patients. Regulation has also received substantially more scholarly attention than benefits or financing policy. Consequently, there is an unfortunate tendency to assume that regulatory politics *is* Medicare politics.

Yet despite all the attention, a crucial fact regarding the development of Medicare regulatory policy—examined here predominantly through the lens of payment policy—is often overlooked. The United States is commonly portrayed as exceptional in health care policy, driven by a political culture that privileges individualism, cherishes the market, and is suspicious of centralized government power. It is hard to imagine a more inhospitable environment for public policy to control health care spending. But over time, Medicare adopted payment policies for physicians and hospitals similar to those used in Canada and Western Europe to control costs, policies that empowered the federal government at the expense of interest groups. The ostensible constraints of American political culture on the regulation of medical care did not stop Medicare from moving in the same direction as other national health systems. The rhetorical veneer of Medicare regulation did take on a technocratic color that distinguished American efforts to slow the pace of spending on public medical care programs. And Medicare lacked some crucial instruments of cost control, such as limiting technological diffusion, employed by health systems abroad.

Yet, ultimately, Medicare moved to control program spending in an assertive manner that defied conventional assumptions both of American political culture and a weak state beholden to social interests. Moreover, Medicare's embrace of stronger controls on payments to hospitals and physicians was thoroughly bipartisan, supported by Democrats and Republicans, liberals and conservatives. Indeed, policy reforms that could have ignited ideological controversy and partisan divisions instead generated quiescence and consensus. How and why this quiet revolution in Medicare regulation of medical providers happened is the focus of this chapter.

The chapter proceeds in three sections. I begin by reviewing the origins and structure of the regulatory policies that Medicare adopted at its start. The second section analyzes developments in Medicare regulation from 1966 to 1994. Here I focus on three major reforms of Medicare regulation: professional standard review organizations (1972), the prospective payment system for hospitals (1983), and the Medicare fee schedule for physicians (1989). Finally, I conclude by analyzing the politics of regulation in view of Medicare's experiences.

THE ORIGINS AND STRUCTURE OF MEDICARE REGULATION

The initial character of Medicare regulation was permissive. Both the formal structure and the implementation of program regulations reflected a conciliatory posture toward the medical industry. In this sense, Medicare's experience resembled that of national health insurance programs in other countries, which generally started on financial terms favorable to medical providers and carried over the same physician payment practices that had existed prior to their enactment.[1]

In Medicare, hospitals and physicians were essentially reimbursed for whatever charges they billed Medicare and were not subject to direct administrative supervision by the federal government. Medicare financed the entry of the elderly into mainstream medicine, but it did not attempt to radically alter the organization or practice of American medicine. The embrace of the status quo was hardly a state secret. The 1965 Medicare statute openly announced the permissive nature of program regulation of medical providers. In section 1801, "Prohibition against Any Federal Interference," the new law declared that "Nothing in this title shall be construed to authorize any Federal officer or employee to exercise any supervision or control over the practice of medicine or the manner in which medical services are provided, or over the selection, tenure, or compensation of any officer or employee of any institution, agency, or person providing health services; or to exercise any supervision or control over the administration or operation of any such institution, agency, or person."[2] The conflict over Medicare's enactment explained the reluctance of the federal government to exercise regulatory authority over the medical industry. That conflict was shaped by the AMA's charges that federal health insurance for the elderly was "socialized medicine" and would inexorably lead to excessive federal interference in private medical practice. During the debate over Medicare's enactment in the late 1950s and early 1960s, the AMA warned that its physician members might refuse to participate in the new program. The threat of a physician strike or boycott against Medicare was given credibility by organized medicine's bitter anti-Medicare rhetoric.[3]

The architects of Medicare consequently designed their proposals for federal health insurance for the aged to temper the hostility of the medical industry (leaving insurance for physician services out of Medicare legislation until 1965) and counteract the charges that Medicare would impose federal control over private medicine, allegations that might erode public support for the program as well.[4] In so doing, they hoped to enhance Medicare's legislative prospects and avoid a potential boycott of the program by medical providers. The primary purpose of Medicare regulation, then, was not to exercise federal power to reorganize the health care system. Nor was the aim to create a fiscally responsible payment policy. Rather, regulation was crafted to reassure medical providers that federal health insurance did not constitute a threat to their professional sovereignty.

Regulations for reimbursing hospitals for treating Medicare patients embodied the commitment to placate the medical industry. Hospitals were paid retrospectively for the services they provided to Medicare beneficiaries on the basis of "reasonable costs."[5] By the 1960s, reasonable-cost reimbursement had become the industry norm.[6] The incorporation of this norm into Medicare rested on an explicit political calculus. Medicare's political sponsors intended to soften the opposition of hospitals by adopting for Medicare the same payment practices used by private insurers—regardless of the cost implications. By relying on the hospital industry's standard for reimbursement, Medicare assured hospitals that the federal government would not disrupt or deviate from the existing operations of the private medical system.

Medicare regulations for paying physicians were designed with the same purpose as those for hospitals: political conciliation.[7] Physicians were to be reimbursed retrospectively for treating Medicare patients on a fee-for-service basis, according to their "reasonable charges."[8] At the time of Medicare's enactment, many local insurance plans paid physicians for their services on the basis of negotiated fee schedules. Aides to Wilbur Cohen argued that Medicare should adopt Blue Shield fee schedules for paying physicians, especially since the 1965 legislation gave physicians the option of billing patients for amounts above what the government reimbursed.[9] Given that safety valve, paying reasonable charges without any predetermined fee schedules meant Medicare was "giving away the store."[10] However, the idea of a national fee schedule operated by the federal government remained anathema to the AMA.[11] Physicians viewed such a fee schedule as an illegitimate instrument of federal power. The same calculus of mollifying the AMA that had earlier dictated limiting Medicare to hospitalization insurance mandated that if the federal government was to pay for physician services, it should do so in the way least objectionable to doctors.

It was therefore not surprising that when physician insurance was added unexpectedly to the final Medicare legislation in 1965, the program did not establish a nationwide fee schedule for physicians. Instead, the adoption of a reasonable-charges standard and unfettered fee-for-service payment promised to minimize federal control of physician reimbursement while maximizing physician income. Reasonable charges meant that physicians were to be reimbursed by Medicare for comparable services at the same levels at which they were paid by private insurers for their non-Medicare patients. The Medicare statute declared that "in determining the reasonable charge . . . there shall be taken into consideration the customary charges [made by the physician] for similar services . . . as well as the prevailing charges in the locality for similar services."[12] The policy of paying customary and prevailing charges (used by the Aetna insurance plan that part B was based on) proved to be a recipe for both general medical inflation and escalating Medicare expenditures. The idea of adding physician services to Medicare was not seriously studied before 1965, and when it was added, "no one knew what doctors were customarily charging."[13] Medicare's system of paying the going community rate provided physicians who were then charging below that rate with a strong incentive to raise their prices, an opportunity they did not pass up. And as more doctors raised their fees, the prevailing community rate moved ever higher, leaving Medicare with a growing bill.

In contrast, then, to a predetermined fee schedule, physicians maintained considerable autonomy in setting charges and, crucially, billing patients for amounts beyond the fee reimbursed by Medicare was permitted. As with hospitals, Medicare adopted a payment policy for physicians that emphasized conciliation over financial control.[14]

MEDICARE ADMINISTRATION

Medicare's administrative structure reinforced the tight connection between program regulation and prevailing practices in the health care market. Not only did the substance of Medicare regulations mirror that of private insurance, but much of the actual authority to administer the program rested with the insurance industry. Federal Medicare administration was lodged in 1965 within the Bureau of Health Insurance (BHI) of the Social Security Administration (SSA), an inevitable outcome given SSA officials' prominent role in developing the program and the linkages between Medicare and Social Security. However, the SSA's administrative authority over Medicare was circumscribed by the program's reliance on private agents to implement the program. The 1965 Medicare legislation provided for the contracting out of Medicare administrative functions to private organizations.[15] These organizations, known as "fiscal intermediaries" for hospitals and "carriers" for physicians, served as administrative buffers between the government and medical providers.

In practice, the use of private intermediaries guaranteed Blue Cross and Blue Shield plans, which controlled the largest share of the American medical insurance market in the 1960s, a privileged position within Medicare. The intent of contracting out Medicare administration was to allow hospitals and physicians to participate in federal health insurance through private administrative agencies with whom they already had established relationships. In most cases, this meant Blue Cross and Blue Shield, since the two organizations enjoyed close ties with the hospital industry and physicians, respectively.[16] The carriers and intermediaries were to handle much of the day-to-day operation of Medicare, including provider reimbursement, claims processing, and auditing.[17] Consequently, the federal government ceded a substantial amount of the regulatory authority potentially available to the private sector.

The position given to Blue Cross and Blue Shield in Medicare also reflected the special status accorded to "the Blues" in the U.S. health care system. Since their birth in the 1930s, the Blues were regarded as uniquely

American institutions that were exemplars of the "third sector:" voluntary, nonprofit organizations with a commitment to serving the community, they were viewed as occupying a reasonable medium between the government and market.[18] Blue Cross and Blue Shield themselves worked hard to promote the "voluntary way" and their image as guardians of the public interest, in part to defuse pressures for national health insurance.[19] Their special status as voluntary nonprofits made the Blues an excellent fit for federal policymakers looking to alleviate concerns over federal power by contracting out administration to the private sector. Blue Cross and Blue Shield, it was believed, were not only technically equipped to administer Medicare, but also uniquely qualified to carry out this new public mission.[20]

Administrative arrangements were thus crafted to make Medicare politically, and later operationally, feasible. As with hospital and physician payment regulations, the structure of Medicare administration represented a political concession to the medical industry. The concession had two purposes. The first was to win the support, or at least to mute the opposition, of the hospital industry to enactment of federal health insurance for the aged. As the legislative debate over Medicare took shape in the late 1950s and early 1960s, an important distinction emerged among the anti-Medicare constituency. While physicians and the AMA were implacably opposed to Medicare proposals, the opposition of the hospital industry and its organizational representative, the American Hospital Association (AHA), was not as rigid. Hospitals viewed Medicare as an attractive financial opportunity that would pay for elderly patients they had been treating without full compensation. Medicare's political strategists sought to exploit the ambivalence of a hospital industry caught between financial incentives to support federal health insurance and professional incentives to align with the AMA against it. In order to attract the AHA, Medicare planners offered the lure of guaranteeing a role in program administration for Blue Cross. In 1962 a federal task force formally recommended that federal hospital insurance use Blue Cross as an administrative agent.[21]

The second purpose of the concession to private administration was to reassure medical providers as well as the public that the introduction of Medicare would not result in their subordination to a federal bureaucracy, an important fear to allay given the AMA's charges that the program represented socialized medicine. "Medicare advocates," Lawrence Jacobs observes, "persistently strove to design new administrative arrangements for the program that would not arouse the public's uneasiness over state interference. Their solution was to forge a new state role but on an administratively weak foundation."[22] Indeed, those involved in planning the program always assumed that Medicare would preserve an administrative role for private intermediaries.[23] There was precedent for decentralizing federal administrative authority in social insurance. Under the disability insurance program enacted in 1956, the SSA contracted out to state agencies to make individual eligibility determinations. The reliance on state administration for disability insurance was a concession to medical providers and conservative legislators who opposed centralized federal control of the program.[24] Medicare's planners adopted the same strategy of administrative devolution, with the concomitant fragmentation of regulatory authority, though in federal health insurance the devolution was directed predominantly to the nonprofit side of the private sector, rather than to state governments.

However, the incorporation of Blue Cross and Blue Shield within Medicare administration in 1965 was not solely a matter of political calculus about mollifying the medical profession and public opinion. Another critical factor was logistical, reflecting the administrative dilemma the SSA faced in implementing the statute by the program's scheduled start-up date, July 1, 1966. Administering health insurance is a profoundly more complex task than public pension management. Pension administration requires serving only beneficiaries, while administrators of health insurance programs must also deal with medical providers and the dynamic market for medical services. Implementation of Medicare required the SSA to complete a series of new, daunting tasks, including the establishment of reimbursement procedures, data-processing systems, and utilization review boards to monitor the quality of medical care provided to Medicare patients. Social Security did not provide an analogue for any of this. In 1965, program officials believed the federal government was not organizationally capable of implementing Medicare by its scheduled start-up date without the assistance of Blue Cross.[25] As Robert Ball, SSA commissioner at the time of Medicare's passage, noted about federal health insurance, "no other Social Security amendments have approached the scope of these amendments.[26] If the federal government was to process Medicare bills without relying on private insurers, Ball argued "there was no way to launch the program without long, long lead time and tremendous build-up of (government) personnel."[27]

The lack of existing federal capacity in health care administration consequently made Medicare dependent on private insurers at the program's inception. However, even if such capacity had existed in 1965, it is likely that program architects would still have given Blue Cross and Blue Shield a central role in Medicare administration for political purposes. Notably, Medicare never seriously contemplated substituting government administration for the Blues, long after the federal government had sufficient expertise, time, and experience to develop its own capacity in administering health insurance.

Regardless of the motivation, private insurers occupied a privileged position within Medicare administration. The consequences for program policy were not difficult to anticipate. According to a 1962 memorandum from a federal task force on program administration, "A considerable price would be paid in order to get the initial public relations advantages with professional groups that might come from using Blue Cross, e.g., loss of direct control with providers so that the Federal Government would not have detailed knowledge of problems and because of this, the loss of ability to react quickly to problems of administration, budget program, etc."[28] Yet strategic calculations trumped fiscal concerns (it was hardly a close call), and when physicians' insurance (part B) was unexpectedly incorporated as part of the 1965 Medicare legislation, the same logic prevailed. Rather than establish direct federal control, Medicare permitted private organizations (predominantly Blue Shield) to serve as carriers to handle reimbursement, claims processing and payment, and other administrative responsibilities for physician services.

The concern with placating the medical industry similarly shaped administrators' positions after Medicare's enactment while drafting and implementing program regulations. Here the SSA's role in administering Medicare had a profound impact on the character of program regulation. As an agency, the SSA's core mission was claims payment: getting Social Security checks out to beneficiaries on time. That mission was not simply an affirmation of efficiency, though the SSA prided itself on being the most efficient of public agencies. Rather, the mission represented a commitment to social insurance, which meant treating program beneficiaries as legitimate claimants. Indeed, protecting beneficiaries became the core value of social insurance administration.[29] When the SSA established the Bureau of Health Insurance to administer Medicare, that bureaucratic culture persisted—hardly surprising, since BHI was staffed with SSA officials. Social insurance privileged claims payment over cost control, and the SSA's experience lay in paying benefits, not in delivering medical care.[30] The Bureau of Health Insurance therefore identified its primary mission as ensuring that Medicare beneficiaries received access to program coverage. Offices of the SSA around the country became contact points for Medicare beneficiaries. The type of benefit may have varied between pensions and medical care, but the SSA's administrative orientation did not.

That orientation was brought into sharp relief during the first years of Medicare's operation. The vagueness of the statutory language governing

Medicare regulation of hospitals and physicians—including the provisions that required that hospitals be paid "reasonable costs" and physicians be reimbursed for "reasonable charges" for treating Medicare patients—left considerable discretion to program administrators. Administrators of the Bureau of Health Insurance had to define the precise meaning of Medicare regulations, including payment policy concerning medical providers, quality standards for hospitals participating in the program, and requirements that hospitals establish utilization committees to review the care received by Medicare beneficiaries.[31]

In implementing these regulations, Judith Feder argues, Medicare administrators consistently pursued a strategy of avoiding conflict with medical providers. Their goal was to secure the cooperation of hospitals and physicians and thus guarantee a "proper takeoff" for Medicare.[32] In practice, this strategy produced a series of policies favorable to the medical industry. Some hospitals were certified to participate in Medicare even though they did not meet program standards. The BHI was also reluctant to use its power to terminate certification, relying instead on an "educational" approach to hospital regulation. On utilization review, the SSA similarly did not enforce utilization review standards to monitor medical necessity and quality of care. And in writing reimbursement rules, the BHI adopted lenient measures that did not impose any real fiscal constraints on providers, permitted hospitals generous capital depreciation allowances, and initially even gave hospitals a 2% bonus on their Medicare charges.[33]

These policies were all developed in the name of mollifying the medical industry, and over time they were institutionalized as administrators proved averse to altering their terms. Above all, SSA officials valued political consensus and feared conflict. They were unwilling to risk changing established procedures if that change would trigger conflict among key parties or threaten program disruption.[34] Consequently, the BHI became vested in a Medicare status quo that reflected decisions made during the program's implementation. That status quo—which also prevailed in the private insurance industry at the time—embodied payment policies that were inherently inflationary and uncontrollable, and eventually it proved untenable.

Here, as elsewhere in Medicare regulation during the program's early years, policymaking in search of fiscal control of program payments was subordinated to the overriding goal of securing the program's acceptance among medical providers and thereby a successful start for Medicare. Medicare regulation was an instrument of conciliation, driven by the presumption that protecting Medicare beneficiaries required ensuring that hospitals and physicians participate in the program, even if that meant that the terms of participation were largely dictated by medical providers themselves. The federal government wrote hospitals and physicians a blank check for Medicare payments, and they were only too happy to indulge by billing Medicare at increasingly costly rates.

DEVELOPMENTS IN MEDICARE REGULATION, 1966–94

Professional Standard Review Organizations

It did not take long for Medicare's fast-rising expenditures to attract attention. The first substantial reform of Medicare came in the 1972 Social Security amendments with the creation of professional standard review organizations (PSROs). Motivated by concern over higher-than-expected utilization rates for Medicare services and unnecessary or inappropriate medical care, federal policymakers sought to strengthen the review of medical care provided to beneficiaries. The origins of PSROs were in the 1969–70 policy activism of the Senate Finance Committee. During those years, the Finance Committee held a series of hearings critical of the implementation of Medicare regulations and the performance of program administration. The committee also issued, in 1970, a landmark report—*Medicare and Medicaid: Problems, Issues, and Alternatives*—detailing problems in Medicare and offering recommendations for its reform that anticipated future changes in the program.[35]

The hearings and the report, framed by higher-than-expected expenditures in Medicare and the impending bankruptcy of the hospitalization insurance trust fund, blamed many of Medicare's problems, including the perceived pervasive practice of giving Medicare patients unnecessary care, on widespread fraud and abuse by the medical industry.[36] The Finance Committee alleged that Medicare was beset by "gang visits" during which physicians saw as many as fifty federal patients in a day "regardless of whether the visit is medically necessary or whether any service is actually furnished"; the "unbundling" into multiple charges of physician services that previously had been billed as only a single charge; and the concentration of huge, and by implication illegitimate, government payments to some medical providers.[37] The committee argued that Medicare's private administrative intermediaries and carriers had failed to stem these practices, and that program administrators within the SSA, as a consequence of their priority on establishing comfortable administrative relations with the medical industry, had not enforced compliance with existing Medicare regulations.[38]

These stories and the higher-than-anticipated utilization of Medicare services persuaded the Finance Committee staff, as well as a bipartisan cross-section of committee members including chairman Russell Long, that Medicare required stronger regulation of the medical care received by federal patients. The existing process of utilization review established in 1965, which mandated that hospitals participating in Medicare establish in-house panels to review patient care, was viewed as hopelessly ineffective, subject both to noncooperation by medical providers and neglect by Medicare administrators. By 1970, then, the Senate Finance Committee was moving toward legislation to create more powerful regulation of the medical care received by Medicare patients.[39]

At the same time, the Nixon administration was considering similar proposals. In 1969, the administration proposed "program review teams" composed of physicians, medical care professionals, and consumers to review the care given to federal patients. The review teams were to be given the power to deny federal payment for medical care deemed unnecessary by their audits.[40] The AMA quickly "saw the handwriting on the wall."[41] Federal regulation of medical practice represented a threat to the core principle of professional sovereignty: medical treatment was exclusively a private matter between physicians and their patients. If government regulators actively challenged the medical care provided to Medicare patients, a significant amount of that sovereignty would be lost. However, the financial problems in Medicare made federal reform of medical care regulation a strong likelihood. Faced with the momentum generated by the Senate Finance Committee and the Nixon administration, the AMA decided to meet the pressures for strengthened regulation by presenting its own reform plan.

The resulting 1970 AMA plan proposed that the federal government contract with state medical societies to perform peer review of the medical services received by Medicare and Medicaid patients. However, since state medical societies were instruments of organized medicine, the proposal minimized the threat to professional sovereignty. The AMA brought its plan to Wallace Bennett, the second-ranking Republican on the Senate Finance Committee, hoping that Bennett's sponsorship would stave off more stringent regulation.[42] Yet while Bennett took up the plan, he departed from the AMA's blueprint in several important respects. Bennett had the plan analyzed by the Senate Finance Committee staff, which in 1970 served both Democratic and Republican committee members. The staff concluded that "the virtue of the AMA plan was that it conceded the problem. Its failing was that it was totally self-serving—in effect, turning responsibility for review over to state medical societies with virtually no accountability.[43] Bennett and the Finance Committee staff reformulated a plan that retained the reliance on physician-operated boards as monitors of Medicare utilization but that also attempted to create a stronger mechanism establishing the accountability of physician boards to the federal government.[44]

In July 1970, Bennett proposed the Professional Standards Review Organizations Act. The organizations it proposed were to review the appropriateness and quality of all medical care provided to federal patients, especially hospital stays and admissions, in order to assure that only medically necessary services were provided.[45] By detecting inappropriate, unnecessary, and fraudulent care, and disallowing payment for such care, PSROs, it was hoped, would reduce federal Medicare expenditures. As in the AMA proposal, physicians were to be the regulators of medical care practice. Bennett's plan assumed that "only physicians are . . . qualified to judge whether services ordered by other physicians are necessary."[46] The review organizations were to be composed of doctors, not federal officials, or consumer representatives, as the Nixon administration had earlier suggested. However, the Bennett proposal rejected the AMA's recommendation that state medical societies have the exclusive right to operate the review organizations. Instead, PSROs could contract with local organizations of physicians that were not limited to the medical societies. Moreover, the government would retain the right to terminate contracts with review organizations that were judged to be ineffective, in contrast to the perpetual monopoly the AMA plan would have given to medical societies.[47]

The Bennett proposal also called for the establishment of a set of professional norms of medical practice to guide utilization review. The idea was to define standards of medical care—what now are termed practice guidelines—that could then be used to identify inappropriate medical treatments. The absence of any such standards had hindered the operation of Medicare's existing utilization review program. Without such criteria, how could specific episodes of medical care be judged to be unnecessary? The norms were also to serve an educational purpose in familiarizing physicians with contemporary medical practices.[48] The AMA, though, saw Senator Bennett's proposals for national norms, along with other changes that Bennett made to their original plan, as precisely the threat to professional sovereignty that they had sought to preempt. As a consequence, the AMA switched from sponsor to opponent of PSROs and lobbied vigorously against the Bennett legislation with the same warnings against "bureaucratic medicine" that had guided earlier campaigns against Medicare and national health insurance.[49]

Congress enacted the PSRO bill in 1972 with bipartisan support, but the opposition of the AMA weakened PSROs' legislative form and impact on the health care system.[50] Review of outpatient care was prohibited, national norms were left out, and restrictions were placed on government ownership of PSRO data.[51] Nor were the PSROs as rigorous in their oversight of medical providers as once had been promised. Partly due to budgetary constraints, in practice PSROs only audited inpatient hospital care, though their statutory authority allowed for broader review of medical care in other settings. Moreover, much of the responsibility for review was simply contracted to hospitals, instead of outside organizations. Finally, the failure to establish national norms of care created ambiguity in defining what constituted medically unnecessary care, leaving widespread regional variations in practice.[52]

Professional standard review organizations lacked any significant political constituency. Doctors saw the review boards, even in attenuated form, as a threat to professional sovereignty. Hospitals regarded PSROs as overly bureaucratic institutions of federal regulation. And subsequent analyses of PSRO performance found that they did not significantly reduce Medicare expenditures. According to the Congressional Budget Office, they actually cost more to operate than any savings they produced.[53] Both the Carter and Reagan administrations attempted (unsuccessfully) to phase out PSROs as ineffective and wasteful.[54] They were transformed into peer review organizations (PROs) in 1982 by Republican Senator David Durenberger. Peer review organizations were to monitor Medicare hospital admissions to make sure beneficiaries were not undertreated or discharged too soon under the program's new prospective payment system, as well as to deny payment for unnecessary care. But this reincarnation of PSROs produced the same result: PROs rarely sanctioned doctors and did not generate any significant savings.[55]

The failure of PSROs, though, was not simply an unintended outcome of implementation. From the beginning, the design of PSROs raised serious doubts about their potential effectiveness as regulatory institutions.[56] Given the belief that Medicare providers were themselves responsible for escalating costs, it made little sense to entrust regulation of medical practice to physicians. Since more Medicare costs meant more income for physicians, and there were no financial incentives to curb spending, what incentives did they have to slow Medicare spending? Moreover, strong norms existed in the medical profession against open criticism of the care provided by other doctors, a critical obstacle to a system of physician self-regulation.[57]

Yet the limited regulatory design of PSROs made sense politically, given the reluctance of Congress and the Nixon administration to break completely with Medicare's 1965 accommodation of the medical industry. Professional standard review organizations were a first step in asserting federal independence from medical providers, but they were a halting first step. The emphasis on regulating fraud and abuse and inappropriate care was politically convenient since, from this perspective, Medicare's problems could be solved by cracking down on a few "bad apples" and high-spending outliers in the medical profession, rather than the more far-reaching step of changing how all medical providers were paid through adoption of a predetermined fee schedule.

To be sure, the 1972 Social Security amendments contained provisions related to the direct regulation of provider reimbursement, including limits on hospital payments and the authorization of demonstration projects in alternative methods of reimbursement.[58] Yet the 1972 reforms re mained focused on the regulation of medical practice and consequently avoided any fundamental challenge to the structure of the Medicare reimbursement system. The limited scope of this regulatory response is explicable, in large part, in terms of Medicare's budgetary profile. Despite the program's financial problems, Medicare still claimed a relatively small share of the federal budget (in 1970, 3.5%).[59] Moreover, American politics at the time was not driven by the preoccupation with budgetary deficits that would define the 1980s. As a result, policymakers could afford to overlook the flaws of the PSRO strategy, since fiscal pressures were not yet sufficiently strong to compel a stronger federal response.

The Prospective Payment System

The willingness of federal policymakers to abide by the 1965 accommodation that limited the scope of Medicare regulation ended in the 1980s. Medicare payment policies had been based on private insurance standards. But by the 1980s, private insurance plans still offered open-ended payments to hospitals and physicians, and American health care spending was accelerating at record rates.[60] The government could not afford to wait for the private sector to change. In 1983, Congress enacted the prospective payment system (PPS) for hospital reimbursement. The rapid rate of increase in Medicare expenditures, the approaching bankruptcy of the hospitalization insurance trust fund, and the rise of the federal budget deficit as a national issue led to the direct regulation of payments to medical providers.

The adoption of the PPS was the outcome of two processes: the technical development of prospective payment as a method and the political development of the commitment to contain Medicare hospital costs.[61] The technical roots of the PPS reached back to the 1970s. Reasonable-cost reimbursement, under which Medicare paid hospitals retrospectively for the costs of treating federal patients, had long been viewed by some policymakers as both fiscally irresponsible and inefficient. It gave the government little power to control its own expenditures and provided hospitals with no incentives to economize on their costs. The 1970 Senate Finance Committee report proposed that Medicare move in the direction of prospective payment, which would set predetermined rates for hospital reimbursement, rather than reimburse hospitals regardless of their costs, and the 1972 Social Security amendments authorized federally funded experiments in hospital payment reform.[62]

That authorization set the stage for state experiments in hospital reimbursement. By 1976, six states—Connecticut, Maryland, Massachusetts, New Jersey, New York, and Washington—had adopted mandatory rate-setting programs for hospitals.[63] Though the programs differed in form, they all embraced the idea of setting predetermined limits on what hospitals could charge (i.e., prospective payment). In general, these rate-setting states initially were more successful than other states in holding down growth in hospital costs, providing a working model for federal regulatory reform.[64]

The influence of the New Jersey experience with prospective payment on Medicare hospital policy proved especially critical. New Jersey used diagnostic-related groups (DRGs) as the basis for their PPS.[65] Diagnostic-related groups, developed at Yale University in the early 1970s by Robert Fetter, John Thompson, and Richard Averill, were designed as an internal management tool for hospitals.[66] These groups were formed by classification of patients according to medical diagnosis, and it was hoped that this would enable hospitals to improve monitoring of their resource use by comparing cases within the same diagnosis. However, DRGs also enabled comparisons between hospitals, a feature that made them attractive as a foundation for prospective payment.[67] New Jersey, with federal financial and administrative support, adopted DRGs in 1978, and in 1983 they became the basis for the Medicare PPS.[68]

The technical development of prospective payment by private researchers, state health agencies, and the federal Medicare administration was accompanied by the development of a political commitment to containing Medicare expenditures. Medicare spending per enrollee marched upward throughout the 1970s, and hospital spending represented the largest share of the Medicare bill. In 1982, hospital services accounted for 70% of all federal Medicare expenditures.[69] The political origins of prospective payment were in the failed efforts by the Carter administration to enact hospital cost containment legislation. From 1977 to 1979, the

Carter administration pushed proposals that mandated limits on the rate of growth in hospital costs, not just for Medicare, but for all hospital charges. The administration identified passage of such legislation as a precondition for introducing national health insurance.[70]

However, the Carter administration's proposals for hospital cost containment never passed Congress, failing for the final time in 1979. The Carter proposals were hindered by the active opposition of the hospital industry and the general skepticism in Congress at the time toward regulatory approaches to public policy.[71] Yet the defeat of the Carter plan actually sowed the seeds for the subsequent adoption of Medicare regulation. As part of its campaign to defeat the legislation, the hospital industry promised to restrain voluntarily the growth of hospital costs. The Voluntary Effort, as it was known, appeared in its first year (1978) to be a success, as the national rate of hospital spending slowed. But during the next three years, hospital costs rose at rates far exceeding the limits promised by the hospital industry; without the immediate threat of regulation, the industry had no incentive to curb its profits.[72] Congressional policymakers, including key supporters of the Voluntary Effort such as Richard Gephardt and Dan Rostenkowski, were now convinced that hospital costs could not be restrained without federal regulation. Confronted by the impending exhaustion of the hospitalization insurance trust fund, they turned their attention to Medicare reform.

By 1981, a convergence had emerged between the technical development of prospective payment and the political development of the desire to contain Medicare hospital costs. However, this convergence between problems and solutions was not accompanied by a favorable political context.[73] The newly elected Reagan administration committed itself to downsizing the federal government and to lessening the burden of government regulation on the private sector. These political and ideological commitments were hardly conducive to the enactment of prospective payment in Medicare, which amounted to a system of administered pricing, seemingly precisely the type of federal regulation that the administration targeted for elimination.[74]

The Reagan administration favored a "procompetitive," market-based approach to Medicare reform whereby program beneficiaries would be moved into health maintenance organizations and given vouchers to shop for private insurance.[75] However, despite their resonance with the administration's antigovernment ideology, market-based proposals for Medicare reform did not advance very far during the Reagan years (though in 1982 an optional Medicare HMO program was enacted that, while its growth and significance proved initially small, became quite consequential for program policy and politics in later years). Instead, the administration turned to the regulatory strategy of prospective payment.

Why did the Reagan administration end up supporting regulatory rather than market-based Medicare reform?[76] There are three explanations for this incongruous development. The first is that fiscal exigency simply overwhelmed ideology. It was widely believed within the administration that market-based approaches to Medicare reform would not produce immediate budgetary savings, since they required the structural reorganization of the health care delivery system, a long-term process. Given the administration's short-term goals for reducing domestic spending, a market approach to Medicare reform was not viable.[77] In order to curtail government spending on Medicare, federal regulatory authority over medical providers consequently had to be strengthened. The irony, then, of the Reagan administration's promarket political philosophy was that in health care the realization of this philosophy actually required the empowerment of the federal government to do more, not less.[78] In order for conservatives to reduce government spending, they had to expand federal authority.[79]

The second reason that the Reagan administration ended up advocating regulation was that prospective payment picked up an important ally within the administration: Secretary of Health and Human Services Richard Schweiker. Schweiker had been ranking minority member on Subcommittee on Health of the Senate Finance Committee, and he came to Health and Human Services committed to restructuring Medicare hospital payment.[80] Influenced by the failure of the hospital industry's Voluntary Effort, Schweiker favored introducing a system of prospective payment for Medicare. His lobbying for prospective payment within the administration, as well as in Congress, helps to explain its adoption in a seemingly unfavorable political context.

The third explanation for the unexpected ascendance of Medicare regulation during the Reagan administration was a feature of prospective payment that lent itself to a broad political coalition. The DRG system paid hospitals per case, according to a standard rate that reflected the diagnosis of patients.[81] If hospitals treated a patient for less than the predetermined rate, they could keep the difference between their costs and the federal payments, while if they treated a patient at costs exceeding federal reimbursement, they would have to absorb the financial loss. Diagnostic-related groups thus evoked the symbolism of the market by ostensibly providing hospitals incentives to become more efficient producers of medical care. As in the private market, more efficient producers would be rewarded with higher profits, a departure from the reasonable-cost reimbursement practice of paying all hospital costs regardless of their merit. The market imagery inherent in the DRG-based prospective payment attracted the Reagan administration and congressional conservatives, while liberals found favor in the system's regulatory promise. In practice, prospective payment may have been an administered pricing system, but its simultaneous rhetorical claim to competition and efficiency enhanced its political legitimacy.[82]

With the approval of the Reagan administration, Congress adopted prospective payment in 1983 without substantial controversy and with broad bipartisan support.[83] The prelude was the 1982 Tax Equity and Fiscal Responsibility Act (TEFRA). The act, which was the product of congressional health subcommittees, provided for strict limits on Medicare hospital reimbursement.[84] The proposed limits were seen as a "doomsday device," intended to signal that Congress was serious about Medicare reform and that the hospital industry should therefore come to the bargaining table.[85] Organizations representing the hospital industry, "recognizing that the status quo had been lost," accepted prospective payment as a preferable alternative to TEFRA.[86] Prospective payment went through Congress "at the legislative equivalent of the speed of light,"[87] running the gamut from introduction to final passage in an astounding six weeks. The most consequential reform of Medicare regulation in program history was enacted with hardly any political attention or public debate and, even more surprisingly, scarcely any opposition from the medical industry.

The absence of opposition from the medical profession to the 1983 Medicare reforms highlighted the changed character of American health politics and the weakened position of organized medicine. Professional standard review organizations had posed less of a threat to the medical industry than prospective payment but provoked a much stronger reaction. Yet PSROs, too, had been hailed as a regulatory breakthrough, only to fail to live up to their promise of stronger regulation in implementation. However, the evidence in its first decade of operation was that the implementation of the PPS was substantially stronger than that of PSROs. Implementation of the 1983 Medicare reforms was influenced more by federal policymakers than by the hospital industry. Table 5.1 shows the hospital payment-to-cost ratios for Medicare, Medicaid, and private payers. The ratio measures the degree to which payments from insurers cover the costs of treating their patients. In 1981, before the enactment of the PPS, the payment-to-cost ratio for Medicare was .96; the federal government, in other words, covered 96% of the costs of treating Medicare hospital patients. By 1990, that ratio had fallen to .89, and the federal government was paying substantially less for Medicare patients than pri-

Table 5.1 Hospital Payment-to-Cost Ratios for Medicare, Medicaid, and Private
Payers

YEAR	MEDICARE	MEDICAID	PRIVATE
1980	.96	.91	1.12
1981	.97	.93	1.12
1982	.96	.91	1.14
1983	.97	.92	1.16
1984	.98	.88	1.16
1985	1.01	.90	1.16
1986	1.01	.88	1.16
1987	.98	.83	1.20
1988	.94	.80	1.22
1989	.91	.76	1.22
1990	.89	.80	1.27
1991	.88	.82	1.30
1992	.89	.91	1.31
1993	.89	.93	1.29

Source: Prospective Payment Assessment Commission, *Medicare and the American Health Care System: Report to Congress* (Washington, D.C.: Prospective Payment Assessment Commission, 1995).

vate insurers were for their hospital admissions, reflecting a trend towards tighter Medicare regulation of hospital payments.[88]

Hospital operating margins, defined as the percentage difference between Medicare hospital payments and the costs allocated to Medicare patients, support the same conclusions.[89] A negative margin means that costs for patient care exceed Medicare payment as measured by the hospital; a positive margin means that hospitals are paid more than their costs by Medicare. Once again, the trend was toward more stringent application of prospective payment, illustrated by the steady decline, from 13.4% in 1984 to −2.4% in 1991, in average PPS operating margins for hospitals treating Medicare patients.[90] In contrast to PSROs, then, the implementation of the PPS asserted regulatory power, rather than merely symbolic power, over the medical industry. In simple terms, the deficit politics of the 1980s generated a willingness to break with Medicare's accommodation of the medical industry that did not exist in the previous decade.[91]

The increasingly assertive stance of the federal government in Medicare regulation paralleled an important administrative development. In 1977, Secretary of Health, Education, and Welfare Joseph Califano moved Medicare administration out of the SSA and merged it with Medicaid administration in a new agency, the Health Care Financing Administration (HCFA). The main reason for the move, in the context of a broader reorganization of Health, Education, and Welfare, was a desire to place health financing programs in the same organization, enabling the integration of program activities and planning. Califano hoped the integration would generate significant administrative savings, though this aspiration was never met.

The real significance of HCFA instead lay in its contribution to transforming Medicare from a social insurance program into a health financing program. The establishment of an agency outside the SSA loosened the program's roots in Social Security. Social insurance administration that emphasized claims payment to protect beneficiaries was replaced with a new mind-set that came to privilege cost containment as the primary administrative task. In HCFA, Medicare was no longer part of a universe of social insurance programs but rather gained a new identity as a health financing program—one in need of stronger spending controls.[92]

The idea that the federal government should aggressively use its purchasing power in Medicare to leverage discounts in program payments was not a primary motivation for the creation of HCFA. But HCFA's creation facilitated the use of this leverage. The establishment of the new agency coincided with new regulatory measures to control Medicare's rate of expenditure growth. These measures, beginning with the PPS, not only transformed Medicare policy, they also gave HCFA an identity as an agency concerned with health care cost containment. However, it is critical to note that the same budgetary pressures would have exerted pressure on the SSA even if Medicare had not been removed from its purview. Fiscal pressures, not administrative changes, were clearly at the core of the shift in Medicare payment policies. Medicare payment reform would clearly have been enacted regardless of the program's administrative location. But given the SSA's social insurance identity, concern for beneficiary welfare, organizational culture of claims payment, and investment in the status quo, it is plausible that the SSA might not have embraced the new cost control role as much or as quickly as HCFA did. That role would only expand as the scope of the program extended to other payment areas.

The Medicare Fee Schedule

Having reformed Medicare regulation of hospitals, federal policymakers turned their attention to physicians. The relative success during the 1980s in slowing Medicare expenditures for hospital care contrasted with increasing rates of federal spending for physician services. During that decade, Medicare physician expenditures rose at a rate three times that for hospital payments.[93] The reform of Medicare hospital regulation was partly responsible for the growing disparity, since it led providers to move medical care to outpatient settings that were not regulated by prospective payment. Congressional policymakers worried not only about the effects of rising Medicare spending for physician services on the budget, but also about the consequences for program beneficiaries from rising premiums, copayments, and balance billing (the amount of a physician's bill beyond what the government deems "reasonable" for federal reimbursement).[94]

In 1984, Congress instituted a fee freeze on Medicare physician payments that was extended through 1986. Despite the freeze, Medicare spending on physician services rose during this period by an average annual rate of 11.6%, in large measure due to increases in the volume of services billed to the program.[95] The growing bill for Medicare physician expenditures, limited success of the 1984–86 fee freeze, and continued pressures from the budget deficit propelled congressional interest in creating a new system for Medicare regulation of physician reimbursement. As it had been for hospitals, the original bargain of granting physicians a blank check was abandoned.

While much of the political impetus for Medicare hospital payment reform had come from Congress, the technical development of prospective payment was concentrated in the executive branch. In contrast, Congress provided not only political support for physician payment reform, but the actual design of the new regulatory system as well. During 1984–85, the Reagan administration was divided over the type of physician payment reform it wanted, as was HCFA.[96] As a consequence, Congress, particularly Representative Pete Stark's (Democrat, California) Ways and Means health subcommittee, took the lead in pushing forward on physician payment reform.[97]

The preferred congressional option for physician regulation was a national fee schedule. Democratic health policymakers, such as Stark, favored a regulatory approach to Medicare physician payment reform, rather than the market-based options, such as encouraging HMO enrollment, that were being considered by the Reagan administration. In 1986, Congress created the Physician Payment Review Commission (PPRC) to help in developing a fee schedule. The PPRC was, in essence, a congressional bureaucracy to aid in health policymaking. It followed the model of the Prospective Payment Assessment Commission (ProPAC), which had been created in 1983 to help Congress monitor the implementation of hospital payment reform, though the PPRC expanded on this precedent by establishing an active role in policy formulation rather than just oversight.[98]

The PPRC built on research, under the guidance of the Harvard economist William Hsiao, previously commissioned by the Health Care Financing Administration into the viability of a resource-based relative value scale (RBRVS). The idea behind RBRVS was to develop a standard for paying doctors based on objective measures of the complexity, time, and resources involved in physician services, in order to eliminate unjustified disparities in the payment levels of various medical specialties. Federal policymakers assumed (an assumption embodied in Hsiao's work) that recalibration of physician payment based on "objective" measures of relative value would result in smaller payments for specialized medical care providers, such as surgeons, and somewhat higher payments for primary care physicians. By reducing the "value" of specialized medical services, RBRVS held out the promise of reducing federal physician expenditures through creation of a system of financial incentives favoring less expensive primary care.[99]

In 1989, as part of that year's Omnibus Budget Reconciliation Act, Congress adopted RBRVS as the basis for a Medicare fee schedule for physicians. A predetermined schedule of fees reflecting the "relative value" of medical services replaced the existing system of payment to physicians for their reasonable charges. In addition, the legislation provided for volume performance standards that would reduce physician payments in subsequent years if spending targets were exceeded, and new limits on how much physicians could balance bill Medicare beneficiaries in excess of federal reimbursement rates.[100] The legislation also established the federal Agency for Health Care Policy and Research to develop national practice guidelines for physicians and to sponsor research into the cost effectiveness of medical procedures, a return to the type of cost containment strategy embodied by PSROs.

The similarities between the adoption of the prospective payment system for hospitals and the establishment of the Medicare fee schedule for physicians were striking. As in the case of prospective payment, Medicare physician payment reform was enacted with bipartisan support, a minimum of visibility, and, for the most part, the acquiescence of the medical industry.[101] Moreover, in both cases regulatory reforms that amounted to the introduction of administered pricing systems were enacted with the support of conservative Republican presidential administrations (the Medicare fee schedule was signed into law by President Bush). Finally, in both the prospective payment system and the Medicare fee schedule, regulation of medical providers was wrapped in the imagery of science, technical proficiency, and objectivity. Both systems promised to enhance efficiency in Medicare through implementation of formulaic corrections to extant payment methods. Like DRGs, RBRVS represented a system of predetermined reimbursement rates and thus provided the basis for prospective Medicare payments similar to those employed by European countries.[102] However, instead of a straightforward embrace of the federal government's regulatory power, the prospective payment system and Medicare fee schedule relied on "objective" measures of resource use as the basis for payment.

James Morone has explained the roots of this peculiar form of regulation in American political culture. Morone notes that "because Americans distrust both politics and politicians, they tend to seek solutions which do not rely on either."[103] Instead of empowering political leaders to regulate medical providers, "Americans constantly search for mechanistic, self-enforcing, automatic solutions which might operate without further politics."[104] The shrouding of Medicare regulation in scientific precision hence reflects a traditional American hope that efficiency and expertise can substitute for political power.

Despite the technical imagery of Medicare regulations, it was politics, not science, that guided their implementation. The regulation of physician payments followed that of hospitals, toward a pattern of strengthened federal authority over medical providers. In the five years before the enactment of the Medicare fee schedule, part B (physician) expenditures rose at an average annual rate of 10.3%; in the five years after its enactment, the average annual rate dropped to 5.6%.

Over time, Medicare payments fell as a percentage of private rates, indicating a slowdown in the rate of growth in federal payments for physician services.[105] In 1993, Medicare fees for physician services stood at only 62% of private sector rates, down from 71% in 1989.[106] The regulation of payments for physician services, then, demonstrated some degree of success in slowing Medicare expenditures, reflecting the growing independence of federal policymakers from the medical industry. Physicians no longer had absolute control over their income from Medicare. Increasingly they were subject to the whims of federal regulators, at the same time that their ability to recoup losses by balance billing Medicare beneficiaries was reduced. The same budgetary politics which had shaped the implementation of the prospective payment system since 1983 also governed the future operation of the Medicare fee schedule. As the pressure to find budgetary savings in Medicare intensified, federal regulation of payments to physicians tightened.

THE POLITICS OF REGULATION

One prominent academic theory of regulation predicts that government regulators will be "captured" by the well-organized and resource-rich interest groups they are regulating.[107] From this perspective, government regulation operates to benefit private industries, which exploit their concentrated interest in shaping regulation to dominate the political process at the expense of diffuse, unorganized consumers. Public policy becomes an instrument of private interests.[108]

This view, particularly pervasive in economics, has helped fuel the movement for deregulation and, in medical care, has sown doubts that the United States could effectively operate a national health insurance system.[109] The Medicare experience in the 1980s, however, directly contradicts capture models of regulation. The enactment of the prospective payment system and Medicare fee schedule, which amounted to an administered pricing system empowering the federal government, stand out as instances of government independence from the concentrated economic interests of the medical industry. Driven by budgetary pressures, federal policymakers in essence recaptured Medicare regulation from the medical profession, which had shaped Medicare's initially permissive payment policies. It has long been held that the more technical policymaking becomes, the more interest groups control policy as complex issues fade into low-visibility arenas where groups can exert political influence far from public view.[110] But the implementation of Medicare's new regulatory regime has not been dominated by hospitals and physicians. Rather, as table 5.2 demonstrates, the federal government has used prospective payment and the physician fee schedule as effective instruments to reduce Medicare payments to providers: after the introduction of Medicare prospective payment in 1983 and the fee schedule in 1989, the rate of growth in Medicare spending declined.[111] Policy complexity and low-visibility politics in Medicare payment policy have not resulted in interest group power.

Indeed, the politics of Medicare regulation appears to turn the old dictum that the symbolic benefits of regulation go to the public, while the tangible benefits are conferred on powerful industries, on its head.[112] The scientific imagery of the Medicare regulatory reforms of the 1980s was constructed, in part, to assure hospitals and physicians that they would be paid on the basis of a fair, objective payment system, not according to the arbitrary decisions of federal policymakers.[113] Yet, in practice, federal officials disregarded the promises they made to providers during the enactment of these reforms and ignored the legislatively mandated formulas for Medicare reimbursement. In the case of the prospective payment system for hospitals, Congress enacted annual increases in reimbursement that were lower than those required by the payment formula in the 1983 statute.[114] Contrary to conventional expectations, then, in Medicare the symbolic benefits of regulation went to the producers (medical providers), while the government has kept the tangible benefits (financial savings) for itself.

Table 5.2 Annual Increase in Medicare Expenditures, Deflated by Consumer Price Index

FISCAL YEAR	INCREASE IN HOSPITALIZATION INSURANCE (%)	INCREASE IN SUPPLEMENTARY MEDICAL INSURANCE (%)
1968	44.6	103.2
1969	19.0	13.0
1970	−2.8	13.3
1971	7.3	−2.6
1972	8.7	7.3
1973	5.3	2.5
1974	8.0	10.6
1975	18.1	16.6
1976	10.8	16.0
1977	6.0	9.0
1978	9.1	9.1
1979	3.5	9.2
1980	5.2	8.1
1981	9.3	9.5
1982	10.7	11.8
1983	7.1	14.0
1984	4.6	7.0
1985	11.5	8.0
1986	−0.1	12.6
1987	−0.9	15.7
1988	0.0	8.1
1989	5.5	4.5
1990	9.3	7.2
1991	−0.8	4.4
1992	14.1	3.7
1993	9.0	4.6
1994	9.2	8.0

Source: Office of the Actuary, Health Care Financing Administration, 1995.

When confronted with the force of deficit politics, the power of medical providers in program politics dramatically receded. Put simply, too much money was on the line given federal budgetary circumstances to abide a regulatory system dominated by hospitals and physicians. The politics of Medicare regulation exemplified a state-centered model of regulation in which government authority operates independently of social interests. Medicare politics in this period simply cannot be explained from the capture perspective.[115]

Notably, Congress played a central role in recapturing Medicare regulation and in implementing policies that saved the government money at the expense of interest groups. This role was unexpected. Conventional wisdom held that Congress was driven by interest group politics and lacked the expertise to keep up with increasingly technical policymaking that advantaged bureaucracies such as HCFA, which ostensibly had an unmatched capacity and expertise to play on the technocratic field of Medicare payment reform.[116] After the adoption of DRGs, James Morone and Andrew Dunham declared that "the locus of health politics has changed to the bureaucracy."[117]

Yet it was Congress, rather than HCFA, that was the primary influence on Medicare regulation and payment policy. Congress's ability to shape Medicare regulation despite its increasingly technical character is explained by three factors. First, Congress responded to its information disadvantage in payment policy by creating its own sources of expertise— namely, the Prospective Payment Assessment Commission in 1983 (for hospital payment policy) and the Physician Payment Review Commission in 1986. These congressional health bureaucracies, which augmented the already established General Accounting Office, Congressional Budget Office, and Office of Technology Assessment, provided lawmakers with policy knowledge independent of the executive branch and HCFA, enabling members of Congress to draft policy proposals and monitor the implementation of Medicare regulatory reforms.[118] In other words, the prospective payment system and Medicare fee schedule raised the costs of congressional participation in Medicare regulation, but Congress raised its policymaking resources.

The second reason that Medicare regulation has not been characterized by a pattern of bureaucratic dominance is that for all the complexity of prospective payment and the fee schedule, each system has crude budgetary instruments that can be manipulated without much expertise. In the case of hospital payment, moving the annual update factor up or down controls the overall level of program payments; for the Medicare fee schedule, the conversion factor offers similar opportunities for legislative intervention.[119] Consequently, Medicare payment regulations are not entirely inaccessible to nonexpert lawmakers.[120]

Moreover, the size and rate of growth of Medicare gives it an importance in the federal budgetary process that does not permit Congress to ignore its operations. Deficit politics led congressional policymakers to intervene in the details of regulatory implementation. In the case of the prospective payment system, Congress took back some of the regulatory authority to set payment rates that the statute had originally given in 1983 to the secretary of health and human services.[121] The breadth and depth of this policymaking activism contravenes arguments that Congress becomes involved in policymaking only when there are electorally motivated opportunities to distribute benefits to constituents.[122] Congress, then, is

influential in Medicare regulatory policy, but for fiscal rather than electoral reasons. Budgetary politics was the core feature of Medicare regulatory policy.

This is not, of course, to argue that Medicare policymaking is solely influenced by Congress. Medicare policy is made through "issue networks,"
in which members of the program's administration, the presidential administration, and the legislature and their staff collaborate on ideas and
strategies. And HCFA played an essential role in shaping policy. But it is
to argue that during the 1980s, because of the primacy of deficit politics,
the independence of congressional fiscal interest in budgetary stringency,
and most critically, the institutional position of Congress in the budget
process, Congress was at the center of these networks.[123] And as long as
Medicare regulatory policy is budgetary policy, congressional influence
over federal health regulation will remain strong.[124]

CONCLUSION

Medicare regulation has experienced a series of dramatic shifts. Throughout these changes, though, there has been one constant: bipartisan consensus. The ideas about what Medicare should do to slow down program
spending changed radically over time from monitoring excessive utilization, fraud, and abuse to establishing prospective payment controls and
administered pricing. Yet it is noteworthy that in each of Medicare's policy regimes, Democrats and Republicans have generally agreed on the
solution du jour. As a result, during Medicare's first three decades there
was far less conflict and controversy surrounding payment and regulatory
policymaking than one might have anticipated. The relative absence of
controversy and the bipartisan nature of regulatory politics is amply
demonstrated by Republican support for centralized controls over hospitals and physicians in the 1980s, regulatory controls shrouded with market language and enacted with a minimum of debate. In regulatory policy,
as in policymaking for financing and benefits, the Medicare consensus
governed the program.

The dynamics of Medicare regulation reveal that American health
politics is not as exceptional as is usually believed. Health economist
Uwe Reinhardt has noted that post–World War II health policy in
industrialized democracies can generally be divided into two eras: the
expenditure-driven policies of 1945–70, during which governments regarded increasing health expenditures as a public policy achievement and
therefore did little to control the open-ended costs of medical care, and the
period from 1970 to the present, when in the face of stagnating economies

and fiscal pressures, governments have turned to budget-driven health policies to control rising costs.[125] During the past two decades, Canada and Western European nations have been increasingly aggressive in controlling spending in their national health care systems, generally moving, for example, from lenient expenditure "targets" to "caps" that set harder limits (with penalties for excess billings) on sectoral expenditures. Over time, the trend has been toward global budgets that prospectively limit governments' annual health care bills.

Medicare, albeit with less force, moved in the same direction of budget-driven health policymaking during the 1980s. Stripped of their technocratic language and scientific veneers, DRGs and RBRVS were essentially blunt instruments of prospective budgeting and price regulation. And as the decade progressed, the scope of the Medicare program subject to prospective payment and budgeting expanded. These reforms brought Medicare closer to the "international standard" in controlling the costs of medical care.[126]

Under the politics of consensus, Medicare looked more and more like other national health systems in its form of cost control. But two dramatic differences between the international standard and Medicare remained. In contrast to other industrial democracies, the United States did not adopt a global budget for Medicare, a ceiling on total program expenditures. A global budget would have required a dramatic altering of Medicare's budgetary entitlement status and would also have been viewed as incompatible with beneficiaries' individual entitlement to coverage, though the right to health care and budgetary constraints seem to coexist comfortably in other nations. Moreover, unlike other countries, Medicare is a public program that buys services in a predominantly private health system. If Medicare fees fall too low, there is a danger that providers will refuse to accept Medicare patients and exit the program, turning instead to privately insured patients for revenues. Universal health systems such as the one in Canada, where the government is the single purchaser of medical care (monopsony), face no such barriers, enabling them to impose lower payment rates than Medicare can in the United States.

A second distinction relates to technology. In Canada and Western Europe, technological diffusion is centrally controlled by the government. As a result, these nations generally have lower rates of expensive medical technology such as magnetic resonance imaging than exists in the United States, where a free market driven by hospital competition leads to wide diffusion of medical technology. Given that technology is the most prominent factor driving up the long-term costs of medical care, this is a critical instrument of cost control—and one that Medicare lacks. With the absence of a broader national health system, there is no way for Medicare to control technological diffusion.

As a consequence of its inability to control technological diffusion and the absence of a global program budget, Medicare remained vulnerable to unanticipated increases in program spending, a vulnerability that set the stage for the political turbulence Medicare entered in 1995.

Medicare Politics

PATTERNS AND EXPLANATIONS

There is no single politics of Medicare. (handwritten annotation)

There is no single politics of Medicare. That is the inescapable conclusion of my analysis of Medicare's political development from 1965 to 1994. No public opinion, interest group, cultural, or institutional theory alone can explain Medicare's political experience. That will disappoint scholars who look to one or another of these theories to explain everything, or at least most things, about American politics. But, quite simply, the reality of Medicare politics defies explanation by any single theory. Ultimately, it is more important to present Medicare as it really is than to fit it artificially into a model for the sake of proving that model's ostensible superiority.

The diversity of Medicare politics is generated by the very nature of the program. In the past, Medicare politics has often been identified exclusively with issues of regulation and payment policies for physicians and hospitals. This study expanded on that narrow vision by illuminating Medicare across three policy areas: benefits, financing, and regulation. My purpose in taking this tack was to provide a more complete analysis of Medicare politics than previous studies and to generate a narrative that, while not comprehensive in capturing all of Medicare's history, provided a representative picture of Medicare politics in its first three decades.

Yet if three separable, if not always independent, policy arenas can be identified, it follows that each arena may have distinctive political dynamics and internal logics, and those dynamics and logics may conflict. A compelling example of the need to attend to different strains within Medicare politics was provided in 1989. At the same time that the repeal of catastrophic health insurance in response to protests from the elderly made Medicare appear susceptible to the influence of social forces, Congress adopted the Medicare fee schedule for physicians, a powerful statement of autonomy from private interests and the end of a twenty-five-year policy of accommodating the medical profession. In one instance (in benefits policy), Medicare appeared at the mercy of societal pressures, in the other (in regulatory politics), independent—all in the same year. There could hardly be more persuasive evidence of the capacity of Medicare politics to move in two directions at once and the difficulty of explaining the program from any one theoretical perspective.

THE POLITICS OF MEDICARE POLICY

Given the scope and complexity of Medicare, the program's political diversity is inevitable. Nevertheless, it is possible to discern patterns of political influence across the program's first three decades and to understand how (and under what conditions) different political forces have shaped Medicare policy.

I outline here a series of hypotheses about Medicare politics derived from political science literature on public policy, the welfare state, and American politics. The hypotheses reflect differing assumptions about the influence of elections, political parties, public opinion, interest groups, state actors, political institutions, and ideas on public policymaking. I compare their predictions about Medicare politics with the actual outcomes observed in this study. This chapter is intended for political scientists: some readers may wish to read ahead to chapter 7, which resumes the narrative of Medicare's political history by exploring the end of consensus and Medicare politics in 1995–2002 before returning to the political analysis in this chapter.

ELECTIONS AND PARTIES

One school of thought in political science argues that public policymaking is explained by the response of political actors to electoral incentives. According to these theories, politicians act in order to maximize their chances for reelection. Electoral theories of policymaking are especially prevalent in the literature on Congress, which emphasizes members' pursuit of individual goals in the context of a decentralized political environment.[1] When applied to broadly based welfare state programs such as Medicare, the implication is that electoral incentives produce generous benefits, since increasing benefits is popular with the public and promotes reelection. Alternatively, elections can be viewed as the "mainsprings" of policy change.[2] Elections may provide public mandates on policy issues or alter the partisan balance of the government, triggering a shift in the direction of public policy.

Theories of electoral influence on public policy suggest three hypotheses about Medicare politics. First, changes in Medicare policy should correspond to changes in electoral outcomes and to shifts in the partisan alignment of the government. Second, the desire of incumbent politicians for reelection should produce a bidding contest to expand Medicare benefits. And third, elections should generate public mandates regarding Medicare policy that are acted on by Congress and the president.

I find only limited evidence to support electoral theories of Medicare politics. The first hypothesis—that Medicare policy should change in response to electoral outcomes—rests on a presumption of party divergence.[3] The expectation is that the Democratic and Republican Parties will formulate and implement different Medicare policies, reflecting divergent party ideologies and philosophies about government, regulation, health policy, and the role of markets in public programs. As the balance of the partisan alignment becomes more Democratic, Medicare policy should become more liberal, moving toward expanded benefits, lower costs for program beneficiaries, and stronger, more centralized regulation of medical providers. As the partisan balance shifts toward the Republican Party, Medicare policy should move in a conservative direction, with less centralized regulation of medical providers, reduced benefits, and higher costs for elderly beneficiaries.

There have been differences in party positions on Medicare. Republican presidents have been more eager to impose higher cost sharing on Medicare beneficiaries than Democrats, and Democrats in Congress have been more eager than their Republican counterparts to expand the program. Yet, in the end, the differences between the two parties on Medicare have been far less impressive than their commonalities. Democrats and Republicans formed a de facto political consensus that favored the maintenance of Medicare as a government-operated insurance program. In the era of consensus, from 1966 to 1994, financing, benefits, and regulatory policies took on a decidedly bipartisan character; for instance, the Medicare regulatory reforms of the 1970s and 1980s, from professional standard review organizations to the Medicare fee schedule, were all noteworthy for their support from both Democrats and Republicans.

Moreover, the substance of Medicare policy has often moved against the direction predicted by party ideology. The largest expansion of Medicare benefits in program history, the 1988 catastrophic health insurance legislation, was initiated not by a liberal Democrat, but by the conservative Reagan administration. The introduction of the Medicare prospective payment system for hospitals in 1983 and the Medicare fee schedule for physicians in 1989, which together amounted to a federally controlled system of administered pricing for Medicare providers, was endorsed by two conservative Republican presidents, Ronald Reagan and George Bush. Partisan alignments, then, generally did not yield predictable changes in the content of Medicare policy during the program's first three decades.

There is, however, a critical caveat. From Medicare's enactment in 1965 through 1994, the Republican Party did not control the House of Representatives, the Senate, and the presidency at the same time. Nor did Republicans control both houses of Congress at any one time. As a consequence, it is unclear what Medicare policy would have looked like under unified Republican control or even Republican control of Congress.[4]

The second electoral hypothesis—that Medicare should induce politicians to enter a bidding contest to expand its benefits—rests on a presumption of party convergence.[5] The assumption is that the popularity of Medicare provides both Democratic and Republican politicians with common electoral incentives that operate regardless of ideology. To the extent that both parties have supported the maintenance of Medicare, this prediction has been substantiated. Electoral incentives clearly helped to preserve the Medicare consensus. However, with the exception of catastrophic insurance, electoral incentives did not produce the expected bidding contest among incumbent politicians to increase Medicare benefits. Instead, the dominant pattern in Medicare benefits has been the absence of benefits expansion, a "negative consensus" on restraining program growth. The desire for reelection has been overwhelmed by the desire to contain the costs of a program widely viewed as fiscally uncontrollable, contradicting theories that assume the predominance of electoral incentives in shaping politicians' behavior.[6]

The third hypothesis—that Medicare policy should reflect public mandates expressed in elections—provides the most direct link between electoral incentives and public policy. In the case of Medicare, it is also the least compelling. In order for electoral mandates to have a direct impact on public policy, three conditions must be satisfied: the electorate must be offered a choice of policy options, voters must respond to this choice in an identifiable way, and elected officials must shape policy to conform with the choice of the electorate.[7]

Under any circumstances, it is difficult to establish that all three conditions have been met. Voters choose elected officials on the basis of multiple considerations, including party affiliation, economic conditions, candidate personality, and ideology. It is therefore always difficult to infer what choice the electorate has made on a given issue or to identify a public mandate for a specific policy action.[8] In Medicare, however, the notion of electoral choice has been even more elusive, because the electorate has not often been presented any choice about program policy. Medicare was rarely a first-order issue in presidential or congressional campaigns from 1965 to 1994.[9] Questions such as what the scope of Medicare benefits should be, how Medicare should be financed, and what regulatory policies Medicare should adopt for medical providers were not debated with any degree of prominence in American elections. Voters were not asked these questions, and consequently they gave no answers.

Medicare policymaking has therefore proceeded apart from any electoral mandates generated by the public. Critical changes in Medicare policy, such as the enactment of the prospective payment system in 1983 or the 1993 removal of any limits on earned income subject to Medicare payroll taxes, have been enacted without ever having received attention as campaign issues. In fact, from 1965 to 1994 there was not a single national election that reasonably can be interpreted as a public referendum on Medicare policy, let alone a mandate.

PUBLIC OPINION

Elections are not the only potential instrument of popular influence on public policy. Such influence is also expressed through public opinion. Scholars from the public opinion tradition argue that policymakers are sensitive to mass preferences because they are exposed to an institutionalized polling apparatus and because attention to public opinion is politically valuable. The prevalence of opinion polls in contemporary politics makes them difficult to ignore and enables politicians to measure public support for their positions on various issues. Policymakers may therefore respond to the established preferences of the public or to what they anticipate as likely public reactions to public policies.[10] Theories of public opinion produce two hypotheses about Medicare. First, the direction of Medicare policy should be dictated by the preferences of public opinion. And second, public responses anticipated by politicians should shape and constrain developments in Medicare policy, including decisions on program reform.

Clearly, public opinion has set limits on Medicare politics. Public support for Medicare has been consistently high, ranking it in the top tier of American welfare state programs in terms of favorable opinion.[11] The

Medicare consensus was so strong from 1965 to 1994 partly because it rested on a firm foundation of public support. As a consequence, there have been identifiable boundaries to Medicare politics; proposals to end the program as a universal entitlement or to drastically reduce its benefits have been rare. However, within these boundaries, the influence of public opinion on Medicare policymaking has been weak. Polling data have shown strong popular support for increasing Medicare benefits, as well as some evidence of public willingness to pay higher taxes for specific proposals to raise benefits.[12] Yet the program's benefits remained mostly static for three decades.

Nor has public opinion influenced the content of Medicare regulatory policies. Changes in how Medicare pays doctors and hospitals have been made without public debate. There is no indication that the public has had any preferences regarding the substantive content of regulatory policies that have been adopted or that these policies have reflected policymakers' anticipated reactions of public opinion. It is difficult, if not impossible, to detect the public's influence in professional standards review organizations, the prospective payment system, or the Medicare fee schedule.

There has been a common theme to the comparative irrelevance of mass opinion in Medicare benefits and regulatory policy. In both cases, public understanding of the particulars of Medicare policy has been low, the details of existing program structure and proposed reforms beyond the scope of public knowledge. Even the segment of the public closest to the program, elderly beneficiaries, has shown inconsistent knowledge of Medicare. These limitations on public knowledge weakened the ability of the public to influence Medicare policy. Medicare thus provides a strong challenge to public opinion theorists who portray a "rational public" sufficiently informed to develop stable preferences and influence public policy.[13]

Even if public knowledge of Medicare policy is low, it is possible that politicians calculate probable public responses in setting program policy. One area where anticipated public opinion clearly has influenced Medicare policy is in the targeting of program cutbacks. The issue is how to distribute the costs of Medicare cutbacks across social groups. In making that choice, it is arguable that policymakers were constrained by the anticipated public preference for imposing such costs on medical providers, rather than on beneficiaries. Opinion polls on health care reform have shown strong public support for controlling medical care spending by regulating payments to hospitals and doctors.[14] Medical providers, then, have been the popular choice to shoulder the brunt of program cuts in spending.[15] And indeed, the vast majority of Medicare cutbacks have fallen on doctors and hospitals, not elderly and disabled beneficiaries. Of course, if this choice of budgetary targets reflects the existing preferences of policymakers, then public opinion reinforces these preferences, rather than serving as their source.

Medicare financing policy presents another intriguing case. It is the area of Medicare policy where anticipated public opinion is expected to matter the most because of the focus on taxes.[16] Indeed, there have been policy episodes in which anticipated public reactions have apparently influenced financing policy. The proposals for expanding Medicare hospitalization coverage that culminated in the 1988 Medicare Catastrophic Coverage Act were not financed through an increase in payroll taxes because policymakers argued that there was a "political limit" on public willingness to accept such an increase. Similarly, chronic shortfalls in the Medicare hospitalization insurance trust fund have been met by policymakers' reluctance to increase the level of Medicare payroll taxes, presumably for "fear of adverse public reaction."[17]

And yet even these apparent instances of indirect public influence are open to question. Anticipated public reactions leave political actors substantial discretion in defining the nature of mass preferences. To cite public reluctance to accept new payroll taxes for Medicare expansion as a justification for an alternative financing scheme is not the same as responding to actual preferences. The distinction is crucial because of evidence that a gap exists between public and elite preferences on Medicare policy. The public is more supportive of increases in Medicare benefits and more sympathetic toward the elderly than members of Congress.[18] Intergenerational equity concerns are thus more pronounced at elite than popular levels.

Given the disparity between elite and popular opinion, policymakers' justifications of their Medicare positions as reflective of public preferences must be considered with caution. In the case of payroll taxes, it is likely that a public supportive of expanding Medicare benefits would have accepted new taxes to pay for catastrophic insurance or to restore the financial health of the trust fund if such an option had been recommended by a consensus of political elites. That it was not offered reveals the ability of politicians to maneuver around mass preferences and shape policy choices so as to influence the substance of public opinion.[19] Under conditions of low public understanding, politicians not only enjoy substantial freedom to adopt their preferred policies, but also hold the power to define public understandings of policy problems, as well as the responses "required" by those problems. Even on issues of Medicare financing that have lent themselves to anticipated public reactions, Medicare policy has not clearly followed mass opinion.[20]

The gap between public opinion and policy outcomes in Medicare benefits and financing policy raises an important question: Is Medicare policymaking democratic?[21] After all, Medicare policy operated from 1965 to 1994 in a political environment bounded by consensus, where even important reforms had low visibility and were decided on far from the public eye. Strong bipartisanship and the absence of controversy meant there was often little public debate and even less public input in Medicare policymaking. And there is evidence that major policy decisions—namely, the refusal to expand benefits and the reluctance to increase payroll taxes—contravened public opinion.

Inasmuch as the Medicare consensus on benefits and financing policy followed the wishes of political elites rather than the public, there appears to be a gap in the democratic responsiveness of Medicare policy. Yet such a judgment must be qualified. On the most important issue in Medicare policy—maintaining the program as a universal social insurance program operated by the federal government—policymakers were in step with the public. Public opinion mattered the most where core values and program structure were in question—a legacy from the debate over Medicare's enactment in the 1950s and 1960s.[22]

But even in the policy areas where a gap persisted between public opinion and elite actions, that policymakers flouted public will is not entirely clear. On financing policy, for example, there is evidence that the public would have accommodated higher taxes. Yet public opinion data do not necessarily reveal anything about the intensity of opinion; to say that a majority of the public supports a particular policy action is not necessarily to say anything about how strong that support is. Did the public intensely desire higher payroll taxes? Were there mass demonstrations to raise the Medicare payroll tax? In both cases, the answer is no. And given the political axiom that you do not win votes by raising taxes, that politicians did not respond to "soft" preferences to raise payroll taxes appears less undemocratic than on initial examination. In short, to argue that a permissive majority of the public would have accepted higher payroll taxes for Medicare is not the same as saying a public groundswell for higher payroll taxes developed and policymakers defied it.

A stronger case for Medicare's failure to respond to public preferences can be made in benefits policy. The public never liked the limits on Medicare coverage and displayed consistent support for expanding program benefits. Since benefits expansion is a more palatable prospect than higher taxes, it is reasonable to assume public opinion was more intensely held on benefits than financing policy. Here political elites' stronger fiscal and intergenerational equity concerns dampened public will. But it is critical to note that the development of private insurance policies to supplement Medicare, especially among higher-income beneficiaries, eroded political pressures from elderly Medicare enrollees for coverage expansion. With reduced pressures from beneficiaries, public opinion favoring benefits expansion could be viewed by a reasonable politician in a different— and less demanding—context. Again, the story is more complicated than a simple picture of political elites defying democratic pressures.

Still, it is clear that the public was not widely engaged with Medicare policy from 1965 to 1994, and that raises critical issues regrading democracy and public policy. The Medicare consensus generated a politics that was quiet, bipartisan, and usually operated outside the public sphere. The political scientist E. E. Schattschneider argues that democracy flourishes when there is a wider scope of political conflict that draws the public into policy debates.[23] As policy debates become more public, mass opinion has a greater influence on public policy, and the power of interest groups, who dominate low-visibility processes in which their machinations are invisible to the public, wanes. Martha Derthick similarly argues that Social Security policy through the 1970s was dominated by a small group of "program proprietors" who restricted public debate on the program, disguised the true costs of benefits, deprived the public of information about choices in Social Security reform, and consequently created a program where growth became "inexorable."[24] She concludes that improving Social Security policy and making it more democratic depends on having a high-visibility, public debate that breaks the program free from the control of program executives.

My examination of Medicare did not find a similar pattern of program policy dominated by a narrow circle of "proprietors," perhaps because early financial difficulties ensured a broader pattern of policymaking involvement.[25] Certainly, Medicare's benefits growth has been anything but inexorable, and reforms have slowed the rate of increase in program spending. Moreover, while public debate is arguably a condition necessary to a more democratic form of Medicare policymaking, judging by the past it clearly is not sufficient.

The most public debate in Medicare during its first three decades, regarding the catastrophic health insurance legislation, generated more heat than light. Public education and deliberative democracy had to take a seat next to demagoguery and misinformation, a pattern repeated in spades during debate over the Clinton health plan in 1993–94. There are good reasons to want policymakers to engage in public education, the public to participate in policy debates, and citizens to understand clearly the trade-offs and issues associated with policy decisions.[26] Yet, as health reformers found out in 1994, there is simply no guarantee that a more visible public debate will produce these democratic outcomes, rather than undemocratic exercises in public manipulation or confusion.

INTEREST GROUPS

Interest group theories depict public policy as the outcome of pressures directed at the state by private interests. Public policy is portrayed as reflecting not the will of the public, but rather the power of well-heeled interest groups. These interests have a concentrated stake in policy outcomes that induces high levels of political mobilization unmatched by the disinterested general public. Pressure groups also possess electoral, economic, and informational resources that are valuable to elected officials, leading to policymaking patterns of "servicing the organized."[27] They have, in other words, both the motive and means to influence public policy. As a result, public policy may in fact be beyond public control. Instead, government may be dominated by private interests in a series of policy subsystems.[28]

In Medicare, two groups have been widely cited as powerful influences on federal policy: the elderly and the medical profession. Theories of interest group influence predict that these groups, including the AMA and AARP, should dominate Medicare policy.[29] However, claims of interest group control of public policy are not substantiated in Medicare. Medicare policy has deviated substantially from the preferences of relevant pressure groups. In the case of the elderly, there has not been a consistent pattern of expansion in Medicare benefits, and over time, out-of-pocket costs for elderly beneficiaries have increased substantially. As a consequence, political organizations representing the elderly have failed to secure some of their primary goals. On the other hand, groups representing the elderly have exerted more influence on efforts to cut back Medicare benefits. The power of political organizations representing the elderly has thus been primarily defensive in nature. They have not succeeded in compelling Medicare policy to develop according to their preferences, but they have enjoyed more success in keeping Medicare policy from moving against their preferences.[30]

Interest groups representing medical providers have, on average, exerted less influence over Medicare than groups representing the elderly. After 1972, Medicare moved away from professional self-regulation, which conceded authority to the medical profession, to adopt regulatory reforms that increased the power of the federal government over hospital and physician reimbursement. And while medical providers shaped the implementation of earlier reforms such as professional standard review organizations in their favor, their influence over implementation of subsequent regulatory reforms such as the prospective payment system waned.[31] Medicare regulation in the 1980s led to federal payment rates for hospitals and physicians that were substantially lower than those for the private sector. Consequently, interest groups representing hospitals and physicians have not even enjoyed the limited defensive power asserted by groups representing the elderly.

In the cases of both the elderly and the medical industry, the limited influence of interest groups on Medicare policy is explained largely by fiscal conditions. Early on, Medicare gained a reputation as an "uncontrollable" program that required containment and reform, not expansion. Low economic growth in the 1970s and high federal deficits in the 1980s further increased the fiscal pressures on Medicare, eventually producing a politics of regulation that empowered the federal government over hospitals and physicians.

The importance of these fiscal conditions to Medicare politics raises important issues about interest group theory and the conditions under which group influence is strong. It should be noted that much of this theory, as represented by the pluralist scholarship in political science of the 1950s and the 1960s, was written in a period marked by an expanding American economy.[32] The changed economic conditions of the 1970s and 1980s, defined by lower rates of growth and, especially, worsening federal deficits, altered the power of interest groups to influence public policy. In such an economic and budgetary climate, there is greater resistance by government officials to granting public concessions to interest groups because such concessions are viewed as unaffordable. The shape of zero-sum politics can hardly be assumed to be the same as that characterized by favorable budgetary conditions. Pluralism consequently depicts less an immutable feature of American politics than the outcome of a distinctive set of economic and fiscal conditions that defined the post–World War II era.

Moreover, political scientists have long held that interest group influence on public policy is strongest under conditions of low public visibility, which enable pressure groups to operate free from democratic constraints.[33] The Medicare experience suggests this axiom needs to be revised to take account of budgetary politics and fiscal constraints. After all, Medicare's reform of payment policies in the 1980s, which marked a substantial defeat for interest groups representing hospitals and physicians, was adopted in a context of low-visibility politics that did not involve the public to any significant degree. Here it is apparent that interest group influence fades not only when subject to the counterpressures of a public audience, but also when enough money is on the line that the policy in question is highly visible and fiscally consequential to politicians—especially under conditions of a federal budget deficit—regardless of public knowledge or participation.

In addition to raising doubts about pluralism, the dynamics of Medicare policymaking contravene rational choice theories of politics. Rational choice, which has become predominant in political science over the past decade, applies microeconomic principles to the study of politics. Rational choice theorists argue that voters are self-interested, public policy reflects the preferences of "rent-seeking" private interests who essentially buy policy with campaign contributions, and public programs in democratic systems grow at unsustainable rates fueled by elected officials' solicitous concern for voters as well as private interests.[34] The Medicare case offers little support for such a perspective. The effective regulation of medical providers by the federal government contradicts the predictions of rent-seeking models of political behavior, which assume the dominance of regulation by producers. And the curtailment of Medicare expenditures, as well as the absence of benefits expansion, run counter to arguments about "government as Leviathan" and uncontrollable public programs. Rational choice substantially underestimates the independence of policymaking from interest group and electoral pressures and consequently explains very little about Medicare politics.[35]

This book's picture of the limited power of interest groups in Medicare clashes with accounts by both journalists and policymakers, who often portray health care politics as a world dominated by pressure groups. The gap between my analysis and what they observe is explained largely by the type of policies in question. I have focused here on the politics of program management in terms of "macropolicies": large decisions about Medicare reform, the transformation of payment policies, the adoption (or nonadoption) of new program benefits. Alternatively, program administrators, congressional staff, and other Medicare policymakers operate in an environment where they constantly make "micropolicy" decisions: how particular regulations affect medical supply companies, how policies influence specific hospitals (and the urban or rural districts of members of Congress where those hospitals are located), whether Medicare will cover a new technology. In such decisions, interest group activity is high; while each decision has a negligible impact on the total Medicare budget, its impact on a particular medical providers' income can be significant.[36] As former Medicare administrator Bruce Vladeck has noted, "Medicare's annual $200 billion is a major prize or more precisely, an enormous aggregation of smaller prizes."[37]

Yet, as budget politics have driven Medicare policy and the program has adopted stronger cost containment measures, interest group posturing for program income has increasingly taken place in a zero-sum environment. Providers battle each other to obtain money, or to be shielded from the largest cutbacks. These internecine battles intensify as Medicare spending is further constrained. And when, as in the case of hospitals, the money at stake in distributing program payments is sufficiently large to attract policymakers' attention, medical providers' interests are subordinated to fiscal goals.[38] Interest group influence on the overall Medicare budget, then, continued to decline during Medicare's first three decades of operation. And while providers and other interests often influenced micropolicy decisions and the distribution of payments, their impact on macropolicy—the overall direction of Medicare reform and payment regulations—declined throughout the 1965–94 period. In sum, visibility and influence in Medicare policy that distributes payments to medical providers have *not* amounted to interest group control of the program.

STATE ACTORS

State-centered theories of politics emphasize the independence of government actors from societal interests and public opinion. Policymakers do not simply ratify the preferences of private groups or the mass public; they adopt policies that reflect their own political, ideological, and strategic motivations.[39] In Medicare, the implication is that policies are made that follow the aims of government actors independent of interest group pressures or public opinion.

I find substantial evidence to support this hypothesis about Medicare politics. Ironically, this finding contradicts not simply interest group and public opinion theories, but also much of the state-centered literature itself. Although early scholarship in the field was devoted to finding an American state and explaining its origins, state-centered theorists of comparative welfare state politics often portray the United States as a "weak state." The absence of an established national bureaucracy, the predominance of antistate liberal values and individualism, and the fragmentation of American political institutions and parties are said to have made the United States vulnerable to interest group pressures and, consequently, less able to pursue independent policymaking.[40]

Yet, contrary to such expectations, federal policymakers have strongly influenced Medicare policy development independently of societal pressures. In benefits policy, federal officials demonstrated independence from social interests and public opinion by refusing to expand Medicare during most of its three decades of operation. In financing policy, policymakers shaped the responses to Medicare bankruptcy crises, taking advantage of the opportunity to enact their preferred policy solutions. And in regulatory policy, state actors legislated and implemented reforms that empowered the government over the medical industry.[41]

From a health policy perspective, this conclusion about the strength of the American state in Medicare policymaking is predictable. Government efforts to control the costs of public medical insurance programs are a common feature of politics in all industrialized nations.[42] The rising costs of medical care generate pressure on public budgets, creating an irresistible incentive for governments to restrain health care expenditures. This frequently leads state officials to act against the interests of medical providers, and sometimes patients. However, despite this common theme in international health policy, the strength of the American state in Medicare is a surprise to much of political science, since the United States is usually viewed as an exceptional case of institutional weakness. The weak American state, riddled with veto points in the policymaking process that provide innumerable opportunities to obstruct change, is allegedly especially vulnerable to interest group pressures and thus exceptionally constrained in its ability to formulate independent policy.

Obviously, the United States is exceptional in one crucial dimension of health politics. America remains the only advanced industrialized country in the world without national health insurance, a disparity that is by now overdetermined by the numerous explanations generated by political scientists.[43] The issue of why the United States has not enacted universal health insurance and its implications for understanding American health politics cannot be overlooked. Yet the politics of legislative enactment should not be confused with that of program management. It is the politics of management, not enactment, that has governed Medicare since 1965. Whatever the ideological or institutional barriers to passing a public health program, once it becomes a law, a new program creates a new politics.[44] In Medicare, this politics has centered on the problem of controlling program costs. And in managing federal health insurance, the United States has not behaved so differently from other countries, paying physicians on the basis of a fixed fee schedule, restricting payments to hospitals, and moving toward prospective budgeting.

This conclusion about the state's role in federal health policy highlights a lesson of Medicare for our understanding of American political institutions. One implication of this study is that scholars have not recognized the potential of Congress to act as an independent political institution and consequently have underestimated the independence of the American state from private interests. Prevailing models in political science conceptualize members of Congress almost exclusively as *politicians*. The Medicare case, however, suggests that scholars need to pay more attention to the role of members of Congress as *policymakers*. As already discussed, Congress has demonstrated substantial independence in Medicare policymaking from public opinion, interest groups, and voters. Members of Congress have managed federal health insurance as state actors, pursuing policies that cannot be explained simply by self-interest or electoral pressures. And they have been involved in the details of policy development to a degree that belies existing assumptions that Congress does not engage in substantive programmatic activity apart from electoral motivations.[45]

What does this imply about the nature of American political institutions? Central to this understanding of the U.S. state as weak are two assumptions:[46] first, that Congress plays a greater role in American policymaking than legislatures in other countries, and second, that this comparatively greater legislative influence weakens the American state because Congress is not an independent political institution, but an instrument of societal influence. This understanding has been reinforced by two scholarly literatures. As already noted, the emphasis on electoral incentives in the congressional literature leaves little room for legislative independence. Yet the literature that argues for the independence of political institutions, state theory, which might be expected to contradict the electoral incentives literature, has not challenged this understanding of Congress. State-centered theorists, working from models of politics derived from European countries, have equated state independence with bureaucratic power, in the process implicitly creating an ideal type of state. Failing to find such bureaucracies and the ideal state in the United States, they have then labeled America a weak polity.[47]

This study suggests that the American state is a more independent force in policymaking than is commonly assumed, but that frequently the source of that independence is Congress, rather than European-style bureaucracies. In part, neglect of congressional independence reflects a misunderstanding of the character of public administration in the United States. In a political system based on the separation of powers, such as exists in the United States, much of the administration of public programs that is traditionally performed by executive bureaucracies instead falls to the legislature. As a result, the incentives to assert state independence in managing these programs that are usually associated with bureaucracies are found in Congress.

The legislative role in American public administration is highlighted by the Medicare case. Not only has Congress pursued independent policy goals; it has created its own congressional bureaucracies to influence Medicare policy, namely the Prospective Payment Assessment Commission and the Physician Payment Review Commission (now merged as the Medicare Payment Advisory Commission). These congressional health bureaucracies add to already established resources such as the Congressional Budget Office, the General Accounting Office, and committee staffs, providing Congress (whose members, after all, often serve terms longer than executive branch bureaucrats) with sources of expertise and policy innovation that are brought to bear in Medicare. The involvement of Congress in Medicare policymaking, especially concentrated on the congressional health subcommittees, has been critical from the enactment of professional standard review organizations to the implementation of the Medicare fee schedule.[48]

Thus, it is misleading and, in the case of Medicare, simply wrong to equate congressional influence over public policy with state weakness. The categories used by state-centered theorists to measure state influence, autonomy and capacity, can be applied to Congress as well as to bureaucracies. The American legislature has a degree of political independence from social pressures and it also possesses the resources to make public policy.[49] This is not to argue that congressional policymaking is consistently or mostly independent of social pressures. But it is to suggest that U.S. public policy cannot be understood without considering the centrality of Congress to the American state and the critical policymaking role of U.S. legislators.[50]

PATH DEPENDENCE

Path dependence is the newest theoretical movement in political science. Path dependence argues for the importance of past decisions and institutional arrangements in constraining public policy options. There are two major strains of path dependence theory; the first emphasizes "policy feedbacks."[51] The core idea is that policies adopted in a specific political context reshape that context, affecting subsequent policy development (a policy feedback effect). Policy decisions are not taken de novo but are inevitably influenced by the legacies of past policies. For instance, in contemplating the adoption of a new prescription drug benefit, policymakers are constrained by the fact that many retirees already have employer-paid supplemental drug coverage. Consequently, a new Medicare drug might be forced to build on top of this existing coverage, rather than replacing it, because of past policy decisions that have made private coverage a popular benefit.

Political scientists have identified three types of policy feedbacks: interest group mobilization, program structure, and political learning. Interest group mobilization predicts that the political organization of private interests will be a consequence, rather than a cause, of public policies. Policy feedbacks involving program structures predict that the internal structure of public policies will shape program politics. And finally, political learning theories predict that policymakers' actions will be shaped by the lessons they draw from existing policies.[52]

How have policy feedbacks affected Medicare politics? Clearly, Medicare provides evidence for the claim that policies can trigger interest group mobilization. While political groups representing the elderly were not a significant force in Medicare's enactment, the enactment of federal health insurance helped to catalyze their subsequent organization. Program structure also has exerted a crucial influence on Medicare policy. In particular, the self-supporting and trust fund structure of Medicare financing has had a substantial effect on program politics by creating the potential for Medicare to "go bankrupt." Finally, political learning has influenced Medicare. The lessons that policymakers learned about the ineffectiveness of Medicare's strategy of self-regulation to control costs led to the subsequent adoption of tighter regulatory systems operated by the federal government.

While there is evidence that policy feedbacks have influenced Medicare policy, it is difficult to gauge the strength of this influence because of the vagueness of the predictions of feedback theories, and problems in identifying all the relevant feedbacks that should be measured. Without knowing the total number of potential feedbacks, it is difficult to assign explanatory power to this variable based only on the feedback effects that are observed to be relevant. What about policy feedbacks that do not matter (such as similar public support for Medicare parts A and B despite different financing mechanisms)? Path dependence has little to say about this. Moreover, the relationship between Medicare and Social Security demonstrates a limitation of feedback analysis. These programs had similar programmatic structures, yet they produced different politics. Feedback effects cannot be deduced automatically from a particular set of institutional arrangements.

A second, and presently more prominent, strain of path dependence theory focuses on the idea, borrowed from economics, of "increasing returns."[53] This perspective emphasizes the stability and inertia of public policy: "particular courses of action, once introduced, can be virtually impossible to reverse."[54] The core idea is that the further a policy travels down a specific path, the more institutionalized it becomes, increasing the costs of change and making it harder to move it off the path. For example, the fact that so many businesses are now dependent on Windows operating systems for their computers makes any effort for a new operating system to gain market share difficult (even if it is more efficient than Windows). Companies would have to pay the prohibitive costs of switching all their computers to the new operating system, replacing software with programs compatible with the new system, and teaching their employees a new computer language. Consequently, the strong incentive is to stay with Windows; exiting that "path" is too costly.

According to path dependence theorists, political institutions and public policies similarly have a "status quo bias."[55] In Medicare, the prediction is that policies will be quite stable, and the longer they are in place, the less likely it is they will change.

This prediction, however, is not borne out. Certainly, Medicare policy has been stable in several key respects; from a beneficiary's perspective, especially, little changed about the program from 1965 to 1994. But other policy areas have been less stable. The adoption of the prospective payment system in 1983, the Medicare fee schedule in 1989, and the Medicare HMO program in 1982 (discussed in the next chapter) all represented dramatic changes in Medicare policy. In the case of payment policy, Medicare moved from a reimbursement policy that gave hospitals and physicians a blank check to one in which the government wrote the check in advance; it is hard to conceive of a more dramatic change. Moreover, the overturning of the status quo in payment policy came two decades into Medicare's operation, directly refuting the claim that the longer a policy is in place, the less likely it is to change.

The failure of path dependence to adequately explain policy reforms in Medicare reveals broader problems with the theory. First, in emphasizing the durability of the status quo, it cannot properly account for changes that take a policy off its predetermined path. Second, it brings history into political science only to take the politics out. Path dependence focuses on "critical junctures" where new policies or institutions are adopted. Consequently, it draws on historical analysis to locate the origins of particular policies in past decisions and series of events. However, having performed this historical exercise, path dependence then projects a deterministic vision of politics according to which policies cannot deviate from their original path. This evolutionary model ignores the contingency inherent in politics and how subsequent changes in political, economic, and social conditions create opportunities to remake public programs.[56]

This problem with path dependence is exemplified by its analysis of why Medicare did not expand into national health insurance. From a path dependence perspective, this failure is not surprising, because "Medicare, unlike the Social Security program it aimed to emulate, covered all elderly Americans in one fell swoop."[57] Medicare thus lacked a rationale for expansion and remained on its original path, restricted predominantly to the elderly. And that path may have hurt the chances for adoption of national health insurance. It is often argued that Medicare fundamentally altered U.S. health politics by taking the elderly out of the coalition for universal health insurance. What would pressure for universal coverage look like if forty million seniors were added to the picture, bringing with them both sympathy and political organization? The balance of health care reform politics could be expected to change in favor of reform. According to this perspective, enacting Medicare actually impeded the adoption of national health insurance, precisely the opposite of what Medicare's designers had anticipated.

This argument leaves much to be desired. There is certainly merit to the notion that a mass population of elderly uninsured would alter the dynamics of health care reform in a way that would make national health insurance more likely. Yet the presumption that Medicare has blocked national health insurance is too blithe. Critics ignore an obvious alternative: the political system in later years could have responded exactly as it did in 1965, by enacting federal health insurance for the elderly and the poor, thereby defusing pressures for national health insurance. In a political system where adopting comprehensive reform is inherently difficult, who is to say that if Medicare had not been established in 1965, the Medicare strategy would not simply have arisen at a later date due to the same political calculus and constraints?

Moreover, national health insurance rose to the political agenda three times before Medicare was enacted, failing all three times. Given all the obstacles to health reform in the United States, it is difficult to single out Medicare for blocking national health insurance when it had a previous history of political failure. And despite the ostensible constraints of Medicare, national health insurance subsequently reached the national agenda in both the early 1970s and 1990s, failing to win enactment for a plethora of reasons (including strategic mistakes by reformers, the absence of liberal congressional majorities, and insurance industry opposition) that had nothing to do with Medicare. Finally, although it covered the elderly in "one fell swoop," Medicare's architects always envisioned it would expand into a national health insurance system. That Medicare did not expand to cover the whole population was not an outcome determined by its initial scope and original path, but the result of contingent political and economic circumstances, as well as Medicare's own financial difficulties.

Path dependence therefore does not offer a satisfying framework for explaining Medicare politics.

IDEAS

Some scholars have emphasized the role of ideas in policymaking. They argue that interest-based and institutional analyses are not sufficient to explain policy outcomes that can be understood only with reference to the influence of ideas.[58] In Medicare, two types of ideas can be expected to influence policy. The first are fundamental ideas about government and its role in social welfare provision, in other words, political culture. The dominant paradigm here is American exceptionalism, which contends that U.S. political ideology is distinguished by its aversion to government power, its commitment to individualism, and its embrace of the private market.[59] The implication for Medicare is that policy should be constrained by these ideological boundaries.

Certainly, the form of Medicare payment regulation, with its emphasis on objectivity and expertise, can be explained, in part, by American political culture. The traditional American distrust of politics leads to a search for regulatory mechanisms that operate as mechanistic, self-executing processes independently of political influence. The prospective payment system and Medicare fee schedule embody precisely this hope that "scientific precision will vanquish politics."[60] This effort to legitimate Medicare regulatory authority in science, rather than to simply treat it as the direct application of political power, is consistent with arguments of American exceptionalism regarding the weakness of the U.S. state.

Yet the extent of federal regulation of Medicare has far exceeded the supposed antistate constraints of American political culture. The imagery of Medicare regulation may be apolitical, but the reality has been a not-so-subtle extension of state power. As in other countries, these regulations have served as mechanisms of the state to assert control over medical expenditures, and the pretense of their scientific basis has been exposed by the transparent connection between Medicare regulation and the federal budgetary process. If the ideas represented by American exceptionalism had governed Medicare policy, there should have been much less empowerment of the state in Medicare policy than has actually emerged. Nor can these ideas explain how Medicare—essentially a single-payer health insurance system—exists in a country whose political culture is often alleged to be incompatible with a system of government-operated medical insurance. In general, then, the boundaries set by American political ideology on Medicare policy have been more flexible than is usually assumed.

A second form of ideas, though, has been absolutely central to Medicare politics. These ideas reflect not the broad dictates of political culture
and ideology, but ideas about particular policy reforms or philosophies
linked to Medicare. After all, the entire program is premised on an idea:
the notion of a social compact between society and seniors that is renewed
from generation to generation. And wherever one looks beyond the crude
limits of exceptionalism, ideas have mattered: the influence of social insurance philosophy on the design of Medicare, the impact of specific ideas
regarding preferred regulatory strategies, and the power of the belief that
deficit reduction was in the public interest. Without reference to the power
of these ideas, Medicare politics is inexplicable.

CONCLUSION

In sum, American political culture, public opinion, and interest groups
have been weaker influences on Medicare policy than anticipated by existing scholarship, while the impact of independent government actors has
been stronger than expected. This conclusion echoes the findings of studies of the politics of social policy in other countries.[61] However, it contradicts the conventional wisdom that American political institutions and
ideology are exceptional, and the related assumption that the role of the
state in health policy is substantially weaker in the United States than in
other countries. Furthermore, the Medicare case revises our understanding of American political institutions by revealing the independent potential of Congress and the distinctive congressional shape of the American
state and public administration.

The analysis of Medicare politics provided in this chapter comes with
one key caveat. The patterns observed in specific policy areas, the distribution of influence from political and social forces, and the outcomes of policy contests all reflected the operation of Medicare from 1965 to 1994.
That period was, as I have argued, characterized by a politics of consensus
that set strong boundaries on the character of program politics. Above all,
the core assumption behind the consensus, that federal health insurance
for the elderly should be provided through a universal government program, went relatively unchallenged. The politics of Medicare in the era of
consensus cannot be generalized as a universal feature of program politics,
because if that consensus had fractured, a very different politics of Medicare could have emerged.

In 1995, that possibility became a reality, and Medicare politics moved
sharply in a new direction.

The New Politics of Medicare

The politics of consensus governed Medicare during its first three decades. Medicare politics during 1965–94 was consensual in two key respects. First, policymaking generally took on a bipartisan character, with major policy changes such as the hospital and physician payment reforms of the 1980s backed by both parties. Even as the preferred policy models for Medicare reform shifted substantially over the years, bipartisan support for changes remained constant as Democrats and Republicans generally moved in the same policy direction. A second feature of consensus was the tacit acceptance of the notion that Medicare should be operated as a universal government program, that federal health insurance for the elderly should take the form, in essence, of a single-payer health system. That view, which I have labeled the Medicare consensus, embodied at its core the liberal philosophies of Medicare's architects and the Great Society era during which the program was passed.

It was not the only programmatic form that Medicare could have taken. Indeed, opponents of the original Medicare legislation advocated a plan whereby the federal government, rather than sponsor its own insurance program, would subsidize beneficiaries to purchase private insurance.[1] That option, however, lost out in 1965. And once Medicare was in operation, its popularity with public and politicians alike meant that its initial program structure and philosophy were institutionalized. The Medicare consensus consequently lived on, with its liberal principles and programmatic institutions, far beyond the liberal era in American politics that receded in the 1970s.[2] The Medicare consensus created a boundary in Medicare politics that was rarely crossed. Not surprisingly, much of the politics of consensus was quiescent; with few high-profile ideological or partisan debates to attract attention, momentous policy reforms were often adopted with scant public notice.

While the politics of consensus defined Medicare from 1965 to 1994, Medicare politics since 1994 has operated on a quite different terrain. Remarkably, the consensus that governed program policymaking in benefits, regulation, and financing broke down in all three areas.[3] This chapter seeks to sketch out the new terrain and to make sense of the central features of what amounts to a new politics of Medicare. Accordingly, this chapter analyzes the political battle over 1995 Republican efforts to reform Medicare, the 1997 program reforms adopted as part of that year's Balanced Budget Act, and the place of Medicare in the 2000 elections and beyond. The issues of Medicare managed care as well as prescription drug coverage are also examined. I explain the forces that led to the fracturing of the Medicare consensus and conclude by examining the issues and circumstances that will shape Medicare's political future.

PRELUDE TO CHANGE: THE CLINTON ADMINISTRATION AND THE 1994 ELECTIONS

The politics of consensus in Medicare came to an end in November 1994. That fall's congressional campaign initially offered little in the way of political drama and played out without much hint of the significance the elections subsequently would have. The Democrats controlled both the Senate and the House of Representatives, and Bill Clinton occupied the Oval Office as the first Democratic president since Jimmy Carter lost his bid for reelection to Ronald Reagan in 1980.

The Clinton administration arrived in Washington in 1993 exuding the confidence and determination to pursue an ambitious agenda that comes with being the champion for a party long out of power.[4] Expectations for the new administration and its promises of change and vigorous reform were high. Most of all, Bill Clinton came to office on the promise of fixing an economy mired in recession. George Bush's image as a do-nothing president out of touch with the pain the economic slowdown of 1991–92 imposed on Americans had helped sow the seeds of his defeat. The Clinton campaign's now familiar slogan—"It's the economy, Stupid!"—represented both a strategic focus and a commitment to an activist agenda to promote economic growth once elected. But the new president was hardly satisfied with economic revitalization alone. Health care had been the second most prominent issue of the 1992 campaign, and Clinton had promised, if elected, to introduce a comprehensive proposal for universal health insurance. Welfare reform, the pledge to "make work pay" for middle-class Americans, "reinventing government" to streamline the federal bureaucracy, and free trade agreements were also on the agenda, while Ross Perot's maverick independent campaign for the presidency had deepened attention to the federal deficit. If the agenda of promises and pressing problems appeared overwhelming, the energetic, youthful president seemed up to the task and indeed cherished the opportunity to change the country's course.[5]

Yet by fall of 1994, only twenty months after Bill Clinton took office, the lofty aspirations and expectations were already shattered. Signs of political trouble were everywhere. The new administration had gotten off to a shaky start, distracted by an unexpected controversy over gays in the military and widely criticized for its handling of the issue, as well as for losing control of the political agenda and sight of its governing priorities. The administration did win a hard-fought legislative victory over its 1993 budget by the slimmest of margins: a vote cast by Vice President Al Gore broke a tie in the Senate after the economic package did not pick up a single Republican vote. But the legislation, constrained by the economic dictates of Wall Street and chairman of the Federal Reserve Board Alan Greenspan, omitted much of the public investment that the president had initially wanted.[6] And a victory on adopting the North American Free Trade Agreement came at the price of alienating the labor movement, a traditional Democratic Party constituency.

The greatest disappointment, though, came on health care reform. Delayed by time spent on other issues, criticized for the "secret" workings of its health reform task force and a complicated plan that proved difficult to explain, attacked by the insurance industry, small business community, and other opponents of national health insurance, and confronted by an increasingly hostile Republican Party and skeptical public, the Clinton administration's Health Security Act failed dismally. The Clinton plan did not make it out of either the Senate or the House. Nor did efforts by congressional leaders to revive a compromise bill succeed. By November 1994, health care reform, the president's primary domestic policy initiative, was dead.[7]

Midterm elections are generally regarded as referendums on the president's performance and the standing of his party. And the president's party usually loses seats in the Senate and House in midterm contests. Democrats, then, had ample reason to be anxious about the 1994 congressional elections, while Republicans looked to make sizable gains. But almost nobody was prepared for the shocking outcome: Republicans took control of both the Senate and the House for the first time since 1954. Many observers blamed the Democrats' defeat on the failure to enact health reform. The Clinton health plan emerged as a convenient foil for Republicans to campaign against the Clinton administration's alleged liberal turn and the excesses of big government. Indeed, health care reform arguably produced, in the words of Theda Skocpol, a "boomerang" effect, as the erstwhile symbol of renewed Democratic activism in social policy unintentionally catalyzed opposition against government, leading to the Republican triumph in the 1994 elections.[8]

MEDICARE POLITICS IN FLUX: THE END OF CONSENSUS

The 1994 congressional elections transformed the politics of Medicare. Indeed, it is not much of an exaggeration to say they changed *everything* about Medicare's political world. In 1995, for the first time in over three decades, a high-profile, partisan, and ideological debate over first principles took place in Medicare. Inasmuch as it returned to the central issue of what form of health insurance the federal government should provide to the elderly, the 1995 contest represented the reopening of the Medicare debate of the 1950s and 1960s. Medicare policy moved from the politics of management, characterized by incremental efforts to enhance program efficiency, to the politics of transformation, characterized by attempts to overhaul a public program's foundation and its core philosophy. The assumptions about the program's future, the boundaries that had defined Medicare politics, and the direction that program reform had taken in the 1980s were all turned upside down. The past was in many ways not a useful guide to Medicare's present, if only because so much of what occurred in 1995 and thereafter was unprecedented in the program's history since enactment.

In retrospect, it is tempting to conclude that the fractured consensus in Medicare was due entirely to the electoral outcomes of 1994. There is obviously a good amount of truth in that view, as well as a historical precedent. The 1994 election results were arguably the most important for the congressional balance of power since 1964—in terms of an ideological, not simply partisan, balance—and just as the 1964 elections enabled the enactment of Medicare, the 1994 elections permitted its remaking, or at least efforts to remake it. But this was not the only important change in Medicare's environment. The following section analyzes the combination of long-term forces, short-term pressures, and unusual circumstances that led to the transformation of Medicare politics.

THE POLITICAL ENVIRONMENT

The most important precipitating factor in Medicare's upheaval was the 1994 congressional elections. Medicare, after all, had never operated under a Republican Congress. The Republican Party had last enjoyed majorities in both the House of Representatives and the Senate in 1954, a decade before the program's enactment. Congressional stewardship of Medicare consequently meant Democratic Party stewardship, except for an interregnum of GOP control of the Senate from 1980 to 1986. If there was a question about how Medicare politics would look under Republican congressional control, it could not be answered during the program's first three decades.

The 1994 elections that brought Republican majorities to both houses of Congress produced a radically new political environment for Medicare. The Republican majorities, led by Speaker of the House Newt Gingrich, were committed to an agenda of assertive conservatism. Their aims were symbolized by the Contract with America, a blueprint of legislative action that Gingrich had shrewdly produced for the election and secured the support of Republican candidates for. This enabled Gingrich both to claim credit for the Republican victory (a dubious claim, given the low level of public knowledge about the contract) and to tie members of Congress to his agenda as Speaker. Although the Gingrich-led Republican majority saw its congressional reign as the continuation of the Reagan revolution, "they were intent on not missing a historic opportunity, as many of them privately believed Reagan had."[9] While Ronald Reagan had helped to redirect political discourse toward conservatism, the new Republican leadership was not satisfied with rhetorical accomplishments. Instead, they sought to dramatically shrink the scope of federal government by redefining the terms of federalism and federal budgeting, including enactment of a balanced budget, and by reshaping (and often dismantling) regulatory and social welfare policies. Journalists Haynes Johnson and David Broder described the confident mood and ambitious agenda of Republicans in 1995: "Not since the New Deal had Washington witnessed such a spectacle. They poured into the capital, eager, determined conservative crusaders who all believed *their* time finally had arrived. Ideologically, they were the heirs of Barry Goldwater and Ronald Reagan, who thirty years before had begun the national movement to replace the liberal welfare state with a radically more conservative model. . . . Now, for the first time, they were America's political majority."[10]

The political world ushered in by the 1994 elections thus stood in stark contrast to the one that Medicare grew up in. Medicare was a programmatic child of the Great Society. Medicare represented liberalism, federal government activism, social insurance, and, by the early 1990s, aggressive government regulation of the private sector. The Republican revolution alternatively promised conservatism, decentralizing federal power to the states, unleashing of market forces, and deregulation. The gap between Medicare's programmatic character and prevailing political winds after the 1994 elections could hardly have been any greater. Medicare was a product of one political time suddenly caught up in another. Given the ideological mismatch between the program and the Republican agenda, it was not surprising that the Republican leadership sought to restructure Medicare into a program that more closely reflected their conservative vision of government.

While Newt Gingrich's Contract with America did not mention Medicare, by the end of the Republican Congress's first one hundred days in 1995, and with an eye on balancing the budget while cutting taxes, the Speaker had decided to prioritize Medicare reform.[11] Gingrich took the unusual step of going around customary committee jurisdictions and taking responsibility for designing Medicare reform himself as chair of a special congressional task force that included members handpicked by the Republican leadership, with the aim of producing party unity on a reform proposal.[12] One Democratic congressman was both impressed and stunned with the political risk the Republicans were taking, as members of Congress marched "in lockstep into the [political] abyss with Newt on Medicare reform almost blindly."[13] The 1994 elections, then, produced a new political leadership for Medicare as well as a new vision for program reform.

But the 1994 electoral triumph of the Republican Party was not the only element in the transformation of Medicare's political environment. The results, and the bitter legislative battles of the following years, represented a longer-term trend toward ideological polarization and partisan division within Congress.[14] As Republican moderates and Democratic conservatives faded out of their respective parties, each party became more internally cohesive and the ideological distance between the parties increased. Roll call votes in 1996 were more divided by party than at any time since 1947, also the last year that had seen so little ideological division within the parties on congressional votes.[15] As Lawrence Jacobs and Robert Shapiro argue, the vanishing moderates in Congress and the polarization of Democrats and Republicans eroded "the vital center" that had long governed American politics through bipartisan coalitions.[16] The resulting polarization was clearly visible in Medicare politics after 1994.

Yet both the Clinton administration and Democrats in Congress were, in 1995, initially surprised by the scope of the proposed Republican changes in Medicare, which was both more radical and more financially ambitious than they had anticipated.[17] The ideological shift in the Republican Party following the 1994 elections caught veteran Democrats in Congress, many of whom were accustomed to working on Medicare policy with moderate Republicans, off guard. They were slow to see the threat to the liberal vision of Medicare that had been institutionalized for three decades.[18] One prominent Democratic congressional staffer on the House Ways and Means Committee recalled not realizing how stridently conservative the new Republican majority was until being introduced to the young daughter of a Republican colleague. When told he worked on Medicare, she immediately launched into a derisive, nursery-rhyme-style chant with the refrain "Medi-scam . . . Medi-scam."[19] Clearly, this was a new political world for Medicare: the days of bipartisan consensus and compromise had ended.

Since Medicare's enactment there had always been an element in Congress uncomfortable with the program and its liberal aspirations. But during the first three decades of Medicare's operations, those voices were faint and not influential, drowned out by the strength of the Medicare consensus. What the 1994 election did was put similar voices into positions of power, transforming the politics of Medicare and triggering a new debate about the program's direction. Thus, the 1994 elections were the most important factor in unraveling the era of consensus in Medicare politics. As Carolyn Tuohy observes, policy changes in health care are often catalyzed by political events that open "windows of opportunity" for comprehensive reform;[20] the 1994 congressional elections opened such a window in Medicare for the first time since 1964.

THE FISCAL ENVIRONMENT

If Medicare grew up in a different political world than 1994 America, the fiscal world it inhabited was equally dissimilar from its early years. Medicare was enacted in 1965 during a period of prosperity and economic growth. And there was broad acceptance of payroll taxes to finance federal programs. Some congressional leaders on Social Security, such as Ways and Means chair Wilbur Mills, voiced concern that payroll taxes not become too burdensome. But in reality, such opposition had little impact, as social insurance benefits were consistently expanded during the 1960s and early 1970s.[21] During Medicare's first financing shortfall, 1970–72, both parties supported rasing the program's hospitalization insurance tax to help redress the shortfall. And through the end of the 1980s, trust fund shortfalls generated a minimum of public controversy and partisanship.

Medicare's fiscal environment began to change with stagflation—low economic growth combined with high inflation—in the 1970s and the rise of the federal deficit as an issue in the 1980s. Preoccupation with balancing the federal budget fundamentally changed Medicare's political position. High rates of growth in program spending, overlooked in fatter financial times, were no longer easily tolerated. Medicare was now viewed as a chief culprit in the federal budget deficit, its expenditures a prime target for deficit reduction.[22] The 1995 Republican budget plan, which called for a balanced budget within seven years, made that link explicit, proposing $270 billion of cuts in Medicare spending, an unprecedented reduction in projected expenditures by 30%.

At the same time as deficit politics took center stage, the politics of the payroll tax had also changed. The Republican Party made opposition to new taxes a political mantra in the 1980s, one that the Democratic Party only weakly challenged in coming years, as exemplified by President Clinton's fiscal gymnastics to avoid paying for his health plan with new taxes. Indeed, a central aim of Bill Clinton's New Democrats was to replace the party's reputation as the party of taxation with an image of the party of prosperity and responsible economic management. The conservative Republican majorities of 1995—still seething over George Bush's betrayal of his "no new taxes pledge" and advancing a tax cut agenda of their own—certainly had no appetite for raising payroll taxes. For Medicare, the consequence was that if a trust fund shortfall appeared, it would not be redressed, as it had in the past, by tax increases. The Republicans were opposed ideologically to tax increases and the Democrats, still trying to escape the stigmatizing "tax and spend" label, were politically unwilling to challenge them. The resulting political cap on Medicare payroll taxes put the program in a financial box. If no additional tax revenue were available, a shortfall in program finances would have to be addressed through cuts or restructuring. Fiscally, then, Medicare's environment was conducive to programmatic upheaval, and the Republican leadership's agenda of tax cuts and a balanced budget—to be funded in no small part through cuts in Medicare spending—made that upheaval a certainty in 1995. Both Social Security and defense spending were considered off limits for spending cuts, so although the Contract with America had not mentioned anything about health care, Medicare (as well as Medicaid) was simply too important to Republican fiscal aims to leave alone, regardless of the possible political fallout.

INTERGENERATIONAL EQUITY

Nowhere was Medicare's changed political environment more apparent than in the transformation of the public image of the elderly. During the 1960s, the elderly were the country's sympathetic social group nonpareil. They were perceived by the public as poorer, less well insured, and sicker than younger Americans.[23] And they were. Indeed, their ability to command public sympathy as a deserving group was the reason Medicare's architects chose to start national health insurance with a program for the aged, though the diversity of the elderly was much greater than the compassionate stereotype of universally poor dependents that their advocates cultivated.[24]

Three decades later the political appeal of the elderly had eroded and their image had been inverted. Public support for programs directed at the aged remained high.[25] However, this support coexisted with a rising discourse of intergenerational equity concerns that recast the elderly, as Robert Binstock argued, as a "scapegoat" in American politics.[26] Policymakers and commentators began to wonder if the federal government had done too much for the elderly at the expense of other social groups and priorities. The success of federal programs had reduced poverty rates among the elderly to levels below that of the general population, though many elders lived just above the poverty line. Poverty rates among the elderly declined from 40% in the late 1950s to 12% in the early 1990s, due in large part to the income maintenance effects of Social Security.[27] And Medicare played a crucial role in providing health security and protecting the elderly from financial ruin brought on by escalating medical care costs.[28]

Yet, ironically, the very effectiveness of these social programs in improving the condition of the elderly made them a target. Critics argued many seniors were now so well off they did not need government assistance: policy success came at a political price. By 1995, over one-third of all federal expenditures went toward seniors.[29] Resentment at the share of the federal budget devoted to the elderly helped feed a new, less compassionate stereotype: that of the "greedy geezer" who was, depending on the story, spending younger taxpayers' dollars on an extravagant retirement, or on expensive high-tech medicine in the final days of life, or perhaps on both, thereby taking potential funds away from public spending on children and needy Americans. The "greedy geezer," in contrast to his or her elderly counterpart in the 1960s, was now viewed as wealthier and better insured than other Americans and, as media images of active elders suggested, increasingly healthy as well. The stereotype was fueled by the repeal of catastrophic health insurance in 1989, as the media zeroed in on the story of more affluent elders selfishly leading the charge against a program that would benefit poorer Medicare beneficiaries (though the actual story of the demise of catastrophic insurance was not so straightforward). The spectacle of seniors beating on the car of Dan Rostenkowski, chairman of the House Ways and Means Committee, could hardly have provided a better (or more misleading) advertisement for the portrait of seniors as selfish and powerful that was being painted in the mainstream press.

Meanwhile, the coming retirement of the baby boomers in the first decade of the twenty-first century increasingly became an object of anxiety in public discourse. Critics such as former commerce secretary Peter Peterson, who helped found a group devoted to budgetary discipline and entitlement control (the Concord Coalition), alleged that Social Security and Medicare would soon represent an unsustainable burden on the federal budget, leaving future generations to cope with enormous public deficits and economic disaster.[30] Medical ethicist Daniel Callahan argued that norms of justice dictated that society ration health care for the aged by setting age limits on eligibility for expensive medical treatments.[31] Political commentators warned that the graying of the population would make the already powerful lobby for the elderly, symbolized by the persistently vilified American Association of Retired Persons (AARP), even more powerful, institutionalizing an imbalanced political system that favored the needs of the elderly over other constituencies. Ken Dychtwald, the commentator on aging, declared that in the twenty-first century "the epicenter of economic and political power will shift from the young to old" as America becomes a "gerontocracy" and deplored the excessive influence of "AARPthink" on political debate.[32] And finally, critics wondered why, in the face of declining poverty rates among the elderly, taxes of working families should finance public health and pension benefits for well-off elders. In particular, they connected the rising fortunes of older persons to the languishing state of American children. The demographer Samuel Preston summarized the zero-sum logic of generational equity: "the gains for one group," he wrote, "at least in the public sphere . . . come partly at the expense of another," meaning that "transfers away from working-age population to the elderly are also transfers away from children."[33]

In sum, the new stereotype of aging casts the elderly as well off, politically powerful, unaffordable, and a source of generational as well as fiscal inequity. There are, to be sure, significant problems with the intergenerational equity story and the dire warnings about the baby boomers.[34] Comparative experience in demography, medical care costs, and pensions suggests a less fearsome outcome of the aging of America than the apocalyptic scenarios predicted by some analysts. Other nations with significantly older populations than the United States spend significantly less on medical care. Nor is spending for seniors necessarily a zero-sum contest with children; were the government not spending on Medicare, there is no more guarantee that the money would go for kids than for tax cuts or building a missile defense shield. Stories about costly high-tech interventions going to the elderly at the end of life are often exaggerated, and the implications of data misunderstood. And the elderly are as divided as other voting groups; they do not vote as a monolithic bloc simply on Social Security and Medicare.

Moreover, the share of national health spending devoted to persons sixty-five and older in the United States is not out of line with the share in other industrial democracies. In 1996, the United States devoted 37% of its health care spending to the elderly, compared to 43% in Japan and 42% in the United Kingdom. And for all the hand-wringing over excess generosity to the elderly, Medicare is hardly a generous program in terms of its benefits, which are quite limited, though it is generous relative to the systems in other nations in its payments to medical providers.[35] Finally, as the ethicist Norman Daniels has observed, if one takes a "lifecourse" perspective, even if the elderly receive more social resources than younger members of society, younger generations too will age and receive more resources, creating an equality of benefits over time and undermining the normative justification for generational equity arguments.[36]

But the intergenerational story need not be accurate in order to be politically influential. And although public opinion studies find mass support for Medicare and Social Security to be consistently high over time, these same studies also find that support for government programs for the aged is noticeably weaker among members of Congress than the public.[37] The social compact that underlies Medicare and commits the government to finance health insurance for the aged remains intact. But the erosion of sympathy for the elderly, and worries over the fiscal and economic impact of the soon retiring baby boomers, has predisposed more policymakers to cut Medicare spending, impose costs on seniors, and challenge the status quo by restructuring existing programmatic arrangements. In 1995, in other words, more than ever before, policymakers were prepared to do something *to* the elderly rather than *for* them.

The rise of intergenerational equity concerns among policymakers was part of a broader pattern in the fracturing of consensus in Medicare. The end of consensus was not driven by public opinion. In this and other areas of change, the impetus for Medicare reform was instead top down. Public confidence in government had dropped precipitously since Medicare's enactment in 1965. In 1994, 77% of Americans believed that the government in Washington did what was right only some or none of the time, compared to 22% in 1964.[38] But there was no evidence of changes in public attitudes on Medicare. Indeed, popular support for Medicare remained consistently high, and the public opposed many of the reforms proposed in 1995.[39] Rather, what had fundamentally changed in Medicare's political environment was the ideological commitments, partisan alignments, and policy beliefs of elites. One of those beliefs was a newfound faith that Medicare must modernize and move to managed care.

THE CHANGING HEALTH CARE SYSTEM

The promise of Medicare was to bring the elderly into the mainstream of American medicine. In 1965, that meant the indemnity, fee-for-service insurance model, along the lines of Blue Cross and Blue Shield, that commanded an overwhelming share of the private insurance market. Alternative delivery systems, such as the prepaid group health plans exemplified by Kaiser Permanente, were rare and geographically limited, and the AMA strongly opposed their inclusion in Medicare.[40] Medicare's adoption of the prevailing model of insurance thereby not only assured retirees continuity in medical care, as well as broad access to mainstream hospitals and doctors, but also reassured the medical profession that the federal government would not disrupt conditions in the private medical market— conditions that clearly favored the profession, including retrospective, fee-for-service reimbursement with few controls over fees; unquestioned physician autonomy in clinical decision making; and the absence of any countervailing power, public or private, that actively challenged physicians' hold over the medical marketplace.[41]

The structure of federal health insurance for the aged essentially remained stable for three decades. The same cannot be said for private health insurance. By 1995, the private health market was in the midst of a dramatic transformation, as "managed care" plans and practices became the dominant form of insurance in the United States.[42] The diversity of health plans, payment practices, and organizational features grouped under the managed care rubric made the term virtually impossible to define. In practice, managed care referred to a wide range of health plans and practices that departed from the traditional American form of health insurance. Managed care overturned many of the features of the traditional health care system: health plans imposed limits on physicians' clinical autonomy, including external review of medical decisions, preauthorization requirements for hospitalization and diagnostic procedures, and physician profiling to detect "inappropriate" or "excessive" care; sought "discounts" from "normal" fees, often in exchange for guaranteed volume; adopted capitation and other payment arrangements, such as bonuses for holding down costs, that put substantial portions of physicians' income at risk; selectively contracted with restricted networks of hospitals and physicians; and provided full insurance coverage to patients only if they saw providers within the plan's network, sometimes requiring a visit to a primary care gatekeeper before granting access to speciality services.[43]

Managed care plans, including health maintenance organizations (HMOs), preferred provider organizations (PPOs), and hybrid point of service plans grew rapidly during the 1990s. In 1992, HMOs' enrollment stood at forty million and PPOs at fifty million; only three years later HMOs covered sixty million Americans and PPOs another ninety million.[44] At the same time, the number of physicians subject to capitation (flat payment per enrollee) and utilization review of clinical decision making rose rapidly. Surely the most striking symbol of change, however, was the steep decline of enrollment in America's traditional health plan, conventional indemnity insurance, from covering 95% of the employer-sponsored market in 1978 to 49% in 1992 and only 14% by 1998.[45]

In fact, by the middle of the 1990s there remained only one significant bastion of "unmanaged" care in the United States: Medicare.[46] During the program's first two decades, there had been halting efforts to expand the role of HMOs in Medicare. The 1972 Social Security amendments authorized federal payments to federally qualified HMOs enrolling program beneficiaries. But the administrative and financial requirements for participation in Medicare were regarded as so onerous by HMOs that by 1979 only one prepaid plan had enrolled in the program. In 1982 policymakers revisited Medicare HMOs and under the Tax Equity and Fiscal Responsibility Act (TEFRA) adopted provisions intended to encourage Medicare HMO enrollment. However, even the program's own sponsors did not expect it to amount to much.[47] Managed care enrollment in Medicare subsequently did grow yet in 1994 stood at only 5% of program beneficiaries.[48]

As a consequence, by 1995 Medicare's managed care enrollment lagged far behind that in the private sector. Medicare had promised to bring the elderly into the mainstream of American medicine, but that mainstream had undergone substantial changes, while Medicare had not. The widening gap between the private sector and federal health insurance was not lost on conservative reformers, who, as Bill Thomas, chair of the Ways and Means Health Subcommittee, bluntly put it, saw Medicare as a "dinosaur" that had been made obsolete by market innovations.[49] The time had come, they argued, to modernize Medicare if it was to survive in future years.

The divergence in insurance structure between Medicare and the private sector created a number of pressures on the program. Medicare is in a unique position internationally. In industrial democracies, government-sponsored health insurance programs commonly operate alongside a small private health sector that acts as a safety valve for more affluent citizens seeking shorter lines or greater amenities. In systems such as the British National Health Service, the size and role of the private sector is a matter of political dispute, but even after some growth in private medical care delivery the public national health service remains the dominant institution in medical care delivery.[50] And in Canada, private insurance for services covered by the national health insurance program is prohibited; a private insurance market exists only for medical services not insured by provincial health plans.

American Medicare's position vis-à-vis the private insurance market is quite different. Since the United States has never enacted national health insurance, Medicare operates as a minority public insurer alongside a larger system of private insurance. One implication for health politics is that whereas in other countries change in the political system is generally responsible for change in the health system because those systems are publicly operated, in the United States there is a greater chance that change in the health system—even in public programs—can be triggered by developments in the private sector. This arrangement, directly opposite to the international standard, creates a distinctive set of potential pressures on Medicare when it diverges from the dominant private model of medical insurance. As managed care advanced in the 1990s, those pressures were fully unleashed.

The first pressure is that of *performance*. If the private insurance model is viewed as outperforming Medicare, for example, in controlling costs or in innovations in delivering care, there will be pressures on Medicare to follow the private sector's lead in health care organization and payment practices. The private sector, in other words, will become the model that Medicare is directed to emulate. As the next section explains, performance pressures were particularly salient in the mid-1990s. In 1995, to the Republican leadership and a number of health care analysts, "fee-for-service [insurance of the type Medicare represented] seemed dead."[51]

The second pressure is that of *consistency*. As the mainstream of medical care moves, there are pressures on Medicare to move as well in order to maintain the continuity between employee and retiree coverage. Concerns can also develop about the administrative costs of maintaining Medicare as a different health insurance system and potential resentment from the public in the context of intergenerational equity issues. For instance, Brookings Institution economists Henry Aaron and Robert Reischauer have written that Medicare must emulate the private sector's move toward managed care because, if it does not, "soon public support may begin to erode for a system of coverage for the aged and disabled that is substantially different than, and therefore more costly, than the health plans that cover the average taxpayer's family."[52] Given that managed care was profoundly unpopular with the American public and that Medicare has always differed from private insurance in important respects, the case that Medicare had to follow the private sector was quite weak. Nevertheless, it remained a compelling reform rationale for some analysts and politicians; a number of conservative Democrats believed that if the rest of the country was in managed care, Medicare beneficiaries should be, too.[53]

Finally, Medicare is subject to the pressures of *expansion*. As insurers exhaust options for growth in the private sector, they look to the public sector to expand their market share. In this context, Medicare clearly represented "the last frontier" for managed care companies, and because of that they fought to expand their enrollment of program beneficiaries, which meant lobbying for reforms that would open Medicare up more widely to private insurers. As Bill Gradison, head of the Health Insurance Association of America, plainly stated about the proposed Republican Medicare reforms of 1995: "the thrust we see in Congress on Medicare and Medicaid is toward privatization. That creates enormous opportunity to offer our services to literally tens of millions of people who are not in the insurance market today."[54]

In all these dimensions, the rise of managed care in the private sector brought about enormous pressures on Medicare to deviate from its single-payer form as a universal government program and consequently helped unravel the Medicare consensus.

THE TRUST FUND CRISIS

Past trust fund shortfalls in Medicare had proved, as I have argued, to be largely noncontroversial, low-profile, and bipartisan affairs. The trust fund crisis of 1995 produced a very different politics. This was a *contested* crisis, the first in program history, and it helped to shatter the consensus that had defined Medicare politics for three decades.

The 1995 trust fund crisis was, in part, happenstance. The Republican leadership was searching for ways to sell its Medicare reform package. In the aftermath of the demise of President Clinton's health plan, the political risk in taking on Medicare should have been abundantly clear. But fiscally, the GOP needed substantial Medicare savings to accomplish its goals of balancing the budget while cutting taxes, and ideologically, Medicare reform was central to Republican efforts to remake the welfare state. Republican Party leaders were wary of the political dangers of tackling the issue, cognizant of President Clinton's political debacle in health reform and fearful of a backlash similar to the one that greeted Ronald Reagan's 1981 Social Security reforms. The 1994 elections had provided the conservative congressional majority necessary to take on the Medicare status quo, but this still seemed insufficient to the daunting political task of passing Medicare reform without incurring a public, and eventually electoral, rebuke. The question remained: how could the GOP convince the country that its vision of Medicare reform would help, not hurt, the program?

As party pollsters tested various Medicare marketing messages, Republican Party chairman Haley Barbour thought he found the answer. In April 1995 he received a copy of the just-released Medicare hospitalization insurance trust fund report. The report, usually an obscure source of mind-numbing actuarial detail, showed that in the absence of corrective action the trust fund would run a deficit beginning in 2002. Politically, the Republican leadership saw the report as a godsend; they could now advance GOP reforms as necessary to "saving Medicare" from "bankruptcy."[55] The trust fund shortfall offered, in other words, a convenient problem to which to attach the solution that the Republican congressional leadership already had in mind. Cutting Medicare spending could now be portrayed as necessary to ensure the program's survival; consistent with this theme, Medicare reform legislation in 1995 was labeled the Medicare Preservation Act.

Indeed, Newt Gingrich believed that defining Medicare reform as a fiscal issue and framing Republican proposals as efforts to "save Medicare" from bankruptcy would catalyze public support.[56] In his mind, this strategy would not only enable the GOP to neutralize Democratic attacks for cutting Medicare, but also empower Republicans to actually take Medicare as a political issue away from the Democrats as they received political credit for fixing the program. Preliminary polls commissioned by the GOP encouraged the Republican leadership to believe (falsely, as it turned out) that their focus on the trust fund crisis resonated sufficiently with the public to protect them from political heat on Medicare.[57] And the success of the Republican leadership in passing a number of its legislative priorities in the first one hundred days of the 1995 Congress gave them a sense that "the wind was behind their sails" as they prepared to reform Medicare.[58]

Focusing attention on Medicare's trust fund problems had the potential to change the dynamics of the Medicare reform debate. Medicare's cost control performance was fairly strong in the 1980s. However, the world of actuaries is one of long-term projections. Federal actuaries compute Medicare financing over periods of twenty-five and seventy-five years. These long-term estimates offer little policy value, given the enormous uncertainty about future rates of medical costs, medical practice and technology, the health of the population, and the impact of program reforms. But for the Republican leadership, these limitations were of no concern, because the actuarial estimates offered an important political advantage: the longer the projection went, the worse Medicare's financial problems looked, in part because such estimates assumed no increases in payroll tax rates, and in part because no public or private insurance program is fully funded seven decades ahead of time.[59]

The outlook for Medicare's trust fund in 2002 may have appeared bleak, but in 2032, it looked downright catastrophic. Among the reasons for the dire predictions were the projections about the retirement of the baby boomers, which allowed Republican (and some Democratic) policymakers to connect Medicare reform to anxiety about the aging of the population and the affordability of entitlements. Suddenly, the concern was not just that the Medicare trust fund would soon go bankrupt, but that Medicare would soon bankrupt the government. Actuarial projections, then, provided an indictment of Medicare on the basis of its future performance and thereby changed the focus of public debate. Medicare reform was now argued to be necessary to save the program (and the federal budget) from an inadequate performance in cost control that had not yet occurred.

If the timing of the trust fund shortfall was convenient for GOP lawmakers, its coincidence with a rise in Medicare spending rates relative to the private sector was pure political manna. The adoption of regulatory reforms during the 1980s had left Medicare with stricter payment policies than private insurers. From 1983 to 1991, Medicare costs rose at rates slower than those in the private sector. As the 1990s wore on the pattern reversed; suddenly, it was Medicare that appeared as the weaker agent of cost control. The spread of managed care arrangements and newly aggressive competition in the health insurance market lowered (temporarily, as it turned out) the rate of increase in private sector health costs. Meanwhile, Medicare costs resumed a higher rate of growth, driven by substantial increases in spending for postacute care and unexpected increases in spending for hospital services. The gap between Medicare and private insurers in cost control was often exaggerated and did not fully take into account differences in services provided and covered populations. Nevertheless, there is no doubt that Medicare's cost containment performance, in relative terms, slipped from its record in the 1980s and thereby provided political ammunition for those favoring program restructuring.[60]

Medicare consequently became financially vulnerable at precisely the same moment it was politically vulnerable. Republican lawmakers pointed to the private sector's lower rates of growth as evidence that Medicare was inefficient, especially in comparison to innovative managed care and competitive contracting strategies. They argued that Medicare's regulatory framework of "price controls," as they derogatorily called them, had failed, and the program should instead adopt successful "market-based" strategies (ironic rhetoric, given that this system of administered pricing had been hailed by Republicans as conducive to fair competition and market efficiency only a decade earlier, and that "price discounts" were a primary tool of managed care).[61]

In large measure, however, the resurgence of Medicare spending arguably was due not to the failure of regulation, but rather to the failure to implement a full-scale regulatory scheme. The 1980s reforms were sectoral, targeting hospital and physician spending. Other sectors, however, such as home health care, were left essentially unregulated. As providers figured out how to shift services (and thus profits) into unregulated areas of the program, an increasing share of program spending was uncontrollable, not subject to prospective budgeting. Moreover, the 1980s regulatory reforms did not impose a prospective limit on total Medicare spending, a global budget of the sort used in Canada. And unlike national insurance systems in other nations, Medicare could not control the diffusion of new technologies. Without a global budget, Medicare was inevitably susceptible to unforseen increases in spending. When there was a high rate of growth in any one program sector, there was no hard cap to compensate by limiting overall program spending. As a consequence of its halfway regulatory reforms, Medicare had in a sense the worst of both worlds: enough regulation to serve as a political scapegoat, but not enough to ensure successful cost control.

From a historical perspective, the Republican leadership's attempt to use the trust fund shortfall in 1995 to push through program reforms was nothing new. During the early 1970s and 1980s, policymakers had pursed the same strategy of taking advantage of trust fund shortfalls to adopt their preferred policy innovations. What was new, however, was the scope of the Republican-sponsored reforms and their impact on beneficiaries. The cuts proposed by the Republican leadership in the rate of growth in Medicare spending rate were substantial: $270 billion over seven years, representing a 30% reduction in projected expenditures over seven years. Previously, the largest cuts adopted in Medicare spending had been the $56 billion over five years in 1993. In 1994, President Clinton had proposed $125 billion in Medicare cuts to help fund his health plan, but that never came to pass.[62] The Republican legislation also proposed a transformation of Medicare's budgetary entitlement status by introducing a hard cap on annual expenditures, as well as a "fail-safe" or "look-back" provision that would automatically cut payments to providers in the traditional Medicare program if spending exceeded predetermined limits. Philosophically, Republican sponsors believed the program cap on the Medicare fee-for-service program represented an important step toward adopting their ultimate goal: a capitated or per person limit on federal spending for Medicare that would essentially convert it into a defined-contribution or voucher program.[63] And finally, the plan called for a restructuring of Medicare insurance by opening the program up to a host of private insurance plans that lawmakers hoped would increase the enrollment of the elderly in managed care at the expense of public Medicare.

The 1995 Medicare proposals thus crossed a threshold in American social policy and were therefore widely seen as threatening to Medicare beneficiaries. Politically, the Republican leadership believed it could not take access to the traditional Medicare fee-for-service program away from the elderly, but they could "wean them from it."[64] When combined with strict limits on spending in the Medicare fee-for-service program, the program cap, and the fail-safe provision that retrospectively reduced payments, Republicans believed that opening the program to more managed care options would inevitably lead beneficiaries to leave public Medicare for HMOs and other private insurance plans.

These reforms thus promised to affect program beneficiaries profoundly—a considerable departure from previous trust fund remedies that had raised taxes and targeted medical care providers. Indeed, until 1995, one of the most enduring features of Medicare was the extent to which, from a beneficiaries' perspective, the program had not changed. As a result, Republicans overreached in their reform effort, miscalculating that the rhetoric of trust fund crisis would inoculate them against political damage. As the Clinton administration had done, the GOP leadership overestimated its ability to reshape public opinion through focus groups, purchase political victory by neutralizing interest groups,[65] and control the debate by polling for sellable language, while it underestimated the inherent political vulnerabilities of its plan and the strength of the opposition.[66] That the size of their proposed tax cuts was roughly the same as the proposed cuts in Medicare spending made the Republican plan particularly ripe for attack, an opening the Democrats aggressively exploited.

The polarizing politics of Medicare reform in 1995 clearly echoed the health reform debate of 1993–94.[67] Just as President Clinton's health reform was saddled with the stigma of forcing Americans into HMOs, so too was the Republican Medicare plan, with the added liability that vulnerable seniors were the sole target. The president and Democrats in Congress forcefully opposed the Republican Medicare reforms as a threat to the integrity of the program and the health of beneficiaries. The Republican cause was not helped by Speaker Newt Gingrich's comments about Medicare, that "we believe it is going to whither on the vine because we think people are voluntarily going to leave it."[68] And as Clinton's health plan had done only two years earlier, the Republican Medicare plan became a political "boomerang," reinvigorating both President Clinton and congressional Democrats.

Despite the controversy, Republican congressional leaders succeeded in passing Medicare reform legislation on almost exclusively a party-line vote: in the House, the legislation passed 231–201, with only six Republicans defecting. The Democrats' so-called Mediscare campaign took is toll, though, and the issue played no small part in rehabilitating President Clinton's political standing and in cementing the Republican Congress's image as extremists. The Medicare reform debate, along with the budget battle that led to the shutdown of the federal government and ultimately to a retreat by Republicans at Clinton's hands, allowed the president to appear as a centrist committed to protecting programs that helped ordinary Americans. When Bill Clinton vetoed the Medicare legislation using the same pen Lyndon Johnson had used to sign Medicare into law, program reform appeared dead. And the Clinton campaign's use of the Medicare issue in 1996 against Republican nominee Bob Dole, who had as a member of the House voted against the original Medicare legislation in 1965 and in 1995 had declared that "I was there, fighting the fight, voting against Medicare . . . because we knew it wouldn't work," did nothing to persuade otherwise.[69]

REFORM RISES FROM THE ASHES: THE 1997 BALANCED BUDGET ACT

Clinton's veto of the legislation and the consequent defeat of the 1995 Republican Medicare reform campaign obscured the fact that powerful long- and short-term forces were undermining the old program consensus. Electoral outcomes had placed ideological opponents of Medicare's liberal model into positions of influence in Congress. The rise of managed care created a powerful constituency in the private sector for ceding Medicare's public insurance function to the market. And Medicare remained a prime fiscal target as momentum for balancing the federal budget increased. Indeed, President Clinton ultimately accepted the notion of a balanced budget within a decade, even as he continued to criticize the Republican map of how to get there.

How much the liberal consensus had unraveled became apparent in the aftermath of the 1996 elections. In August of the following year, the Congress and the president agreed on the Balanced Budget Act of 1997 (BBA).[70] The BBA mandated a wide variety of key policy changes, including a balanced federal budget by 2002. The BBA also kept alive the practice that had been prominent in the previous decade of adopting Medicare reform as part of large-scale fiscal legislation. Among the BBA provisions was a series of Medicare reforms and substantial cuts (of $115 billion over five years) in the rate of growth in Medicare spending over the next decade.[71] The legislation also established the National Bipartisan Commission on the Future of Medicare to consider the program's future. But the centerpiece of the reforms was the creation of a new Medicare + Choice option that opened Medicare up to a variety of new private insurance plans, including medical savings accounts, commercial fee-for-service plans, provider-sponsored organizations, and the full gamut of managed care plans.

The changes in Medicare attracted, in comparison to the high-profile Medicare debate of 1995, relatively little public attention or press scrutiny.[72] Indeed, most of the coverage of the 1997 reforms focused on controversial measures that were passed by the Senate but ultimately omitted from the final legislation—provisions to raise Medicare's eligibility age from sixty-five to sixty-seven and to introduce income-relate beneficiary premiums by charging higher-income seniors more for Medicare—though the fact that these measures were adopted by the Senate was a significant development in Medicare politics in and of itself.[73]

The dearth of attention to what did pass in 1997 was largely a function of the bipartisan agreement on the need for reform. There simply was no echo of the deeply partisan and highly charged 1995 atmosphere in deliberations over the BBA. In a telling show of bipartisanship, in June 1997 the House Ways and Means committee approved the Republican-sponsored Medicare reforms 36–3, while the Senate Finance Committee voted for them 20–0, a far cry from the polarizing partisanship and party-line voting on Medicare reform in 1995. The final conference report containing the Medicare legislation similarly cleared the House of Representatives 346–85 and the Senate 85–15. One prominent participant declared that after the ill will of the 1995 Medicare debate, enactment of the BBA was "a bipartisan miracle."[74]

Yet for all the apparent bipartisanship, the stakes were still high; taken together, the 1997 Medicare reforms arguably represented the most important changes in the program since its inception. The scope of agreement on these reforms, and the consequent absence of public debate, was remarkable, since the Medicare BBA provisions resembled, in some key respects, the GOP plan that had died amid all the controversy just the year before. As one Republican drafter of the 1995 legislation argued, the 1997 reforms, when compared to those proposed two years earlier, were "more similar than different."[75]

Why the abrupt political turnabout? First, the BBA omitted or altered several key provisions that had been the focus of Democratic Party objections, including a hard cap on Medicare spending that would have transformed the program's budgetary entitlement status, as well as the fail-safe provision that would have triggered automatic spending cuts in the program. Democrats widely viewed such a cap as threatening the ability of seniors to access quality medical care and as incompatible with Medicare's social contract. Moreover, they believed (with good reason, given stated Republican aims and the probable impact of the proposed reforms) that the program cap and fail-safe provision would starve traditional Medicare of beneficiaries and providers, who would both have financial incentives to operate in managed care plans.[76] Managed care organizations, in turn, would be guaranteed a larger piece of program spending.[77] In short, traditional Medicare would be devastated by the spending cap. Without its omission, broad Democratic support for the legislation simply would not have been forthcoming in 1997. In addition, the spending cuts adopted in 1997 were less than those initially sought by the Republican leadership, making them more palatable to Democratic members of Congress as well as the president, who viewed the 1995 cuts as unrealistically high.[78]

The BBA was consequently not as ambitious as the 1995 GOP Medicare reform proposals. Still, by embracing Medicare + Choice, Republicans saw the BBA as "moving the ball a great deal down the field" towards their goal of a competitive Medicare market.[79]

Second, as the electoral glare of 1996 receded, the extent to which President Clinton and the Republican Congress shared common ground on crucial elements of health reform became clear. The president's opposition to the 1995 legislation focused on the size of spending cuts, not the proposed structural changes in Medicare insurance that opened the program up to private insurers. The Republican Medicare proposals ironically (or hypocritically, as the Clinton administration believed) followed an approach similar to the blueprint for health reform proposed by the Clinton health plan: managed competition, which seeks to control health care costs by having patients pay the costs for choosing more expensive health plans that compete in a regulated private market. In the end, the president was hard pressed to oppose a plan for Medicare reform that reflected his own preferred model of health care reform. And as managed care arrangements advanced in the private sector and appeared to outperform Medicare, a growing number of congressional Democrats supported the goal of expanding managed care in the program as a remedy for the program's financing problems and benefits limitations. That the 1997 reforms retained a commitment to a Medicare fee-for-service option—beneficiaries would not be financially penalized for staying in traditional Medicare—made it easier for the Clinton administration and liberal Democrats in Congress, who both believed there should not be undue pressures on beneficiaries to leave traditional Medicare for managed care, to support this version of competition.[80]

Moreover, the 1997 reforms represented something of a legislative wishing well: different interests and political factions saw in the legislation what they wanted to—and their wishes were quite different. For Republicans, conservative Democrats, and the managed care industry, the 1997 Medicare reforms represented an important move toward transforming Medicare into a competitive market, a managed competition system that embraced managed care. Liberals saw it differently. Pete Stark, for example, a key Democratic congressional figure on Medicare policy, predicted that the legislative provisions intended to accelerate managed care and introduce competition into Medicare "wouldn't amount to a hill of beans."[81] Stark and other Democrats were therefore willing to vote for legislation that they did not believe would work as Republicans intended. The BBA thus had broad political appeal, since its impact was sufficiently uncertain to ensure that multiple and even conflicting political interests could find it acceptable.

A third, and perhaps the most crucial, reason for the success of Medicare reform in 1997 was that deficit pressures continued to shape Medicare politics. President Clinton's acquiescence to adopting a balanced budget was a major turning point. While the president regarded the proposed Republican cuts as excessive, Medicare spending reductions were still essential to balancing the budget. The president and congressional Democrats may have had a different vision of how to end the federal deficit than Republicans, but reducing Medicare spending remained crucial to that vision.

Fourth, the BBA omitted any proposals to limit federal contributions to health insurance for the poor by block granting (i.e., capping payments to states) Medicaid. The 1995 Medicare reform bill had also targeted Medicaid, and the president strongly opposed Republican efforts to block grant the program and loosen government regulations on nursing homes.[82] Immediately after his 1996 reelection, President Clinton was politically stronger than at any point since 1993, and congressional Republicans were forced to compromise with him on the issue.[83]

Finally, without controversies over spending cuts and the budgetary cap, the rhetorical appeal of the 1997 reforms was difficult to oppose. After all, the legislation's managed-competition-like provisions promised to offer Medicare beneficiaries more choice while at the same time generating budgetary savings and more competition among insurers. The reforms thus combined the assurance of fiscal control with the symbolism of individual empowerment and market efficiency, a powerful appeal in the confines of American political culture that legislators find difficult to resist.

In short, the BBA represented at least a temporary reinstatement of political consensus in Medicare. It also offered a programmatic direction for Medicare that radically departed from the old program consensus. Put simply, the 1997 legislation marked for many observers the unraveling of Medicare as single-payer insurance and the transformation of Medicare from a health insurance *program* into a health insurance *market*. That was a profound change in Medicare's operations. Writing about the significance of the 1997 reforms, health policy analyst Lynn Etheredge declared the transformation of Medicare into a "consumer-choice design" similar to the Federal Employees Health Benefits Program (long a favorite of managed competition advocates), a "watershed" in federal health policy that "ratif[ied] the market paradigm as national policy."[84] Etheredge summarized the conventional wisdom among many supporters of the legislation as well as analysts, concluding that the BBA brought Medicare: "into the mainstream of managed care plans and competitive markets. Through a national political process it ratifies market-oriented approaches as the new national health policy for dealing with health care costs. This is a political recognition of just how well the market-oriented approach has been working."[85]

By opening Medicare up to a host of new private insurance options, the BBA had the potential to fundamentally alter Medicare's character as a public, federally operated insurance program. Public Medicare was now to take its place among dozens of private plans competing for beneficiaries in a new Medicare insurance market. And over time a substantial number of program beneficiaries were expected to leave traditional Medicare and enroll in managed care organizations and other private plans offered under Medicare + Choice. The Congressional Budget Office forecast that, by 2002, the BBA would result in 27% of all Medicare beneficiaries' being enrolled in managed care plans, a number projected to increase to 35% by 2005.[86] Beneficiary movement out of traditional Medicare was to be facilitated by raising payments to managed care plans in rural counties that had little success in attracting Medicare beneficiaries, reducing geographic variation in payments, and loosening some regulations on health plans.[87] If the legislation worked as planned, then, the philosophy underlying Medicare as well as program operations would be transformed. Medicare would shift from a single-payer government insurance program to a federal subsidy program for private insurance. And over time, many expected that the majority of beneficiaries would no longer enroll in public Medicare (though, as previously noted, some congressional liberals and health policy analysts believed these provisions would not work as planned and consequently would not transform Medicare).

This vision of Medicare closely resembled what opponents of Medicare had proposed in 1965, with the role of government cast as subsidizing beneficiaries' purchasing of private insurance, rather than operating a government insurance plan. Medicare had in essence come full circle back to the original debate over its enactment, but with a realignment of political forces that favored market advocates. And the features of the new Medicare market as envisioned by the BBA—competing private insurance plans, a regulated marketplace, an organized shopping period for enrollees—clearly embodied the principles of managed competition.[88] Yet while the imprint of managed competition on Medicare was strong, in one crucial respect the Medicare reforms diverged from traditional managed competition, and consequently the new program philosophy did not completely supplant the old Medicare consensus.

The BBA did not legislate what the Republican leadership had originally wanted to do: convert Medicare into a defined-contribution system. Under such a system, the federal government would give Medicare enrollees a fixed dollar amount to choose a health plan. If Medicare beneficiaries chose a plan that cost more than the value of the government voucher, they would have to pay the difference themselves. A defined contribution, or voucher, is a core element in managed competition since, according to the theory, it generates savings, allows budgetary certainty, promotes innovation, and creates incentives for people to choose low-cost (and presumably more efficient) health plans. In the case of Medicare, managed competition advocates anticipated that the impact of a defined-contribution incentive would be to hasten the departure of enrollees from public Medicare to lower-cost managed care plans.

By the mid-1990s, a wide range of health policymakers and analysts, as well as the Congressional Budget Office and the American Medical Association, endorsed the introduction of a defined-contribution system in Medicare.[89] And the idea enjoyed considerable support among Republican congressional majorities and some Democratic conservatives. But the political stigma of "voucherizing" Medicare was still sufficiently strong in 1997 that defined contributions were left out of the reform package. The omission had two key consequences: the first was that it lessened the financial pressure on beneficiaries to leave public Medicare, since that program was expected to be more expensive than lower-cost managed care insurance plans. This in turn ensured large enrollments in the public sector of the program in the short term, meaning that traditional Medicare would remain predominant in the new Medicare market. The second consequence was that without defined contributions, the BBA lacked the key cost control mechanism of managed competition. Even though the BBA contained much of the managed competition infrastructure, without defined contributions and cost consciousness imposed on Medicare beneficiaries, the competitive dynamics of the system were not fully unleashed.

Yet, as already noted, the BBA mandated substantial cuts in the rate of growth in Medicare spending over the next decade. Where, then, did the $115 billion savings come from, if not from the dynamics of competition? Herein lay the ultimate paradox of the 1997 legislation: while the BBA represented a historic milestone in bringing managed competition to Medicare, at the same time it continued the recent process of moving Medicare closer to the single-payer model. The 1997 legislation substantially increased the scope of Medicare subject to prospective budgeting by reining in payments for home health care and skilled nursing facilities.[90] With the addition of these two sectors to prospective payment, Medicare was now closer than ever to having a program or global budget by default. The legislation also linked the growth in payments for physician services to changes in the gross domestic product, a potentially stronger brake on program expenditures that resembled cost control instruments used in other industrial democracies.

These new regulatory reforms, as well as reducing payments to providers under already established regulations, generated the savings in program spending, not the procompetitive elements of the legislation.[91] In this the BBA echoed a familiar theme from Medicare politics during the 1980s. In 1997, as in 1983, when the prospective payment system for hospitals was adopted, the rhetoric was all about markets and competition. But the reality was that the savings were all from regulation. The secret of the BBA was that the move to competition was not projected to save Medicare any money. Given budgetary pressures for Medicare savings, Republicans and Democrats once again embraced more regulation and lower payments to providers as the best way to achieve short-term budgetary goals. In 1997, as in 1983, policymakers talked right, but ultimately moved left.[92]

In the short term, at least, Medicare was characterized by a dual personality, moving in two directions at once, embracing the market while continuing the development of its traditional component toward a global budget. The new market vision thus did not replace the traditional liberal consensus. The new coalition in Medicare politics was not sufficiently strong to undo Medicare's existing arrangements, so it had to build market arrangements on top of them. Market and regulatory instruments now shared an uneasy coexistence within the same program. Consequently, the ultimate shape of Medicare as a public program was by no means clear. Would the program's original status as government insurance endure, or would Medicare transform into a full-fledged market of private insurers? Political and economic circumstances in the coming years would determine which direction Medicare would move in. The first of those circumstances was the work of the National Bipartisan Commission on the Future of Medicare.

THE BIPARTISAN COMMISSION

Congress established the National Bipartisan Commission on the Future of Medicare in the 1997 Balanced Budget Act. Its mandate was to go beyond that year's reform package and comprehensively examine Medicare's future, including financing, eligibility, and benefits. The commission was to make recommendations to Congress by March 1999 on how to strengthen the program to meet the coming challenges of the baby boom generation set to retire into Medicare beginning in 2010. The Medicare commission recalled the 1981 National Commission on Social Security Reform, created by President Reagan after his proposals for changing Social Security became embroiled in controversy and beset by Democratic opposition at a heavy political cost.[93] The Social Security commission considered changes as the program faced an imminent financing shortfall: without action, the Social Security trust fund was scheduled to fall short of paying out program benefits obligations in 1983. That shortfall was eventually averted by bipartisan agreement on a broad range of reforms, though the agreement did not result from the operations of the commission, which deadlocked along partisan lines only to have a smaller group of key actors work out a compromise plan.[94]

Medicare's short-term financial condition was not as dire as Social Security's had been in 1982. As the commission convened in 1998, the program's trust fund was predicted to be insolvent in 2008, six years later than forecast in 1997, as a result of the savings generated by the BBA, whose fiscal impact turned out to be even larger than anticipated. Nevertheless, the aspirations and underlying logic of establishing the Medicare commission were similar to those of its Social Security predecessor: to provide Congress and the administration political cover for making politically difficult decisions and tough policy choices about a popular entitlement program. That cover included the bipartisan character of the commission and, because its operations were outside the normal congressional process, its ostensible immunity from interest group pressures. In the immediate aftermath of the BBA's passage, congressional leaders asserted that the legislation was a short-term, incremental fix and that the newly minted commission would tackle longer-term solutions and fundamental Medicare reform.

The National Bipartisan Commission on the Future of Medicare first met in April 1998. John Breaux, Democratic senator from Louisiana, headed the commission, which was cochaired by Bill Thomas, a California Republican who also chaired the House Ways and Means Subcommittee on Health. The board's seventeen members were variously appointed by President Clinton, Speaker of the House New Gingrich, Senate majority leader Trent Lott, House minority leader Richard Gephardt, and Senate minority leader Tom Daschle. In all, there were eight Democratic and eight Republican appointees, with Senator Breaux, who as a fiscal conservative was acceptable to Gingrich and personally liked by Clinton as a fellow Southern New Democrat, jointly agreed upon by both parties.[95] Commission members, taken from both Congress and the private sector, represented a diverse ideological spectrum, from conservative icon Senator Phil Gramm to liberal stalwart Senator Jay Rockefeller.

From the beginning, though, the commission focused exclusively on one vision for Medicare reform—that of transforming the program into a system of managed competition in which private insurers such as HMOs would compete for enrollees with traditional Medicare, and beneficiaries would pay higher costs if they remained in traditional Medicare. This plan (now benignly renamed "premium support," a marketing label that enabled both disassociation from Bill Clinton's ill-fated "managed competition" scheme and the controversial "voucher" tag) promised to fundamentally reshape Medicare by converting it from a *defined-benefit* program in which the federal government operated its own insurance plan to a *defined-contribution* program in which beneficiaries would be provided with a fixed sum to purchase insurance.[96] That change would dramatically alter the nature of Medicare's entitlement. It also had the potential to transform the politics of Medicare, unraveling the universal coalition of beneficiaries behind the program along with its insurance pool, as seniors increasingly were segmented across private health plans and the collective philosophy underlying Medicare was replaced by individualism.

The focus on premium support was predictable. John Breaux, the commission's chair, had backed managed competition plans during the 1993–94 health care reform debate, and cochair Bill Thomas was an established advocate of adopting such a system in Medicare. Republicans had already attempted to turn Medicare into a full-fledged managed competition model in 1995, and the BBA created the infrastructure for such a system while introducing incentives to promote managed care. Moreover, as a result of conditions put on Republican appointees by Newt Gingrich, the commission did not consider raising revenues, either through payroll taxes or general revenues. In early private discussions, commission leaders agreed to put the need for more revenues on the table, but that promise was not kept.[97] The refusal to consider raising the payroll tax or other revenue sources put Medicare into a tight political and financial box, privileging restructuring plans such as premium support that promised to slow down program spending. Without relying on new revenues, and in the context of a growing ratio of retirees to workers, restructuring was made to appear to be the only feasible way to make up Medicare's financing gap and alleviate the financial burden of the baby boomers' enrollment in the program.

Support for reforming Medicare into a premium support system, however, was much broader than the confines of the Republican Party. As epitomized by Breaux, conservative Democrats liked the appeal of the market dynamics, while entitlement "hawks" concerned about the fiscal impact of the baby boomers, such as Democratic commission member Senator Bob Kerrey of Nebraska, were drawn to the cost savings that premium support promised.[98] In addition, by 1998 a wide array of health policy analysts inside and outside government had endorsed premium support as a model for Medicare reform. In particular, a lengthy list of health economists backed the idea, notably including not just longtime pro-market advocates such as Stuart Butler of the Heritage Foundation, but also Brookings Institution economist Henry Aaron and former Congressional Budget Office director Robert Reischauer, both associated with Democratic Party thinking on budgetary and social policy issues.[99]

For many economists, whose views predominate among health policy analysts in the United States, the march to support market-based reform in Medicare was irresistible. Managed competition and its applications to Medicare appealed to basic axioms in economics: the superiority of markets over public programs and government regulation, the benefits of efficiency and innovation that follow from competition, and the virtues of consumer choice.[100] And although there were obvious limitations to applying this logic to health care generally, and Medicare more specifically, the changed political environment after the 1994 Republican revolution perhaps led some analysts to throw these cautions to the wind in order to remain politically relevant.[101] As the bipartisan commission convened in 1998, market reform in Medicare appeared to be picking up intellectual as well as political momentum.

The commission conducted a yearlong series of meetings, task forces, and analyses on a wide range of subjects. On many of these issues, Chairman Breaux and cochair Thomas proposed controversial solutions, recommending raising the eligibility age from sixty-five to sixty-seven and introducing an "affluence test" on Medicare for beneficiaries with incomes over sixty thousand dollars.[102] But the centerpiece of the Breaux plan, and the focus of commission debate, remained the proposal to reform Medicare into a competitive market. The final Breaux-Thomas plan, released in March 1999, called for restructuring Medicare along the lines of the premium support model. Breaux argued for the necessity of radical change because of the financial implications of the changing ratio of workers to retirees—expected to drop from 3.9 in 2000 to 2.2 in 2040[103] —and because "Medicare is still a 1965 health care delivery system trying to keep pace with 21st Century medicine."[104] Furthermore, he argued that adopting premium support would enhance the quality of medical care for beneficiaries, improve their choice of health insurance options, generate additional benefits, and slow down program spending substantially. Commission staff estimated that, over the next three decades, the plan could cut projected Medicare spending by 1% a year, ultimately producing $500–$700 billion of savings by 2030. Those cost savings represented the central promise of premium support; after all, the commission's charge was to produce recommendations to put Medicare on a firmer financial footing for coming decades. Breaux and others pointed to the favorable experience of the Federal Employees Health Benefits Program during the early 1990s as evidence that a federally operated system of managed competition would generate savings.[105]

Yet the market-based proposal had an ideological valence that trumped its fiscal appeal. Said Senator Phil Gramm about the Breaux-Thomas plan, "it's going to save money, but I'm for it even if it doesn't save a dime."[106] That view reflected the frustration some commission members felt with what they perceived as ineffective and overly micromanaged regulatory policies by the Health Care Financing Administration (HCFA), which operated Medicare and made its payments to hospitals, physicians, and other medical providers. Premium support promised to reshape Medicare administration by creating a new Medicare board to supervise the program and diminishing the role of HCFA, viewed as both hostile to HMOs and lacking expertise in private health plans, in administering Medicare managed care.[107] It also offered the opportunity "to breathe innovation into the otherwise bureaucratically stiff system that is too often controlled by a politically motivated Congress."[108] Premium support thus reaffirmed the "technological wish" embodied by the prospective payment system for hospitals in the 1980s, the aspiration to adopt a policy system that would operate rationally and according to an automatic logic (of the market, in this case) that was self-regulating, without political interference, resulting in efficient and desirable outcomes. Medicare reform would not only cut costs, it would, according to this view, reduce a regulatory role that the federal government had taken too far in health care.

There was, however, hardly consensus on the commission as to the virtues of a Medicare program modeled on a competitive market. The ideological valence of premium support worked in both directions. Former HCFA administrator Bruce Vladeck joined other commission members in criticizing commission staff estimates of savings from the Breaux-Thomas plan as exaggerated and having little impact on the long-term solvency of the hospitalization insurance trust fund. He sardonically remarked that the promised result of financial savings and simultaneous benefits expansions relied on the appearance of the "premium support fairy."[109] Commission critics also warned that the plan could segment the Medicare market by income, with low-income beneficiaries stuck in low-cost, low-quality managed care while wealthier beneficiaries opted for private fee-for-service plans. They also admonished that premium support would endanger public Medicare, since healthier beneficiaries would be more likely to opt out of the program, and private plans might "cherry-pick" (select) healthier enrollees, leaving public Medicare with a sicker and more expensive population, while unraveling the program's insurance pool.[110] Finally, liberal members viewed the commission staff, which was tightly controlled by Bill Thomas, as inadequate to the task, and staff projections of savings from the Breaux-Thomas plan consequently had a serious credibility problem within the commission.[111]

The vote on the final Breaux-Thomas plan broke down mostly along predictably partisan and philosophical lines, with Republican appointees supporting the proposal and Democratic appointees, with the anticipated exception of Bob Kerrey, opposing it. But the outcome was still in doubt. With Kerrey's vote, premium support had ten votes on the seventeen-member commission; however, according to its grounds rules it required a supermajority of eleven to forward its recommendations on to Congress. Indeed, that supermajority rule had been insisted on in 1997 by a White House working group partly because they did not trust the Democrats on the Senate Finance Committee, who they believed might appoint "entitlement hawks" predisposed to Republican reform ideas.[112] The supermajority requirement also served the purpose of ensuring that major reform could not be recommended on a narrow partisan vote, a precondition for selling it to the public.[113] The key for Breaux was to persuade at least one of two swing voters on the commission, Clinton appointees Stuart Altman and Laura Tyson. Altman and Tyson were both economists and therefore were naturally predisposed to remake Medicare into a competitive market. Indeed, both the White House and Democrats on the commission and in Congress were worried that Tyson and, in particular, Altman would "flip" and support Breaux's premium support model.[114] However, as the price for their support Altman and Tyson insisted that a new prescription drug benefit be made universally available to all Medicare beneficiaries, in private plans as well as traditional Medicare.

Prescription drug coverage in Medicare reemerged as an issue for the first time since the catastrophic insurance episode of 1989 when President Clinton called for its adoption in his 1999 State of the Union address. He also called for dedicating 15% of the newly discovered surplus over the next decade—$670 billion—to Medicare, a provision Altman and Tyson supported. However, in offering a Medicare drug benefit, Breaux risked losing conservative commissioners, who, as Phil Gramm warned, were "reluctant to sign onto a brand new benefit when we have not dealt with the financial predicament of Medicare."[115] But as the commission proceeded, Democratic members became more vocal and insistent about a Medicare drug benefit.[116]

What the White House desired as an outcome was not entirely clear, though some commission members believed from the start that many in the Clinton administration were rooting for a deadlock and did not want an eleventh vote for premium support.[117] However, the president clung to the notion that the commission could reach a compromise, and three of his four appointees were open to a managed competition model for Medicare.[118] Indeed, liberal Democrats worried that, as with welfare reform, the president had signed on to a reform process that would ultimately end up beyond his control.[119]

Breaux, reputed to be a formidable deal maker, fought for the eleventh vote all the way until the end of the commission, ultimately maneuvering to win Altman and Tyson's support by offering to mandate Medigap plans to offer prescription drug coverage and to subsidize drug coverage for low-income Medicare beneficiaries. Breaux, though, did not endorse a universal drug benefit for all Medicare beneficiaries, nor did he change his opposition to dedicating a portion of the surplus to Medicare. The limited drug benefit proved insufficient for Altman and Tyson, however, and the "drugs for competition" grand bargain failed to materialize. The commission disbanded, with President Clinton disavowing its plan to raise the Medicare eligibility age and its failure to provide an adequate drug benefit and Senator Breaux and Representative Thomas promising to introduce legislation mirroring the commission model in Congress.[120] Medicare reform remained elusive, as the ideological and political contest between the old Medicare consensus and the resurgent market model endured.

THE 2000 ELECTIONS: SURPLUS POLITICS AND PRESCRIPTION DRUGS

In 2000, Medicare commanded more attention in a presidential election than at any time since 1964. In a contest between the incumbent Democratic vice president, Al Gore, and the Republican governor of Texas, George W. Bush, that lacked (until election night) both excitement and compelling candidates, Medicare emerged as a first-order issue. However, as the 2000 campaign season got underway, the fiscal environment of Medicare had fundamentally changed, and with it Medicare's place in American politics. In 1998, for the first time in three decades, the Congressional Budget Office announced a federal budget surplus, forecasting a surplus of $131 billion for 2000 and $381 billion by 2009.[121] The surplus arrived as a result of the unprecedented period of economic growth in the 1990s, which filled federal tax coffers, and the budgetary policies pursued by President Clinton and Congress. And it heralded a new era in Medicare politics, one in which the deficit pressures and zero-sum politics of the 1980s and 1990s would give way to the politically friendlier, and costlier, contours of surplus politics. The trust fund outlook for Medicare was also brightening. In 1997, Medicare's hospitalization insurance trust fund had been predicted to become insolvent in 2001; by 1999 Medicare trustees had pushed back the date of insolvency to 2015; and by 2000, it stood at 2025, the best fiscal situation Medicare had been in since 1974.[122] The improved finances of the program were due to surging revenues from the growing economy and the success—even more than anticipated—of the 1997 reforms in slowing down Medicare spending. In 1998 Medicare spending grew by only 1.5% and in 1999, it actually declined for the first time in program history. The idea that Medicare faced a trust fund crisis, which had driven program politics since 1995, now seemed far-fetched, as well as far off.

Two of the most important pressures for fiscal restraint in Medicare, then, federal deficits and trust fund shortfalls, were nowhere in evidence in 2000. As a consequence, the politics of Medicare in that year's election revolved around something that had rarely happened in the program's history: a bidding war to expand benefits. The potential benefit that became the subject of Al Gore and George W. Bush's attention was prescription drug coverage. The rise of prescription drug coverage as an issue in Medicare politics was made possible by surplus politics, but that was not its only impetus. The long-standing gap between Medicare's lack of outpatient drug coverage and the standard of coverage in the private sector was widening. Medicare HMOs, an important source of drug benefits for 15% of program beneficiaries, were increasingly adopting tight restrictions on such coverage, for instance, instituting low ceilings on the maximum amount that could be covered or dropping drug coverage altogether. Similarly, Medigap and supplemental insurance plans that covered prescription drugs were raising premiums to levels many beneficiaries could no longer afford, and employer-sponsored drug coverage for seniors promised to follow a similar trajectory. The erosion of prescription drug coverage for seniors was due largely to an explosion in drug costs. Though small as a percentage of overall health care spending in the United States, spending on medications rose by 15% in 1998, making pharmaceuticals the fastest-growing component of national health spending.[123] The increasing costs made Medicare's omission of coverage for outpatient medications all the more glaring.

Beyond the financial pressures that underlined the widening gap between Medicare and the private standard, the medical implications of that gap seemed to grow as well, with the promise of a new generation of drugs for treating arthritis, blood pressure, depression, heart disease, and numerous other conditions reinforced by an avalanche of advertisements and celebratory media stories about the latest medical discovery that made access to these "miracle" drugs seem like a basic human right. The promised benefits of drugs soon to be generated by research on the human genome only upped the ante, as some observers boldly, and undoubtedly precipitously, imagined sizable gains in average life expectancy and even "life without disease."[124] William Schwartz, a prominent health policy analyst and physician, declared the United States on the threshold of a "medical utopia," arguing in a fit of hyperbole typical of the times that "our exploding knowledge of the genetic mechanisms of disease begins to make plausible the once impossible dream of a largely disease-free existence . . . the possibility of a broad-based victory over disease and a dramatic increase in the human lifespan in the not too remote future must be taken seriously."[125] The prospects, then, of a genetic revolution on the horizon made extending drug coverage to Medicare imperative. John Breaux, chairman of the National Bipartisan Commission on the Future of Medicare, captured the emergent conventional wisdom when he declared that "drugs are as important today as a hospital bed was in 1965."[126] The data were overwhelming: in 1996, 80% percent of seniors took medications, and seniors got an average of twenty prescriptions filled in a year.[127] In a 2000 survey by the Kaiser Family Foundation, 76% of the public supported "guaranteeing prescription drug coverage to everyone on Medicare, even if it means more government spending to pay for it."[128] Modernizing Medicare now entailed benefits expansion as an integral part of program restructuring.

By 2000, Medicare's promise to bring the elderly into mainstream medicine therefore appeared to require adding a drug benefit to the program.[129] What form the benefit would take was an entirely different matter. While both presidential candidates had joined the bandwagon of expansion of Medicare benefits—Bush more reluctantly than Gore—they offered contrasting plans. Gore proposed a drug benefit that resembled a plan proposed earlier in 2000 by the Clinton administration. It was voluntary, was universally available to all Medicare beneficiaries, and would add coverage to the traditional Medicare program, at an estimated cost of $338 billion over ten years. Bush, after suffering politically earlier in the campaign without a proposal, eventually countered with a plan that initially provided block grants to states to assist low-income Medicare beneficiaries with drug costs as well as enrollees with "catastrophic" costs that totaled more than six thousand dollars annually; in subsequent years, coverage would be made available through private insurers participating in Medicare, at an estimated cost of $158 billion over ten years.[130] The cost differential was explained by the fact that benefits were not as generous and the eligibility not as comprehensive as that envisioned in the Gore plan. Yet in reality, the insurance protection offered by both plans, which left beneficiaries responsible for considerable costs and paled in comparison to standard benefits in the employer-sponsored market, was likely to disappoint seniors. In addition, candidate Bush tied his prescription drug plan to a commitment to comprehensively reform Medicare along the lines recommended by the bipartisan commission. Gore proposed to strengthen Medicare's trust fund by devoting a share of the federal budget surplus to a much-talked-about "lockbox."

Once again the philosophical divide over Medicare's direction stood in full view. In 1988, when the catastrophic insurance legislation added prescription drug coverage to Medicare (a benefit later repealed), there was consensus that the drug benefit should be added to Medicare as a universal federal benefit. How much Medicare politics had changed was underscored by the fact that in 2000, only a decade later, no such consensus existed.

Gore's proposal harkened back to Medicare's roots, with a commitment to universalism, government-provided benefits, and social insurance, though significantly, the Gore proposal called for voluntary enrollment rather than the mandatory enrollment conventionally associated with social insurance arrangements. The logic of insurance pools and adverse selection suggested, strictly from a policy perspective, that mandatory enrollment for a prescription drug benefit was a sensible course.[131] The political logic, however, with roughly two-thirds of seniors already having some drug coverage (through employer-sponsored plans, Medicaid, Medigap, and Medicare HMOs—in this case the legacies of past decisions not to provide federal coverage constrained contemporary possibilities and politics) and the potential stigma of a "coercive" government plan argued for voluntarism, and so Gore chose the more convenient route of modified universalism.

In contrast, the Bush plan relied on market forces and the private sector for benefits expansion, rejecting the notion that the federal government should directly provide the benefit through public Medicare. The Gore-Bush debate on drug coverage anticipated the partisan divisions on the issue that carried over into the next Congress. Prescription drug coverage thus became another front in the war over the future of Medicare between the old Medicare consensus and the new vision of a Medicare market.

Gore's argument was more popular with the public, but Bush won the election, and despite Bush's controversial proposals for Social Security and Medicare reform, Gore carried the vote of those sixty and older by only 51%-47%.[132]

THE BUSH ADMINISTRATION AND MEDICARE, 2001–2

George W. Bush came into office without any public mandate. Al Gore actually received more popular votes in the 2000 election, and Bush achieved a narrowed and delayed victory in the Electoral College only after a divided Supreme Court voted 5-4 to stop a recount of the controversial Florida vote. Nevertheless, Bush's agenda on entitlements remained ambitious. He convened a commission to study Social Security reform whose membership tilted strongly to privatization, hoping it would lay the groundwork for his own proposals to introduce private accounts into Social Security. Similarly, in Medicare the Bush administration came to office committed to comprehensive program reform that would overhaul Medicare along more market-friendly lines.

The first political priority in Medicare, however, was prescription drug coverage. The issue had resonated strongly enough with voters that Congress felt compelled to pass some sort of new benefit by the next election. Yet by the summer of 2002 there had been little progress in breaking the stalemate on the issue. The lack of progress was partly due to external circumstances. The September 11, 2001 terrorist attacks on Washington, D.C., and New York City transformed the national political agenda. Domestic issues gave way to foreign policy and defense concerns, and the Bush administration made the war on terrorism its first priority. Attention to the prescription drug issue, and other domestic issues, was postponed. In addition, the 2001 recession, the economic fallout from September 11, and the fiscal impact of the tax cuts sponsored by the Bush administration meant that by 2002 the federal budgetary surplus had disappeared. Medicare drug coverage could no longer be paid for "for free."

Nevertheless, with the 2002 elections approaching and congressional candidates eyeing elderly voters, both parties maneuvered to push plans for a Medicare drug benefit. Congressional Republicans and Democrats regarded the Bush administration's initial proposals to create a discount card for seniors to purchase prescription drugs and a limited subsidy for low-income seniors as inadequate to the task. However, the parties remained far apart on the design and scope of a Medicare drug benefit, with Democrats generally favoring a universal benefit that subsidized coverage for all beneficiaries and more comprehensive coverage of prescription drug expenses, at a greater cost to the federal government. Republicans focused on a more limited benefit with subsidies targeted at lower-income beneficiaries, resulting in a less expensive plan. The political salience of the issue meant that some sort of Medicare drug benefit might emerge by 2004, but how the distance between Democratic and Republican proposals would be bridged and the ultimate shape of reform remained unclear.

Meanwhile, while attention centered on the Medicare prescription drug debate, policymakers continued to ignore another critical problem: what to do about long-term care for the elderly. As the baby boomers approached retirement, there was less political willingness to tackle long-term care in 2001 than there had been a decade before. As had been the case for much of the past three decades, the high and unpredictable costs of long-term care kept it off the agenda, despite public support for reform. Prescription drugs provided politicians a cheaper and more focused way to do something for the elderly.

The Bush administration originally sought to link enactment of a Medicare drug benefit to broader program reforms such as those proposed by the bipartisan commission. However, in 2002 the immediate prospects for major, market-driven Medicare reform looked bleak. First, President Bush lacked sizable enough conservative majorities in the Senate and House to enact such reform. Second, the financial condition of Medicare's hospitalization insurance trust fund was better than it had been in three decades. In 2002, government trustees pushed the estimated date of trust fund exhaustion back to 2030.[133] There was therefore no compelling basis to argue for a crisis in Medicare that necessitated radical reform, as the Republican leadership had done in 1995. Third, Medicare's experience with managed care since the 1997 introduction of Medicare + Choice did little to promote the idea that the program should move further in a market-oriented direction.

Indeed, in 2002 Medicare + Choice appeared to be a clear policy failure, and its future was in doubt. The anticipated entry of medical savings accounts, provider-sponsored organizations, and other new health plans into Medicare never materialized.[134] And instead of accelerating managed care's development in Medicare, Medicare + Choice's first five years were characterized by HMO withdrawals from Medicare, cutbacks in the extra benefits (such as prescription drugs) offered by managed care plans, and a decline in the number of Medicare beneficiaries enrolling in managed care plans. Plans enrolling nearly one million Medicare beneficiaries withdrew from the program in 2001, and HMOs providing care to another 536,000 beneficiaries pulled out of Medicare in 2002.[135] These trends continued unabated despite Congress's enactment of so-called provider givebacks that paid heath plans more. Efforts to experiment with a competitive bidding model also stalled. In short, the theory of Medicare managed care and competition ran head-on into a sobering reality.

When the BBA was passed, the managed care industry had expected it to promote Medicare HMO enrollment. They badly miscalculated, in part because the market rhetoric distracted attention from cuts that were made in Medicare payments to health plans.[136] In addition, Medicare tried to accelerate its managed care enrollment at precisely the time when the industry was beginning to fall on hard financial times; the retreat of managed care was not limited to Medicare. In 2002, the actual percentage of Medicare beneficiaries enrolled in managed care plans stood at 14%, roughly half the projected enrollment of 27% that the Congressional Budget Office had predicted in 1997. The Medicare + Choice experience only strengthened the opposition of congressional critics of Medicare managed care. Whether administration and congressional policies to turn around Medicare + Choice through higher plan payments would succeed was unclear.

A third constraint on Medicare reform was the performance of the private insurance market. By 2002, the private sector no longer appeared an attractive model for reform. Premium increases for health insurance had returned to the double-digit inflation of the 1980s, and managed care no longer seemed capable of controlling costs. Moreover, the two public systems operating managed competition that had been cited as models for Medicare, the Federal Employees Health Benefits Program and the CalPERS insurance plan for California state employees, were experiencing staggering increases in their premiums, reversing the successes of the mid-1990s. The inability of such competitive systems to control costs weakened the case for adopting a market-based system in Medicare.

CONCLUSION

Nevertheless, the rise of the market in Medicare politics is hardly over. The year 1995 marked the end of the liberal consensus in Medicare, and a debate over the program's core philosophy and purpose has reopened for the first time since 1965. The question now is what will emerge in its aftermath as the new framework for program politics. Clearly, the political contest over Medicare during 1997–2002 did not settle the issue, and as the deadlocked bipartisan commission revealed, there is no easy consensus in sight.

Changes in the partisan and ideological balance in Congress that favor conservatives, a recovery in the Medicare + Choice system, improved performance in private sector cost control, and, especially, rising costs in Medicare and a downward turn in its trust fund balance in the context of budgetary deficits could revive the possibilities for major reform of Medicare into a competitive market. Alternatively, further erosion of Medicare + Choice, a strong performance by Medicare in controlling spending, and a divided Congress with no clear conservative majority would make such reform unlikely. In this circumstance, Medicare reform is likely to continue on its regulatory path of the past two decades, saving money by tightening federal payments to hospitals, physicians, and other medical care providers.

Medicare's future, then, remains uncertain. What is certain is the transformation of program politics that has taken place. During Medicare's first thirty years, the program was governed by the politics of program management, which focused on rationalizing Medicare. Policymaking centered on technical issues of the most efficient means to pay for Medicare services. Political disputes were contained in a bipartisan consensus in which both parties accepted Medicare's existing structure and the need to control costs. The politics of management, however, has now receded, and with it so has the era of consensus in Medicare. Medicare politics is now transparently a battle of ideas about the role of markets and government in public policy. This is, in many respects, the same debate held in the 1950s and 1960s before Medicare's enactment, replete with the same sharp partisan cleavages, high-visibility politics that reach into national elections, a broad scope of conflict, and an engaged public. The new politics of Medicare is an echo of the past.

As a consequence, after thirty-seven years of policy innovations, political upheaval, changing economic circumstances, and a radically altered health care system, Medicare politics is back where it started.

NOTES

CHAPTER ONE

1. Colette Farley, "Republicans Outline Medicare Plan," *Congressional Quarterly,* September 16, 1995, 2780–81. The details of the Republican proposals, and a comparison with current law, are summarized by the Henry J. Kaiser Family Foundation in *Medicare Provisions of the House and Senate Bills* (November 1995).

2. Linda Killian, *The Freshmen: What Happened to the Republican Revolution?* (Boulder, Colo.: Westview Press, 1998), 163.

3. Barbour's warnings about Medicare as a Republican Achilles heel can be found in Michael Weisskopf and David Maraniss, "Republican Leaders Win Battle by Defining Terms of Combat," *Washington Post,* October 29, 1995.

4. On the role of Republican political consultants, including Linda DiVall and Frank Luntz, in the Medicare campaign, see David Maraniss and Michael Weisskopf, *"Tell Newt to Shut Up!"* (New York: Simon and Schuster, 1996), 128–145.

5. For example, Republican leaders sought to assuage physicians' and hospitals' concerns—and those of their organized representatives, the American Medical Association and the American Hospital Association—about Medicare payment cuts by offering legislation that would encourage the spread of provider-sponsored organizations (PSOs), health plans organized and run by medical care providers. At the time, PSOs were increasingly seen by providers as a way for the medical profession to reassert professional sovereignty that had been eroded by the rise of managed care plans.

6. Analysis of the failure of the Clinton administration's health plan has become a cottage industry. See Jacob Hacker, *The Road to Nowhere* (Princeton, N.J.: Princeton University Press, 1997); Theda Skocpol, *Boomerang: Clinton's Health Security Effort and the Turn against Government in U.S. Politics* (New York: W. W. Norton, 1996); Haynes Johnson and David S. Broder, *The System: The American Way of Politics at the Breaking Point* (Little, Brown and Company, 1996); Paul Starr, "What Happened to Health Care Reform?" *American Prospect* 20 (winter 1995): 20–31; and Henry

Aaron, ed., *The Problem That Won't Go Away: Reforming U.S. Health Care Financing* (Washington, D.C.: Brookings Institution Press, 1996). For an account of Newt Gingrich's strategic management of Medicare reform, see Johnson and Broder, *The System*, 573–92.

7. Thomas's description of the Republican Medicare plan as "bold, innovative . . . and radical" is quoted in Colette Farley, "Historic House Medicare Vote Affirms GOP Determination," *Congressional Quarterly*, October 21, 1995, 3206. The statement that transforming Medicare was part of the Republican "mandate of the year" (1995) is found in "Medicare, Medicaid on Table for Possible Cuts," *Congressional Quarterly*, February 11, 1995, 458.

8. Farley, "Historic House Medicare Vote," 3206.

9. The quote is from Democratic House minority whip David Bonior, ibid., 3210.

10. Eric Painin and Judith Havemann, "House Medicare Tussle over Cuts Turns Real," *Washington Post*, September 21, 1995.

11. Colette Farley, "Democrats Say GOP Surgery on Medicare Goes Too Far," *Congressional Quarterly*, October 7, 1995, 3068.

12. See Pete Stark, "The Politics of Medicare," *Journal of the American Medical Association* 274 (1995): 274–75.

13. Colette Farley, "GOP Scores on Medicare, but Foes Aren't Done," *Congressional Quarterly*, November 18, 1995, 3535.

14. Killian, *The Freshmen*, 169.

15. *1995 Annual Report of the Board of Trustees of the Federal Hospital Insurance Trust Fund* (Washington, D.C.: U.S. Government Printing Office, 1995).

16. The rhetorical strategy of emphasizing the danger of Medicare bankruptcy is discussed in Maraniss and Weisskopf, *"Tell Newt to Shut Up!"* 128–133. Thomas is quoted in Colette Farley, "Using Vouchers for Medicare May Help GOP Cut Costs," *Congressional Quarterly*, July 22, 1995, 2189.

17. In one of the more memorable confrontations of the Medicare debate, during congressional hearings Representative Bill Thomas cited the movie Jurassic Park in warning Health Care Financing Administration chief Bruce Vladeck about the danger of protecting Medicare as a "dinosaur." Vladeck retorted that the real message of the movie was the danger of experimenting with the unknown, a lesson he alleged Republicans were ignoring in their Medicare reform proposals. See Robin Toner, "GOP Moves Health Debate to Medicare," *New York Times*, February 12, 1995. The argument about Medicare's being out of date with the health system and performing poorly in cost control compared to the private sector is made in Bill Thomas, "1965–1995: Medicare at a Crossroads," *Journal of the American Medical Association* 274 (1995): 276–78.

18. Killian, *The Freshmen*, 161.

19. Compare the conclusions of William Schneider, "Who's Really Medicare's Best Friend?" *National Journal*, May 6, 1995, 1138, with those in "Medicare Lies," *Wall Street Journal*, January 22, 1996. See also "The Medicare Debate," *Washington Post*, November 1, 1995; Gerald F. Seib, "Medicare Scare: It's a Fun Game, But Risky Too," *Wall Street Journal*, July 17, 1996; and "The Medicare Argument," *New York Times*, June 4, 1996.

20. The description of the baby boom generation as a "fiscal tsunami" is from Robert D. Reischauer, "Medicare: What to Do?" *Brookings Review* 13 (1995): 50.

21. Ibid. For additional claims that demographic trends make Medicare unsustain-

able in its current form, see Henry J. Aaron and Robert D. Reischauer, "The Medicare Reform Debate: What Is the Next Step?" *Health Affairs* 14 (1995): 8–30; Congressional Budget Office, *Reducing the Deficit: Spending and Revenue Options* (Washington, D.C.: U.S. Government Printing Office, 1996); and Peter G. Peterson, "Will American Grow Up Before It Grows Old?" *Atlantic Monthly* 277 (May 1986): 55–86.

22. See Victor Fuchs, "Perspective on Medicare: Are We Asking the Right Questions?" *Los Angeles Times,* July 1,1996; Peterson, "Will America Grow Up?" and Congressional Budget Office, *Reducing the Deficit,* 447–72.

23. For a comprehensive analysis of the impact of the baby boomers on the United States, see Joseph White, *False Alarm: Why the Greatest Threat to Social Security and Medicare Is the Campaign to "Save" Them* (Baltimore: Johns Hopkins University Press, 2001). The relationship between demography and health care spending internationally is analyzed in Thomas E. Getzen, "Population Aging and the Growth of Health Expenditures," *Journal of Gerontology* 47 (1994): S98–S104. See also Morris L. Barer, Robert G. Evans, and Clyde Hertzman, "Avalanche or Glacier? Health Care and the Demographic Rhetoric," *Canadian Journal on Aging* 14 (1995): 193–224; Robert G. Evans, "Illusion of Necessity: Evading Responsibility for Choice in Health Care, *Journal of Health Politics, Policy, and Law* 10 (1985): 439–67; and Morris L. Barer, Robert G. Evans, Clyde Hertzman, and Jonathan Lomas, "Aging and Health Care Utilization: New Evidence on Old Fallacies," *Social Science and Medicine* 24 (1987): 851–62.

24. Vouchers would give Medicare beneficiaries a flat amount of money to purchase health insurance on the private market, with beneficiaries financially responsible if they chose more expensive plans. This would represent a radical departure from Medicare's current philosophy of guaranteeing a set level of benefits for all beneficiaries and assuring that there is no extra cost for beneficiaries who choose to remain in traditional Medicare rather than join private plans.

25. The classic work on Medicare's enactment is Theodore R. Marmor, *The Politics of Medicare* (Chicago: Aldine, 1973). The political fate of the Truman administration proposals for national health insurance is discussed in Monte M. Poen, *Harry S. Truman versus the Medical Lobby* (Columbia: University of Missouri Press, 1979).

26. For evidence of Medicare's high standing in public opinion, see Fay Lomax Cook and Edith J. Barrett, *Support for the American Welfare State: The Views of Congress and the Public* (New York: Columbia University Press, 1992).

27. Henry J. Kaiser Family Foundation, *Medicare Chart Book* (Menlo Park, Calif.: Henry J. Kaiser Family Foundation, 1995).

28. See, for instance, Karen Davis and Cathy Schoen, *Medicare Policy: New Directions for Health and Long-Term Care* (Baltimore: Johns Hopkins University Press, 1986); David Blumenthal, Mark Schlesinger, and Pamela Brown Drumheller, eds., *Renewing the Promise: Medicare and Its Reform* (New York: Oxford University Press, 1988); and Marilyn Moon, *Medicare: Now and in the Future* (Washington, D.C.: Urban Institute Press, 1993).

29. The impact of the scope of conflict on politics is set out in E. E. Schattschneider, *The Semisovereign People* (New York.: Holt, Reinhart, and Winston, 1960). Schattschneider argues that the wider the scope of conflict, the more influential the public (in his words "the audience") is on political contests and the better off democracy becomes.

30. This distinction draws on the discussion of rationalizing politics in Lawrence D. Brown, *New Politics, New Policies: Government's Response to Government's*

Growth (Washington, D.C.: Brookings Institution Press, 1983). Carolyn Hughes Tuohy likewise distinguishes between "founding periods" and "reformist periods" in *Accidental Logics: The Dynamics of Change in the Health Care Arena in the United States, Britain, and Canada* (New York: Oxford University Press, 1999).

31. Max J. Skidmore, *Social Security and Its Enemies* (Boulder, Colo.: Westview Press, 1999).

32. The "quiet" enactment of significant Medicare reforms during the 1980s is analyzed in James Morone and Andrew Dunham, "Slouching to National Health Insurance," *Yale Journal on Regulation* 2 (1985): 263–91.

33. This approach to analyzing Medicare politics echoes that of Marmor, *The Politics of Medicare*, 1st ed.; and Rudolf Klein, *The Politics of the National Health Service*, 2d ed. (London: Longman, 1989).

34. The best summary of economic thinking on Medicare policy is Marilyn Moon, *Medicare: Now and in the Future*, 2d ed. (Washington, D.C.: Urban Institute Press, 1996).

35. See, for example, Lawrence D. Brown, "Technocratic Corporatism and Administrative Reform in American Medicine," *Journal of Health Politics, Policy, and Law* 10 (1985): 579–99; Judith M. Feder, *Medicare: The Politics of Federal Hospital Insurance* (Lexington, Mass.: D. C. Heath, 1977); David G. Smith, *Paying for Medicare: The Politics of Reform* (New York: Aldine de Gruyter, 1992); and Richard Himmelfarb, *Catastrophic Politics: The Rise and Fall of the Medicare Catastrophic Coverage Act* (University Park: Pennsylvania State University Press, 1995).

36. The closest example is Theodore Marmor, *The Politics of Medicare*, 2d ed. (New York: Aldine de Gruyter, 2000). However, while this book draws attention to selective themes in Medicare's development, Marmor explicitly notes that it is not intended as a comprehensive political analysis or policy history of Medicare's first thirty years of operation.

37. The complete list of interviews is included in the bibliography.

38. At its inception, the designers of Medicare intended the program to cover only part of the costs of health care for the elderly. However, public expectations regarding Medicare's coverage of health costs for the aged have always been far wider than either the original intent or programmatic reality. These expectations have alternatively reflected Medicare's symbolic promise of ensuring freedom from the financial burdens of medical care. It is these public expectations that are, in part, the source of the gap between promise and performance in Medicare.

39. As chap. 3 explains, trust fund dynamics in Medicare hospitalization insurance (Medicare part A) were different from those in Medicare insurance for physicians' services (Medicare part B).

40. On the politics of social insurance, see Margaret Weir, Ann Shola Orloff, and Theda Skocpol, *The Politics of Social Policy in the United States* (Princeton, N.J.: Princeton University Press, 1988): 3–37.

41. By 2002, the federal budget was again in deficit.

42. The rise and decline of liberalism is chronicled in Allen Matusow, *The Unraveling of America: A History of Liberalism in the 1960s* (New York: Harper and Row, 1984).

43. For a full discussion of the separation of politics from policy in Medicare research, see Jonathan Oberlander, "Medicare and the American State: The Politics of Federal Health Insurance" (Ph.D. diss., Yale University, 1995):14–20.

44. See Thomas Rice and Jill Bernstein, "Volume Performance Standards: Can They Control Growth in Medicare," *Milbank Quarterly* 68, no. 3 (1990): 310.

45. For a critique of the rational model of the policy process, see Deborah Stone, *Policy Paradox and Political Reason* (New York: W. W. Norton, 1997).

46. These ambitions are most pronounced among proponents of rational choice theory, though other schools of thought, including historical institutionalism, also occasionally reveal this aim.

47. The tradition of associating different politics with different policies is exemplified by Theodore Lowi, "American Business, Public Policy, Case Studies and Political Theory." *World Politics* 16 (1974): 677–715; James Q. Wilson, *Political Organizations* (New York: Basic Books, 1973), chap. 16; and Marmor, *The Politics of Medicare*, 1st ed., and *Political Analysis and American Medical Care* (Cambridge: Cambridge University Press, 1983).

48. I am drawing here on Marmor, *The Politics of Medicare*, 1st ed., vi.

49. A classic statement of national political culture as a determinant of public policy is Anthony King, "Ideas, Institutions, and the Policies of Governments," *British Journal of Political Science* 3 (1973): parts 1–3.

50. The view that public policy is dominated by pressure groups and private interests is advanced in David Truman, *The Governmental Process* (New York: Knopf, 1951); Theodore Lowi, *The End of Liberalism* (New York: W. W. Norton, 1979); Grant McConnell, *Private Power and American Democracy* (New York: Knopf, 1966); George Stigler, "The Theory of Economic Regulation," *Bell Journal on Economics and Management Science* 2 (1971): 137–46; and Hugh Heclo, "Issue Networks and the Executive Establishment," in *The New American Political System,* ed. Anthony King (Washington, D.C.: American Enterprise Institute, 1978). For more recent accounts of interest group politics, see Beth L. Leech and Frank Baumgartner, *Basic Interests* (Princeton, N.J.: Princeton University Press, 1998); Jeffrey M. Berry, *The Interest Group Society,* 2d ed. (Glenville, Ill.: Scott, Forseman and Little, Brown, 1989); Paul S. Herrnson, Ronald G. Shaiko, and Clyde Wilcox, eds. *The Interest Group Connection: Electioneering, Lobbying, and Policymaking in Washington* (Chatham, N.J.: Chatham House Publishers, 1997); John R. Wright, *Interest Groups and Congress* (Boston: Addison-Wesley 1995); Jack Walker, *Mobilizing Interest Groups in America* (Ann Arbor: University of Michigan Press); and Kay Lehman Schlozman and John T. Tierney, *Organized Interests and American Democracy* (New York: HarperCollins, 1986).

51. The public opinion perspective can be found in Lawrence Jacobs, *The Health of Nations: Public Opinion and the Making of American and British Health Policy* (Ithaca, N.Y.: Cornell University Press, 1993), and "The Recoil Effect: Public Opinion and Policymaking in the U.S. and Britain," *Comparative Politics* 24 (1992): 199–217; Benjamin I. Page and Robert Y. Shapiro, "Effects of Public Opinion on Policy," *American Political Science Review* 77 (1983): 175–90; James A. Stimson, Michael B. MacKuen, and Robert S. Erickson, "Dynamic Representation," *American Political Science Review* 89 (September 1995): 543–65; Paul J. Quirk and Joseph Hinchliffe, "The Rising Hegemony of Mass Opinion," *Journal of Policy History* 10 (1998): 19–50; and John G. Geer, *From Tea Leaves to Opinion Polls* (New York: Random House, 1996). On the impact of anticipated public opinion, see R. Douglas Arnold, *The Logic of Congressional Action* (New Haven, Conn.: Yale University Press, 1990); and John R. Zaller, *The Nature and Origins of Mass Opinion* (New York: Cambridge University Press, 1992).

52. Theda Skocpol, "Bringing the State Back In," in *Bringing the State Back In,* ed. Peter R. Evans, Dietrich Reuschemeyer, and Theda Skocpol (New York: Cambridge University Press, 1985), 12. One of the ironies of the state-centered research in political science that seeks to "bring the state back in" to the study of politics is that, more often than not, in comparative studies it concludes that the United States is a weak state relative to the European "ideal."

53. James Morone provides an excellent summary of the impact of American political culture and institutions on health policy in "American Political Culture and the Search for Lessons from Abroad," *Journal of Health Politics, Policy, and Law* 15 (spring 1990): 129–43.

54. For a review of the impact of American political institutions on health politics in the United States, see Jonathan Oberlander and Theodore Marmor, "The Path to Universal Health Care," in *The Next Agenda,* ed. R. Boorsage and R. Hickey (Boulder, Colo.: Westview Press, 2001): 93–125.

55. The number of opportunities for opponents to block policy action in the United States exceeds the number of "veto points" typical in other democratic countries. See Ellen M. Immergut, *Health Politics: Interests and Institutions in Western Europe* (Cambridge: Cambridge University Press, 1992).

56. See Leon Epstein, *Political Parties in the American Mold* (Madison: University of Wisconsin Press, 1986), and *Political Parties in Western Democracies* (New York: Praeger, 1967).

57. On American national bureaucracy, see Hugh Heclo, *A Government of Strangers* (Washington, D.C.: Brookings Institution Press, 1977); James Q. Wilson, *Bureaucracy: What Government Agencies Do and Why They Do It* (New York: Basic Books, 1989); and James A. Morone, *The Democratic Wish: Popular Participation and the Limits of American Government* (New York: Basic Books, 1990). On the low standing of American bureaucrats compared with their counterparts abroad and the implications for health policy, see David Wilsford, *Doctors and the State* (Durham, N.C.: Duke University Press, 1991): 73–83; and Carol S. Weissert and William G. Weissert, *Governing Health: The Politics of Health Policy* (Baltimore: Johns Hopkins University Press, 1996): 144–181.

58. Weissert and Weissert, *Governing Health,* 3.

59. The classic statement of American political culture as suspicious of centralized government is Louis Hartz, *The Liberal Tradition in America* (New York: Harcourt Bruce Jovanovich, 1955). See also Alexis de Tocqueville, *Democracy in America* (Garden City, N.Y.: Doubleday, 1966); Samuel P. Huntington, *American Politics: The Promise of Disharmony* (Cambridge, Mass.: Harvard University Press, 1981); and Seymour Martin Lipset, *The First New Nation: The United States in Historical and Comparative Perspective* (New York: Basic, 1963).

60. James A. Morone, "The Bureaucracy Empowered" in *The Politics of Health Care Reform,* ed. James A. Morone and Gary S. Belkin (Durham, N.C.: Duke University Press, 1994), 154.

61. Morone, *The Democratic Wish,* 1. Morone goes on to note that "the state and its bureaucracy grew; however they never won a legitimate role at the center of [American] society" (323).

62. Huntington, *American Politics,* 33.

63. Wilsford, *Doctors and the State,* 56.

64. Ibid., 2. Wilsford, who offers the most eloquent statement that the United

States has a weak state in health policymaking, writes, "state autonomy in making health policy has been weak as many health interests, including physicians, have exploited many political openings into the state to their advantage."

65. This view of Congress is articulated in David Mayhew, *Congress: The Electoral Connection* (New Haven, Conn.: Yale University Press, 1974); and Morris Fiorina, *Congress: Keystone of the Washington Establishment* (New Haven, Conn.: Yale University Press, 1977). The electoral perspective has been particularly prominent in rational choice scholarship on American politics. For summaries of this work, see Dennis C. Mueller, *Public Choice II* (New York: Cambridge University Press, 1989); and Mathew D. McCubbins and Terry Sullivan, *Congress: Structure and Policy* (New York: Cambridge University Press, 1987).

66. See the discussion in Morone, "American Political Culture," 132–35, 140–42.

67. The *New York Times* has suggested Canadian-style national health insurance would not work here because American government lacks "the discipline of parliamentary government" necessary "to the task of negotiating with medical providers, setting reimbursement rates that carefully balance the needs of patients, taxpayers and providers." See "The Wrong Medicine," *New York Times,* May 29, 1991. Stanford University health economist Alain Enthoven, a prominent advocate of market-based health initiatives and "managed competition," has similarly argued the Canadian health care system is irrelevant to U.S. reform because American culture and politics are too different. See Enthoven's letter to the editor and responses from Theodore Marmor and Jerry Mashaw in *American Prospect 5* (1991): 20–24. See also Seymour Martin Lipset, *Continental Divide: The Values and Institutions of the United States and Canada* (New York: Routledge 1990). Lipset argues Americans are more individualistic than their more communitarian neighbors to the north. Prominent health policy analysts—both from the left and right of the political spectrum—who have concluded that American values explain the absence of national health insurance include Victor Fuchs, Eli Ginzberg, Robert Evans, and Uwe Reinhardt. See Vincente Navarro's discussion in *The Politics of Health Policy* (Cambridge: Blackwell Publishers, 1994), 171–74. Navarro alternatively emphasizes the weakness of the American working class relative to other nations as an obstacle to national health insurance.

68. The success of Medicare cost-containment mechanisms in slowing down cost increases is documented in Moon, *Medicare: Now and in the Future,* 2d cd., 18–20.

69. "International standard" is a term coined by Joseph White, *Competing Solutions: American Health Care Proposals and International Experience* (Washington, D.C.: Brookings Institution Press, 1995).

CHAPTER TWO

1. Theodore Marmor, "Coping with a Creeping Crisis: Medicare at Twenty," in *Social Security: Beyond the Rhetoric of Crisis,* ed. Theodore R. Marmor and Jerry L. Mashaw (Princeton, N.J.: Princeton University Press, 1988), 178.

2. The classic work on Medicare's enactment is Theodore R. Marmor, *The Politics of Medicare* (Chicago: Aldine, 1973). See also Eugene Feingold, *Medicare: Policy and Politics: A Case Study and Policy Analysis* (San Francisco: Chandler, 1966); Richard Harris, *A Sacred Trust* (New York: New American Library, 1966); Lawrence R. Jacobs, *The Health of Nations: Public Opinion and the Making of American and British Health Policy* (Ithaca, N.Y.: Cornell University Press, 1993); James Sundquist, *Politics and Pol-*

icy: The Eisenhower, Kennedy, and Johnson Years (Washington, D.C.: Brookings Institution Press, 1968): 287–321; Peter Corning, *The Evolution of Medicare: From Idea to Law* (Washington, D.C.: Government Printing Office, 1969); and Sheri I. David, *With Dignity: The Search for Medicare and Medicaid* (Westport, Conn.: Greenwood, 1985).

3. The political history of national health insurance in the United States can be found in Daniel S. Hirshfield, *The Lost Reform: The Campaign for Compulsory Health Insurance in the United States from 1932 to 1943* (Cambridge, Mass.: Harvard University Press, 1970); Roy Lubove, *The Struggle for Social Security, 1900–1935* (Cambridge, Mass.: Harvard University Press, 1968); Ronald Numbers, *Almost Persuaded: American Physicians and Compulsory Health Insurance* (Baltimore: Johns Hopkins University Press, 1978); Monte M. Poen, *Harry S. Truman versus the Medical Lobby* (Columbia: University of Missouri Press, 1979); Paul Starr, *The Social Transformation of American Medicine* (New York: Basic Books, 1982); Rashi Fein, *Medical Care, Medical Costs* (Cambridge, Mass.: Harvard University Press, 1989); and Beatrix Hoffman, *The Wages of Sickness: The Politics of Health Insurance in Progressive America* (Chapel Hill: University of North Carolina Press, 2001).

4. German chancellor Otto von Bismarck adopted health insurance as a ploy to divert the loyalties of the working class from leftist political forces in Germany. The political logic of German social insurance programs, he explained, was "to bribe the working classes, or, if you like, to win them over to regard the State as a social institution existing for their sake and interested in their welfare." Quoted in Numbers, *Almost Persuaded*, 11.

5. Daniel T. Rodgers, *Atlantic Crossings: Social Politics in a Progressive Age* (Cambridge, Mass.: Harvard University Press, 1998), 4. In this pathbreaking work, Rodgers notes that the Progressive Era was unusual in the extent to which American social policy development was influenced by European ideas. Health insurance was one of many policy ideas that crossed the Atlantic in this period. Before 1870, Americans were inwardly focused on their own problems and not attentive to international developments. After World War II, the United States emerged as so powerful that Americans saw no need to learn lessons from abroad. Indeed, the focus was on exporting the American model of democracy and capitalism to other nations.

6. Hoffman, *Wages of Sickness*, 9

7. Numbers, *Almost Persuaded*, 19–20.

8. Starr, *Social Transformation*, 243–44.

9. Ibid.

10. Odin W. Anderson, "Compulsory Health Insurance, 1910–1950," in Feingold, *Medicare*, 86. On the AALL's successful campaign for workman's compensation insurance, see Lubove, *Struggle for Social Security*, 45–65.

11. Quoted in Robert J. Myers, *Medicare* (Bryn Mawr, Pa.: McCahan Foundation, 1970), 5.

12. Quoted in Numbers, *Almost Persuaded*, 52.

13. Anderson, "Compulsory Health Insurance," 76; and Numbers, *Almost Persuaded*, 52.

14. Hoffman, *Wages of Sickness*, 2.

15. Hirshfield, *Lost Reform*, 25.

16. Lambert was Theodore Roosevelt's personal physician and the head of the AMA's Committee on Social Insurance.

17. Harris, *Sacred Trust*, 7.

18. Gompers feared that social insurance would strengthen workers' loyalties to the state at the expense of unions. See Hirshfield, *Lost Reform,* 20. On the reversal of the medical profession, see Numbers, *Almost Persuaded,* 110–14.

19. Harris, *Sacred Trust,* 7.

20. Anderson, "Compulsory Health Insurance," 87.

21. Hoffman, *Wages of Sickness,* 45.

22. Ibid., 178.

23. The stigma of German and Bolshevik association ascribed to compulsory health insurance by its opponents is described in Lubove, *Struggle for Social Security,* 83–89. During the 1918 California elections, a state insurance group opposing a constitutional amendment for health insurance published a bulletin with the kaiser's picture on the cover, accompanied by the caption "Made in Germany: Do You Want it in California?"

24. Rodgers, *Atlantic Crossings,* 256.

25. The most prominent study was undertaken by the Committee on the Costs of Medical Care (CCMC), a privately funded commission of health specialists. See Starr, *Social Transformation,* 261–66, for a description of the CCMC's activities.

26. Ibid., 266.

27. Feingold, *Medicare,* 91.

28. Hirshfield, *Lost Reform,* 135–65.

29. Harris, *Sacred Trust,* 23–30.

30. Ibid., 29–30.

31. Ibid., 36–38.

32. Marmor, *The Politics of Medicare,* 10.

33. Feingold, *Medicare,* 99.

34. Ibid., 261.

35. Harris, *Sacred Trust,* 43–50. For an account of the key role Blue Cross played in campaigning for voluntary insurance as the "American way" and as an alternative to national health insurance, see David J. Rothman, *Beginnings Count: The Technological Imperative in American Health Care* (New York: Oxford University Press, 1997): 16–39.

36. Harris, *Sacred Trust,* 2.

37. Ibid., 53.

38. Marmor, *The Politics of Medicare,* 12.

39. Starr, *Social Transformation,* 286.

40. Marmor, *The Politics of Medicare,* 23. The inner circle of Medicare strategists came to include Cohen, Falk, Ewing, Robert Ball of the Social Security Administration, and Nelson Cruikshank of the AFL-CIO. References herein to Medicare "strategists," "advocates," "designers," and "architects" are to this group.

41. Ibid., 14–15; Harris, *Sacred Trust,* 55.

42. Marmor, *The Politics of Medicare,* 16.

43. Feingold, *Medicare,* 25–26.

44. Sundquist, *Politics and Policy,* 292–93.

45. David, *With Dignity,* 4. Blue Cross traditionally offered "community-rated" premiums that were the same regardless of health status. Commercial insurers cut into their market by "experience rating," that is, offering employed populations rates based on their own premium experience—a lure for healthy, less expensive groups who could thus purchase insurance at a lower premium.

46. Sundquist, *Politics and Policy,* 292.

47. Ibid., 288.

48. Marmor, *The Politics of Medicare,* 15.

49. For a discussion of the roles of welfare and "deservingness" in American political culture, see Michael Katz, *In the Shadow of the Poorhouse: A Social History of Welfare in America* (New York: Basic Books, 1986).

50. Edward D. Berkowitz, *Mr. Social Security* (Lawrence: University Press of Kansas, 1995), 236–37.

51. Harris, *Sacred Trust,* 55.

52. In addition to Wilbur Cohen, Robert Ball, an official in the Social Security Administration, played a critical role in shaping the Medicare strategy. For an account of Ball and Cohen's place in the social policymaking, see Theodore R. Marmor, "Entrepreneurship in Public Management: Wilbur Cohen and Robert Ball," in *Leadership and Innovation: A Biographical Perspective on Entrepreneurs in Government,* ed. Jameson W. Doig and Erwin C. Hargrove (Baltimore: Johns Hopkins University Press, 1987), 246–81. For a biography of Wilbur Cohen, see Berkowitz, *Mr. Social Security.*

53. Jacobs, *Health of Nations,* 89–90.

54. Marmor, *The Politics of Medicare,* 20–23.

55. Sundquist, *Politics and Policy,* 288.

56. Robert Ball, "What Medicare's Architects Had in Mind," *Health Affairs* 14 (winter 1995): 66.

57. Marmor, *The Politics of Medicare,* 21.

58. Ibid., 18.

59. My thanks to Ted Marmor for this observation.

60. Marmor, *The Politics of Medicare,* 23.

61. Sundquist, *Politics and Policy,* 290.

62. Marmor, *The Politics of Medicare,* 29.

63. Feingold, *Medicare,* 101. For an excellent analysis of Wilbur Mills's role in American politics and fiscal policy, see Julian E. Zelizer, *Taxing America: Wilbur D. Mills, Congress, and the State, 1945–1975* (Cambridge: Cambridge University Press, 1998).

64. Harris, *Sacred Trust,* 59.

65. David, *With Dignity,* 12.

66. Feingold, *Medicare,* 51 and 57.

67. See Harris, *Sacred Trust,* 27–47, on the AMA's tactics during the Truman years. The public relations firm of Whitaker and Baxter, which had previously worked against the compulsory health insurance proposals of Earl Warren in California, played a large role in shaping the AMA's strategy in 1949–50.

68. Quoted in James A. Morone, *The Democratic Wish: Popular Participation and the Limits of American Government* (Basic: New York, 1990), 262.

69. Marmor, *The Politics of Medicare,* 23–28.

70. Ibid., 28.

71. Sundquist, *Politics and Policy,* 287.

72. Feingold, *Medicare,* 101.

73. Ibid., 105. The Eisenhower administration plan called for using a .25% increase in the Social Security tax to enhance insurance coverage for the elderly but initially did not detail a specific plan and rejected compulsory insurance.

74. The 1956 amendments to the Social Security Act sanctioned, for the first time, state payments (with federal matching grants) for medical services for recipients of public assistance, known as vendor payments.

75. Myers, *Medicare*, 40–41.

76. The decision by the Kennedy campaign to emphasize Medicare as an issue in the 1960 elections is examined in Jacobs, *Health of Nations*, 94–99.

77. Harris, *Sacred Trust*, 11–12. The origins of Kerr-Mills are discussed in *Sacred Trust*, 10–15. Cohen was famous for his analogy of incrementalism to making a sandwich; he believed American politics required one slice of salami at a time. See David, *With Dignity*, 39.

78. Quoted in Sundquist, *Politics and Policy*, 308.

79. Marmor, *The Politics of Medicare*, 36–37.

80. Harris, *Sacred Trust*, 123.

81. Kennedy's nationally televised address at Madison Garden in New York City was widely regarded by Medicare advocates as a disaster because of the president's lackluster performance. See ibid., 141–45.

82. Harris, *Sacred Trust*, 107.

83. Marmor, *The Politics of Medicare*, 60–62; Feingold, *Medicare*, 137–40.

84. Feingold, *Medicare*, 140–42.

85. Ibid.

86. Harris, *Sacred Trust*, 180. The cosponsors of Eldercare were Representative Sydney Herlong (Democrat, Florida) and Thomas Curtis (Republican, Missouri).

87. Marmor, *The Politics of Medicare*, 69.

88. Zelizer, *Taxing America*, 213. Mills feared "that the Social Security tax could not withstand the high costs of health care."

89. Harris, *Sacred Trust*, 187.

90. Sundquist, *Politics and Policy*, 320. That compromise had originally been contained in a 1961 bill proposed by Senator Jacob Javits.

91. Ibid., 321.

92. In a June 1965 meeting, eight state delegations within the AMA called for boycotting the program, an appeal rejected by AMA president James Appel as "unethical and bad citizenship." See Feingold, *Medicare*, 146–48.

93. Ball, "Medicare's Architects," 62–63.

94. David Rothman accuses Medicare advocates of weakening the case for national health insurance by implicitly arguing that if the Congress passed Medicare for the elderly, the health care system would not need any further reform, thereby ignoring the problems of uninsured younger Americans. This argument ignores the role that policymakers such as Wilbur Cohen played in designing earlier national health insurance proposals as well as their view that Medicare would serve as a cornerstone for national health insurance. See Rothman, *Beginnings Count*, 68–86.

95. Core elements of single-payer insurance include a public insurance program operated by the government rather than subsidized private insurance, universal coverage for the targeted population, and public administrative responsibility for cost control and benefits.

96. The private subsidy approach had been favored by the Eisenhower administration, the AMA, House Republican leadership, and Senator Jacob Javits.

CHAPTER THREE

1. Medicare's impact on increasing access of the elderly to medical services is discussed in Karen Davis and Cathy Schoen, *Health and the War on Poverty: A Ten Year*

Appraisal (Washington, D.C.: Brookings Institution Press, 1978); and Marian Gornick, Jay N. Greenberg, Paul W. Eggers, and Allen Dobson, "Twenty Years of Medicare and Medicaid: Covered Populations, Use of Benefits, and Program Expenditures," *Health Care Financing Review* annual supplement (1985), 13–59.

2. In 1994, Medicare covered 45% of the total health expenditures by the elderly. See the *Medicare Chart Book* (Menlo Park, Calif.: Kaiser Family Foundation, 1995). See also Marilyn Moon, "Will the Care Be There? Vulnerable Beneficiaries and Medicare Reform," *Health Affairs* 18 (1999): 107–17, and *Medicare: Now and in the Future* (Washington, D.C.: Urban Institute Press, 1993).

3. The comparative stinginess of Medicare benefits in an international context is noted by Uwe E. Reinhardt in "Can America Afford Its Elderly Citizens?" paper presented at the Princeton Conference on Medicare Reform, Princeton, N.J., July 1997.

4. "Reasonable charges" referred to the amount of a medical bill the government deemed acceptable for reimbursement. The details of the 1965 Medicare legislation are summarized in Senate Special Committee on Aging, *Health Insurance and Related Provisions of Public Law 89–97, the Social Security Amendments of 1965*, 89th Cong., 1st sess. (Washington, D.C.: Government Printing Office, 1965).

5. Cecil King, quoted in Eugene Feingold, *Medicare: Policy and Politics: A Case Study and Policy Analysis* (San Francisco: Chandler, 1966), 182.

6. For a review of Medicare benefits policy, see Mark Schlesinger and Terrie Wetle, "Medicare's Coverage of Health Services," in *Renewing the Promise: Medicare and Its Reform*, ed. David Blumenthal, Mark Schlesinger, and Pamela Brown Drumheller (New York: Oxford University Press, 1988), 58–89.

7. Bruce C. Vladeck, *Unloving Care: The Nursing Home Tragedy* (New York: Basic Books, 1980), 47.

8. Ibid., 49.

9. Ibid.

10. Schlesinger and Wetle, "Medicare's Coverage," 58–60.

11. Ibid., 61. For a general critique of the American health care system's slant toward financing acute care (including Medicare), see Daniel M. Fox, *Power and Illness: The Failure and Future of American Health Policy* (Berkeley: University of California Press, 1993).

12. Moon, *Medicare: Now and in the Future*, 232.

13. Schlesinger and Wetle, "Medicare's Coverage," 60.

14. Moon, *Medicare: Now and in the Future*, 72–74, 231–32. Home health care covered only patients who were approved by physicians in expectation of rehabilitation. Furthermore, care had to be intermittent, meaning less than daily, and in order to qualify, beneficiaries had to be confined to the house. A 1989 court decision led to subsequent easing of these restrictions.

15. Interview with Robert Ball; interview with Jay Constantine. See also *1971 Advisory Council on Social Security* (Washington, D.C.: Government Printing Office, 1971), 64–66. On Medicare's disabled population, see Sandra M. Foote and Christopher Hogan, "Disability Levels and Health Care Costs of Medicare Beneficiaries under Age Sixty-Five," *Health Affairs* 20 (2001): 242–53.

16. Charles L. Plante, "Reflections on the Passage of the End-Stage Renal Disease Medicare Program," *American Journal of Kidney Disease* 35 (2000): S45.

17. The authoritative story of how coverage for ESRD was added to Medicare is told in Richard Rettig, "Origins of the Medicare Kidney Disease Entitlement," in *Bio-*

medical Politics, ed. Kathi Hanna (Washington, D.C.: National Academy Press, 1991), 176–208. This section draws heavily on Rettig's valuable account. For the perspectives of physicians involved in the campaign for ESRD coverage, see George E. Scheiner, "How End-Stage Renal Disease (ESRD)—Medicare Developed," *American Journal of Kidney Disease* 35 (2000): S37–S44; and Plante, "Reflections," S45–S48. For discussions of the policy issues associated with ESRD, including rising costs and quality of care, see Allan R. Nissenson and Richard Rettig, "Medicare's End Stage Renal Dialysis Program: Current Status and Future Prospects," *Health Affairs* 18 (1999): 161–79; Richard Rettig and Norman Levinsky, eds., *Kidney Failure and the Federal Government* (Washington, D.C.: National Academy Press, 1991); Paul Eggers, "A Quarter Century of Medicare Expenditures for ESRD," *Seminars in Nephrology* 20 (2000): 516–22; and Paul Eggers, "The Medicare Experience with End-Stage Renal Disease: Trends in Incidence, Prevalence, and Survival," *Health Care Financing Review* 5 (1984): 69–88.

18. Rettig, "Medicare Kidney Disease Entitlement," 177–78.

19. Ibid., 179–80.

20. Plante, "Reflections," S45–S46.

21. Scheiner, "ESRD," S39.

22. Quoted in Rettig, "Medicare Kidney Disease Entitlement," 187.

23. Ibid., 188–89; and Scheiner, "ESRD." Glazer experienced ventricular tachycardia and a serious drop in blood pressure during dialysis before the committee. The attending physician quickly clamped the lines and announced the termination of the procedure. Glazer had apparently lied to a physician about his physical condition and past difficulties with dialysis because he saw his participation in live dialysis as critical to the passage of an ESRD program.

24. Rettig, "Medicare Kidney Disease Entitlement," 189.

25. Ibid., 191.

26. Ibid., 193; Plante, "Reflections," S47–S48.

27. See the comments of former Senate Finance Committee staffer James Mongan in Plante, "Reflections," 48. Mongan was involved in designing the ERSD legislation.

28. Ibid., 48.

29. Health Care Financing Administration, *1995 Data Compendium* (Baltimore: U.S. Department of Health and Human Services).

30. At the time of the ESRD program's enactment, it was not anticipated that kidney dialysis would be used by elderly Medicare beneficiaries.

31. James Q. Wilson, *Political Organizations* (New York: Basic Books, 1973), 332.

32. For a critique of Wilson's typology of public policy based on the diffusion and concentration of benefits and costs, see Deborah A. Stone, *Policy Paradox and Political Reason* (New York: HarperCollins, 1988), 221–26.

33. See, for example, Fay Lomax Cook and Edith J. Barrett, *Support for the American Welfare State: The Views of Congress and the Public* (New York: Columbia University Press, 1992), 58–93. A 1981 ABC News—Washington Post poll found that 57% of respondents favored increasing spending on Medicare (*Public Opinion Online*, Roper Center at the University of Connecticut, March 8, 1981).

34. See the polls on long-term care in the Roper Center Public Opinion database, 1980–93. However, consistent with polling data on national health insurance, those majorities dissipated when those surveyed were asked about contributing specific, various amounts of additional income ($50–$100 a month, or $500 a year).

35. For arguments regarding the influence of public opinion on health policy, see Lawrence R. Jacobs, *The Health of Nations: Public Opinion and the Making of American and British Health Policy* (Ithaca, N.Y.: Cornell University Press, 1993).

36. Henry J. Pratt, *The Gray Lobby* (Chicago: University of Chicago Press, 1976). For a review of the political activities of interest groups representing the elderly in the United States, see Christine Day, *What Older Americans Think: Interest Groups and Aging Policy* (Princeton, N.J.: Princeton University Press, 1990). For an international comparison of old-age interest groups, see Henry J. Pratt, *Gray Agendas: Interest Groups and Public Pensions in Canada, Britain, and the United States* (Ann Arbor: University of Michigan Press, 1993).

37. Day, *What Older Americans Think,* 25. In 1983, the AARP expanded its membership to anyone over fifty, and by the end of the decade its members constituted one-third of that age group.

38. Ibid., 25–26.

39. Jeffrey M. Berry, *The Interest Group Society,* 3d ed. (New York: Addison Wesley Longman, 1997), 234.

40. Pratt, *Gray Agendas,* 1.

41. David Mayhew, *Congress: The Electoral Connection* (New Haven, Conn.: Yale University Press, 1974), 130.

42. Theda Skocpol has argued that the decentralized and federalist structure of American political institutions advantages groups that can organize across local political jurisdictions. See Theda Skocpol, *Protecting Soldiers and Mothers* (Cambridge, Mass.: Harvard University Press, 1992), 54–57.

43. Robert H. Binstock and Christine L. Day, "Aging and Politics," in *Handbook of Aging and Social Sciences,* 4th ed., ed. Robert H. Binstock and Linda George (New York: Academy Press, 1996), 362–87. However, most studies do not show significant differences between the elderly and younger populations in their support for Medicare and Social Security; the elderly are often divided among themselves. Some surveys have even found *less* support among seniors than younger Americans for increases in government benefits for the elderly. See Day, *What Older Americans Think,* 47–62.

44. Binstock and Day, "Aging and Politics,", 367.

45. For a discussion, see Moon, *Medicare: Now and in the Future.*

46. Schlesinger and Wetle, "Medicare's Coverage," 60–61.

47. Ibid., 58.

48. Social Security was exclusively financed from payroll taxes until 1983 reforms imposed a tax on higher-income beneficiaries. Medicare part A (hospitalization) is financed through payroll taxes, while part B is funded from general revenues and beneficiary premiums.

49. Martha Derthick, *Policymaking for Social Security* (Washington, D.C.: Brookings Institution Press, 1979).

50. Senate Committee on Finance, *Medicare and Medicaid,* 91st Cong., 1st sess. (Washington, D.C.: Government Printing Office, 1969), 1.

51. Schlesinger and Wetle, "Medicare's Coverage," 69–70.

52. See Richard Fenno, *Congressmen in Committees* (Boston: Little, Brown, 1973); John Manley, *The Politics of Finance* (Boston: Little, Brown, 1970); and Randall Strahan, *New Ways and Means* (Chapel Hill: University of North Carolina Press, 1990).

53. First-dollar insurance covers medical bills without patients' having to pay any out-of-pocket costs for deductibles and copayments.

54. Gail Lee Cafferata, "Private Health Insurance of the Medicare Population and the Baucus Legislation," *Medical Care* 23 (1985): 1087; and Thomas Rice, "An Economic Assessment of Health Care Coverage for the Elderly," *Milbank Quarterly* 65 (1987): 491.

55. In 1980, Congress passed the Baucus amendments regulating the Medigap market. The legislation came in response to concerns over insurance industry practices in selling supplemental insurance, including duplicative coverage, limited benefits, and marketing abuses. The Baucus amendments provided standards for voluntary state certification of Medicare supplemental insurance policies, including requirements for minimum benefits packages. See Cafferata, "Private Health Insurance," 1086–96. Although the amendments cut down on abuses in the Medigap market, comparison shopping between plans was still difficult, and in 1990 another federal law was passed that mandated that any Medigap plan fit one of ten benefits package categories. See Thomas Rice, "Supplemental Insurance and Its Role in Medicare Reform," in *Medicare Tomorrow: The Report of the Century Foundation Task Force on Medicare Reform* (New York: Century Foundation Press, 2002), 195–96.

56. Medicare beneficiaries have traditionally been responsible for paying the amount of physicians' charges beyond what the government reimburses for covered services.

57. Rice, "Economic Assessment," 493; Thomas Rice and Nelda McCall, "The Extent of Ownership and the Characteristics of Medicare Supplemental Policies," *Inquiry* 22 (summer 1985): 190; Michael Morrisey, Gail Jensen, and Stephen Henderlite, "Employer-Sponsored Health Insurance for Retired Americans," *Health Affairs* (spring 1990): 59. In addition to Medigap, the elderly also carry so-called dread-disease policies, which insure against specific diseases, and indemnity policies that provide cash benefits often linked to hospital stays. See Steven Garfinkel, Arthur Bonito, and Kenneth McElroy, "Socioeconomic Factors and Medicare Supplemental Insurance," *Health Care Financing Review* 9 (fall 1987): 22.

58. For analysis of the state of the Medicare supplemental and Medigap insurance markets a decade after the demise of catastrophic insurance, see Nadereh Pourat, Thomas Rice, Gerald Kominski, and Rani E. Snyder, "Socioeconomic Differences in Medicare Supplemental Coverage," *Health Affairs* 19 (2000): 186–96; and Rice, "Supplemental Insurance," 189–214.

59. Rice, "Economic Assessment," 491. For a discussion of employer-sponsored supplemental insurance, see Morrisey, Jensen, and Henderlite, "Employer-Sponsored Health Insurance."

60. Morrisey, Jensen, and Henderlite, "Employer-Sponsored Health Insurance."

61. Rudolf Klein, *The Politics of the National Health Service* (London: Longman, 1989), 156.

62. Ibid.

63. Garfinkel, Bonito, and McElroy, "Socioeconomic Factors," 25–27.

64. See Morrisey, Jensen, and Henderlite, "Employer-Sponsored Health Insurance."

65. Rice and McCall, "Extent of Ownership," 198.

66. Sidney Verba and Norman Nie, *Political Participation in America* (New York: Harper and Row, 1972).

67. Ibid., 13–18. For an examination of the barriers to private long-term care insurance despite public efforts to encourage its provision, see Joshua Wiener, Jane Tilly,

and Susan Goldenson, "Federal and State Initiatives to Jump Start the Market for Private Long-Term Care Insurance," *Elder Law Journal* 8 (2000): 57–102.

68. Joshua M. Wiener, Laurel Hixon Illston, and Raymond J. Hanley, *Sharing the Burden: Strategies for Public and Private Long-Term Care Insurance* (Washington, D.C.: Brookings Institution Press, 1994), 13.

69. Vladeck, *Unloving Care,* 50.

70. Ibid., 51.

71. Teresa A. Coughlin, Leighton Ku, and John Holahan, *Medicaid Since 1980* (Washington, D.C.: Urban Institute Press, 1994), 18–20.

72. Many states also paid for low-income seniors' cost-sharing burden under Medicare.

73. Schlesinger and Wetle, "Medicare's Coverage," 63–64.

74. Ibid., 65.

75. Gail Lee Cafferata, "Knowledge of Their Health Insurance Coverage by the Elderly," *Medical Care* 22 (September 1984): 835–47; Zarrel Lambert, "Elderly Consumers' Knowledge Related to Medigap Protection Needs," *Journal of Consumer Affairs* 14 (winter 1980): 434–51; Nelda McCall, Thomas Rice, and Judith Sangl, "Consumer Knowledge of Medicare and Supplemental Health Insurance Benefits," *Health Services Research* 20 (February 1986): 633–57. Knowledge of Medicare coverage is generally associated with health care utilization; services that are used the least by respondents not surprisingly tend to be those they understand least well.

76. Cafferata, "Knowledge," 846–47.

77. McCall, Rice, and Sangl, "Consumer Knowledge," 642.

78. Schlesinger and Wetle, "Medicare's Coverage," 70.

79. Robert J. Blendon, Drew E. Altman, and John Benson, "The Public's View of the Future of Medicare," *JAMA* 274 (1995): 1646.

80. This section builds on the analysis in Jonathan Oberlander, "Medicare and the American State: The Politics of Federal Health Insurance" (Ph.D. diss., Yale University, 1995), chap. 3. For accounts that similarly cover the catastrophic insurance episode, see Richard Himmelfarb, *Catastrophic Politics: The Rise and Fall of the Medicare Catastrophic Coverage Act of 1988* (University Park: Pennsylvania State University Press, 1995); Julie Rovner, "Congress's Catastrophic Attempt to Fix Medicare," in *Intensive Care: How Congress Shapes Health Policy,* ed. Thomas E. Mann and Norman Ornstein (Washington, D.C.: AEI and Brookings Institution Press, 1995), 145–78; and Moon, *Medicare: Now and in the Future,* 107–37.

81. On welfare state politics in the Reagan era, see John L. Palmer and Isabel Sawhill, *The Reagan Experiment* (Washington, D.C.: Urban Institute Press, 1982); Michael Brown, ed., *Remaking the Welfare State* (Philadelphia: Temple University Press, 1988); and Francis Fox Piven and Richard Cloward, *New Class War: Reagan's Attack on the Welfare State and Its Consequences* (New York: Pantheon, 1982). On the deficit, see Joseph White and Aaron Wildavsky, *The Deficit and the Public Interest* (Berkeley: University of California Press, 1989). The first significant cuts for Medicare proposed by the Reagan administration came in 1982. See Elizabeth Wehr, "Reagan Calls for $4 Billion Cuts In Medicare, Medicaid," *Congressional Quarterly,* February 13, 1982, 244–45.

82. David A. Stockman, *The Triumph of Politics: How the Reagan Revolution Failed* (New York: Harper and Row), 8; cited in Cook and Barrett, *Support for the American Welfare State,* 17.

83. Advisory Council on Social Security, *Medicare: Benefits on Financing* (Washington, D.C.: Government Printing Office, 1984), 46–53.

84. Ibid., 53.

85. Janet Hook, "Senate Confirms Otis Bowen as HHS Secretary," *Congressional Quarterly,* December 14, 1995, 2630. Before Bowen was nominated to Health and Human Services, he had written an article for the *Federation of American Hospitals Review* with his chief aide on the Advisory Council, Tom Burke, setting out the details of a catastrophic insurance plan for Medicare. The article was released while his confirmation was pending. See Otis Bowen and Tom Burke, "Cost Neutral Catastrophic Care Proposed for Medicare Recipients," *FAH Review* (November/December 1985): 12–25.

86. Interview with Otis Bowen, formerly secretary of health and human services, May 15, 1995.

87. Bowen interview.

88. Himmelfarb, *Catastrophic Politics,* 19.

89. Jacqueline Calmes, "Reagan's Address Repeats Familiar Themes," *Congressional Quarterly,* February 8, 1986, 261.

90. Interview with Tom Burke, formerly chief aide to Otis Bowen at Health and Human Services, May 10, 1995.

91. Richard Sorian, *The Bitter Pill* (New York: McGraw-Hill, 1988).

92. Bowen interview.

93. Sorian, *Bitter Pill,* 184–90; Bowen and Burke interviews.

94. Sorian, *Bitter Pill,* 189–90. After an initial meeting in front of the DPC where catastrophic health coverage was assailed, Bowen lobbied cabinet members in order to secure their support, or at least, to mute their opposition (Burke interview).

95. Julie Rovner, "Reagan Sides with Bowen on Medicare Plan," *Congressional Quarterly,* February 14, 1988, 115.

96. David Blumenthal, "Medicare: The Record to Date," in Blumenthal, Schlesinger, and Drumheller, *Renewing the Promise,* 26. However, the basket of medical goods and services Medicare benefits buy now is much more valuable than in the past.

97. Interview with Bill Gradison, formerly member of Congress and the House Ways and Means Committee, May 15, 1995. The conclusion that Medicare coverage had eroded received support from a growing number of academic and government studies that documented the limitations of program coverage. Researchers in the Harvard Medicare Project pointed out in a 1986 study that by the mid-1980s Medicare coverage no longer compared favorably with private health insurance policies, and the gap had widened, as Medicare continued to lack stop-loss and prescription drug coverage, protections that younger employed Americans generally enjoyed. See Blumenthal, Schlesinger, and Drumheller, *Renewing the Promise.*

98. On the electoral advantages of taking positions, see Mayhew, *Congress: The Electoral Connection,* 61–73.

99. On rationalizing politics, see Lawrence D. Brown, *New Policies, New Politics: Government's Response to Government's Growth* (Washington, D.C.: Brookings Institution Press, 1983).

100. *Report of the 1982 Advisory Council on Social Security* (Washington, D.C.: Government Printing Office, 1982), 53.

101. Julie Rovner, "Bowen: Expand Medicare to Cover Catastrophes," *Congressional Quarterly,* November 22, 1986, 2956.

102. *Medicare Catastrophic Coverage Act of 1988* (Chicago: Commerce Clearing House, 1988).

103. Bowen's experience as a family physician influenced this perception of Medicare's problems (Bowen interview).

104. Bowen interview.

105. Bowen interview; Burke interview.

106. Julie Rovner, "Democratic Leaders Slow Pace of Medicare Bill," *Congressional Quarterly*, July 4, 1987, 1437. The meeting included Dan Rostenkowski, Pete Stark, John Dingell, and Henry Waxman.

107. Rovner, "Congress's Catastrophic Attempt," 157.

108. Waxman was chair of the Subcommittee on Health and the Environment of the House Energy and Commerce Committee. Stark was chair of the Subcommittee on Health of the House Ways and Means Committee.

109. Julie Rovner, "House Panel Adds Drug Benefit to Catastrophic Insurance Bill," *Congressional Quarterly*, June 13, 1987, 1263.

110. Fewer than 50% of Medicare beneficiaries below the federal poverty line had Medicaid coverage in 1987, because many states set their Medicaid eligibility requirements at levels below the poverty line. Moon, *Medicare: Now and in the Future,* 112.

111. Rovner, "Congress's Catastrophic Attempt," 153.

112. Ibid., 158.

113. Himmelfarb, *Catastrophic Politics,* 25.

114. Interview with John Rother, director of legislative affairs, American Association of Retired Persons, May 11, 1995.

115. Moon, *Medicare: Now and in the Future,* 123.

116. Interview with Kenneth Bowler, formerly of the staff of the House Ways and Means Committee, April 8, 1991.

117. The Pharmaceutical Manufacturers Association spent three million dollars million opposing the legislation in 1987 (Rovner, "Congress's Catastrophic Attempt," 160).

118. For an excellent analysis of the social insurance contract, see Michael J. Graetz and Jerry L. Mashaw, *True Security: Rethinking American Social Insurance* (New Haven, Conn.: Yale University Press, 1999), 26–46.

119. "New Bills Introduced on Catastrophic Illness," *Congressional Quarterly,* February 28, 1987, 399.

120. Bowen interview.

121. Interview with Bill Frenzel, formerly member of Congress and member of the House Committee on Ways and Means, May 1, 1995; Bowler interview. In the debate over Medicare's enactment in the 1960s, there was considerable sentiment that Social Security taxes could not be raised past 10%—a Rubicon that was soon crossed.

122. Robert H. Binstock, "The Aged as Scapegoat," *Gerontologist* 23 (1983): 136–43; Fernando Torres-Gil, *The New Aging: Politics and Change in America* (Westport, Conn.: Auburn House, 1993); Gradison interview.

123. Quoted in Himmelfarb, *Catastrophic Politics,* 34.

124. House Ways and Means Committee, *1993 Green Book* (Washington, D.C.: Government Printing Office), 1564.

125. Cook and Barrett, Support for the American Welfare State, 21.

126. The classic statement of intergenerational equity can be found in Samuel H.

Preston, "Children and the Elderly: Divergent Paths for America's Dependents," *Demography* 21 (1984): 435–57.

127. Phillip Longman, "Justice between Generations," *Atlantic Monthly* (June): 73–81; Robert J. Samuelson, "Benefit Programs for the Elderly—Off Limits to Federal Budget Cutters?" *National Journal* (October 3): 1757–62.

128. On intergenerational politics, see John Palmer and Isabel Sawhill, eds., *The Vulnerable* (Washington, D.C.: Urban Institute Press, 1988); and Jill Quadagno, "Generational Equity and the Politics of the Welfare State," *Politics and Society* 17 (1989): 353–76.

129. *1993 Green Book,* 1313.

130. See Max. J. Skidmore, *Social Security and Its Enemies* (Boulder, Colo.: Westview Press, 1999), 85–109.

131. For a critical review of the politics of intergenerational equity, see Theodore R. Marmor, Fay Lomax Cook, and Stephen Scher, "Social Security Politics and the Conflict between Generations," in *Social Security in the Twenty-first Century,* ed. Eric Kingson and James Schulz (New York: Oxford University Press, 1997), 195–207.

132. On the myth of the affluence of the elderly, see Marilyn Moon and Janemarie Mulvey, *Entitlements and the Elderly* (Washington, D.C.: Urban Institute Press, 1996), 11–23.

133. Cook and Barrett, Support for the American Welfare State, 72–83.

134. Ibid., 230.

135. *Medicare Catastrophic Coverage Act of 1988,* 31–34.

136. Gradison interview.

137. Julie Kosterlitz, "Working with Stark," *National Journal,* July 5, 1986, 166–69.

138. Bowler interview.

139. Frenzel interview.

140. Theodore R. Marmor, *The Politics of Medicare* (Chicago: Aldine, 1973).

141. Stark and Gradison had discussed taxing the value of Medicare part B as a progressive financing mechanism, but labor opposed the precedent it would have established for taxing fringe benefits. See Rovner, "Congress's Catastrophic Attempt," 157.

142. I am drawing here on the work of John Kingdon. Kingdon has observed, in applying the research of James March and Johan Olson, that in contrast to the expectations of rational policy models, policy solutions are often attached to problems for which they were not specifically developed. See Kingdon, *Agendas, Alternatives, and Public Policies* (New York: HarperCollins, 1984), 91,186.

143. Rovner, "Congress's Catastrophic Attempt," 173.

144. Opposition came from groups representing the elderly that were disappointed by catastrophic insurance's benefits and financing, and from pharmaceutical interests concerned about government regulation that could arise from Medicare coverage of prescription drugs.

145. The only major benefits that were retained were the mandates on the states to expand Medicaid to cover the low-income elderly and pregnant women and children.

146. Morrisey, Jensen, and Henderlite, "Employer-Sponsored Health Insurance," 58.

147. Himmelfarb, *Catastrophic Politics,* 73.

148. Ibid., 77–78.

149. Ibid., 80.

150. Ibid., 61.

151. Rother interview.

152. Thomas Rice, Katherine Desmond, and John Gabel, "Medicare Catastrophic Coverage Act: A Post-Mortem," *Health Affairs* 9 (1990): 75–87; Rovner, "Congress's Catastrophic Attempt," 146.

153. The National Committee to Preserve Social Security previously had been investigated by Congress for fraudulent mailings. The group had sent out letters offering to provide a printout of elderly persons' Social Security records for a fee of ten dollars—something the Social Security Administration provides for free. See Julie Kosterlitz, "Mailouts to the Elderly Raise Alarms," *National Journal*, February 14, 1987, 378–79.

154. Rovner, "Congress's Catastrophic Attempt," 169.

155. Julie Rovner, "Long-Term Care Bill Derailed—for Now," *Congressional Quarterly*, June 11, 1988, 1604–5; Moon, *Medicare: Now and in the Future*, 130.

156. Thomas Rice and Jan Gable, "Protecting the Elderly against High Health Care Costs," *Health Affairs* (fall 1986): 7.

157. *1993 Green Book*, 144.

158. Himmelfarb, *Catastrophic Politics*, 54–56.

159. Ibid., 39.

160. Ibid., 55–56.

161. On corporatism, see Gerhard Lembruch and Philippe Schmitter, *Patterns of Corporatist Policy-Making* (London: Sage, 1982).

162. The district Rostenkowski represented, however, was hardly wealthy.

163. Annetta Miller, Mary Hager, and Betsy Roberts, "The Elderly Duke It Out," *Newsweek*, September 11, 1989. See also Bill Peterson, "Rostenkowski Heckled by Senior Citizens," *Washington Post*, August 18, 1989.

CHAPTER FOUR

1. Peter G. Peterson has been an influential voice in arguing that the aging of America puts the nation at peril. See *Gray Dawn: How the Coming Age Wave Will Transform America—and the World* (New York; Times Books, 1999), and *Will America Grow Up Before It Grows Old?* (New York: Random House, 1996). For similar perspectives, see also Lester Thurow, "The Birth of a Revolutionary Class," *New York Times Magazine*, May 19, 1996; and Richard D. Lamm, "Care for the Elderly: What about Our Children?" in *The Generational Equity Debate*, ed. John B. Williamson, Diane M. Watts-Roy, and Eric R. Kingson (New York: Columbia University Press, 1999), 87–100. For a critique of this perspective that argues the United States can afford the baby boomers without radically reforming Social Security or Medicare, see Joseph White, *False Alarm: Why the Greatest Threat to Social Security and Medicare Is the Campaign to "Save" Them* (Baltimore: Johns Hopkins University Press, 2001); Dean Baker and Mark Weisbrot, *Social Security: The Phony Crisis* (Chicago: University of Chicago Press, 1999); Theodore R. Marmor and Jerry L. Mashaw, "The Great Social Security Scare," *American Prospect* 7 (1996): 30–37; and Theodore Marmor and Jonathan Oberlander, "Rethinking Medicare Reform," *Health Affairs* 17 (1998): 52–68.

2. It is common for political analysts to speak of a "bifurcated" American welfare state, making a distinction between the politics of social insurance programs (Medicare and Social Security) and the politics of welfare programs (Aid for Families with Dependent Children and Medicaid). Social insurance programs, which are universal rather than means tested in their eligibility, are grouped together as enjoying more public support, stronger political constituencies, and better financing and administration. See Maragaret Weir, Ann Shola Orloff, and Theda Skocpol, eds., *The Politics of Social Policy in the United States* (Princeton, N.J.: Princeton University Press, 1988), 6–9, 422–23; Theda Skocpol, "The Limits of the New Deal System and the Roots of Contemporary Welfare Dilemmas," in Weir, Orloff, and Skocpol, *The Politics of Social Policy*, 293–311; Theodore R. Marmor, Jerry L. Mashaw, and Philip L. Harvey, *America's Misunderstood Welfare State* (New York: Basic Books, 1990), 22–128; and Edward D. Berkowitz, *America's Welfare State* (Baltimore: Johns Hopkins University Press, 1991).

3. Medicare's financing arrangements are summarized in Robert J. Myers, *Medicare* (Bryn Mawr, Pa.: McCahan Foundation, 1970), 154–72. See also Nancy J. Altman, "Medicare Financing: The Government's Share," in *Renewing the Promise: Medicare and Its Reform*, ed. David Blumenthal, Mark Schlesinger, and Pamela Brown Drumheller (New York: Oxford University Press, 1988), 160–75; *Medicare and Social Security Law* (Chicago: Commerce Clearing House, 1965); and Marilyn Moon, *Medicare: Now and in the Future* (Washington, D.C.: Urban Institute Press, 1993).

4. The relationship between Social Security benefits and financing is summarized in Robert J. Myers, *Social Security* (Bryn Mawr, Pa.: McCahan Foundation, 1975), 21–177.

5. For an elaboration of the differences between Medicare and Social Security financing, as well as a critique of Medicare financing principles, see Advisory Council on Social Security (1979), "Social Security Financing," *Social Security Bulletin* 45, no. 5 (May 1980): 18–29.

6. Ibid.

7. Martha Derthick has posed exactly this puzzle about the reliance on payroll taxes in Social Security. See Derthick, *Policymaking for Social Security* (Washington, D.C.: Brookings Institution Press, 1979), 228.

8. On the influence of European social insurance models on American reformers, see Daniel T. Rodgers, *Atlantic Crossings: Social Politics in A Progressive Age* (Cambridge, Mass.: Harvard University Press, 1998). For an account of the U.S. social insurance movement, see Theda Skocpol, *Protecting Soldiers and Mothers: The Political Origins of Social Policy in the United States* (Cambridge, Mass.: Harvard University Press, 1992), 154–310; and Roy Lubove, *The Struggle for Social Security, 1900–1935* (Cambridge, Mass.: Harvard University Press, 1968). More generally, on the Progressive period in American politics, see Richard McCormick, *The Party Period and Public Policy* (New York: Oxford University Press, 1986), 263–356.

9. The history, principles, and goals of social insurance are discussed in I. M. Rubinow, *Social Insurance* (New York: Henry Holt and Company, 1916). In one key respect, social insurance differed from private insurance: compulsory participation. See Lubove, Struggle for Social Security, 4–5.

10. Michael J. Graetz and Jerry L. Mashaw, *True Security: Rethinking American Social Insurance* (New Haven, Conn.: Yale University Press, 1999), 16–17. Common sources of market failure include adverse selection, moral hazard, asymmetry of information, and market segmentation by risk.

11. Ibid., 26.

12. Lubove, *Struggle for Social Security*, 1–24. Lubove defines voluntarism as "organized action by nonstatutory institutions." It emphasized private activity, such as charity, as an alternative to government action. Voluntarism was connected to laissez-faire, individualist ideology.

13. Rubinow, *Social Insurance*, 481.

14. Graetz and Mashaw, *True Security*, 19.

15. Derthick, *Policymaking*, 228–31.

16. Rubinow, Social Insurance, 491.

17. Daniel S. Hirshfield, *The Lost Reform: The Campaign for Compulsory Health Insurance in the United States from 1932 to 1943* (Cambridge, Mass.: Harvard University Press, 1970).

18. Theda Skocpol links the political failures of the American social insurance movement to institutional features of the American political system that complicated enactment of reforms (such as the absence of a developed national bureaucracy and the prominent role played by courts) and to the disenchantment with the U.S. Civil War pension system, which was associated with the excesses of patronage democracy. See Skocpol, *Soldiers and Mothers*, 248–310. Daniel Hirshfield and Roy Lubove alternatively emphasize the constraints of American ideology, particularly the tenacity of "voluntarism," which favored private charity and assistance to government programs as a response to social problems, and stressed individual liberty and responsibility.

19. For accounts of the enactment of Social Security, see J. Douglas Brown, *An American Philosophy of Social Security* (Princeton, N.J.: Princeton University Press, 1972); Lubove, *Struggle for Social Security;* and Edwin Witte, *The Development of the Social Security Act* (Madison: University of Wisconsin Press, 1963). For accounts of the subsequent development of Social Security, see W. Andrew Achenbaum, *Social Security: Visions and Revisions* (Cambridge: Cambridge University Press, 1986); Merton C. Bernstein and Joan Brodshaug Bernstein, *Social Security: The System That Works* (New York: Basic Books, 1988); Derthick, *Policymaking;* Eric Kingson and Edward Berkowitz, *Social Security and Medicare: A Policy Primer* (Westport, Conn.: Auburn House, 1993); and Marmor, Mashaw, and Harvey, *America's Misunderstood Welfare State.*

20. *The Report of the Committee on Economic Security of 1935: 50th Anniversary Edition* (Washington, D.C.: National Conference on Social Welfare, 1985), 17. Besides Perkins, the Committee on Economic Security included Attorney General Homer Cummings, Secretary of Agriculture Henry Wallace, Federal Emergency Relief Administrator Harry Hopkins, and Secretary of Treasury Henry Morgenthau. Edwin Witte, a University of Wisconsin economics professor, served as executive director of the CES. Other members of the staff included Robert Myers, subsequently chief actuary for the Social Security Administration, and Wilbur Cohen, one of the designers of Medicare. Assistant Secretary of Labor Arthur Altmeyer, subsequently chief administrator of Social Security, was also active as chair of the CES Technical Board.

21. Ibid., 43–55. See also Brown, *An American Philosophy,* 6–24; and Witte, *Development of the Social Security Act.*

22. Derthick, *Policymaking,* 228.

23. Martha Derthick argues that the public was encouraged to see Social Security as "a vast enterprise of self-help in which government participation was almost incidental" (ibid., 232). In other words, Derthick argues the money in the trust fund was

not regarded as government money, but instead the trust fund was seen as a collection of individual pension accounts accumulated by participants in the system. Derthick almost certainly overstates this case; Social Security was still identified by the public as a government program.

24. Michael Katz, *In the Shadow of the Poorhouse: A Social History of Welfare in America* (New York: Basic Books, 1986). On the importance of perceptions of political culture to the formulation of Medicare, see Lawrence R. Jacobs, *The Health of Nations: Public Opinion and the Making of American and British Health Policy* (Ithaca, N.Y.: Cornell University Press, 1993), 88–90; and Theodore Marmor, *The Politics of Medicare* (Chicago: Aldine, 1973), 14–23.

25. Derthick, *Policymaking,* 231.

26. Ibid., 229.

27. The 2.5% refer to the rate of payroll taxes applied to both employers and workers; the combined tax rate that was regarded as a limit was thus 5%.

28. Ibid., 230.

29. Myers, *Medicare,* 25–28. Roosevelt also advocated self-supporting financing in order to preempt criticism that Social Security would exacerbate budgetary deficits (interview with Robert Myers, formerly chief actuary of the Social Security Administration, July 8, 1995).

30. Marmor, *The Politics of Medicare,* 13–14.

31. Social Security financing had been previously extended, in 1956, to disability insurance, which was funded by a .25% increase in payroll taxes. The campaign for disability insurance served as a prelude to Medicare. See Derthick, *Policymaking,* 295–315.

32. Marmor, *The Politics of Medicare,* 14–23.

33. This same argument was made for Social Security. See Derthick, *Policymaking,* 239.

34. Mills quoted in Julian E Zelizer, *Taxing America: Wilbur D. Mills, Congress, and the State, 1945–1975* (Cambridge: Cambridge University Press, 1998), 206.

35. Ibid., 213.

36. Edward D. Berkowitz, *Mr. Social Security* (Lawrence: University Press of Kansas, 1995), 229.

37. Zelizer, *Taxing America,* 213.

38. On the role of Mills in shaping Medicare's financing provisions, see Eric Patashnik and Julian Zelizer, "Paying for Medicare: Benefits, Budgets, and Wilbur Mills's Policy Legacy," *Journal of Health Politics, Policy, and Law* 26(2001): 8–36.

39. Interview with Robert Ball, former Social Security commissioner, March 25, 2002.

40. Interview with Robert Myers, March 25, 2002.

41. See Senate Committee on Finance, *Medicare and Medicaid: Hearings before the Committee on Finance,* July 1–2, 1969 (Washington, D.C.: Government Printing Office, 1969), *Medicare and Medicaid: Hearings before the Committee on Finance,* February 25–26, 1970 (Washington, D.C.: Government Printing Office, 1970), and *Medicare and Medicaid: Hearings before the Subcommittee on Medicare-Medicaid of the Committee on Finance,* April 14–15, May 26–27, June 2, 3,15–16 (Washington, D.C.: Government Printing Office, 1970); Elizabeth Wehr, "Congress Seeks Elusive Cure for Medicare Financial Ills," *Congressional Quarterly,* April 14, 1984, 841–44; and "Health Care Policy Briefing," *Roll Call,* June 19, 1995.

42. Advisory Council on Social Security (1982), *Medicare: Benefits and Financing: Report of the 1982 Advisory Council on Social Security* (Washington, D.C.: Government Printing Office, 1984).

43. The 1982–84 and 1995 periods of media attention to Medicare crises were identified through a search of Nexis, a computerized database of national newspapers and magazines. Because Nexis does not go back to 1970, it was impossible to confirm media attention to Medicare's financial crisis at that time. The *New York Times* index, which does go back that far, did not indicate media attention in 1969–70 on the same scale as that in the other two cases.

44. For a comprehensive look at trust fund financing in the United States, see Eric Patashnik, *Putting Trust in the U.S. Budget: Federal Trust Funds and the Politics of Commitment* (Cambridge: Cambridge University Press, 2000).

45. For an account of the Social Security crisis, see Paul Light, *Artful Work: The Politics of Social Security Reform* (New York: Random House, 1985). See also Achenbaum, *Social Security,* 61–99; and Bernstein and Bernstein, *The System That Works,* 32–60.

46. Paul Pierson, "Policy Feedbacks and Political Change: Contrasting Reagan and Thatcher's Pension-Reform Initiatives," *Studies in American Political Development* 6 (fall 1992): 360.

47. Ibid., 69.

48. The board of trustees for the hospitalization insurance trust fund is composed of six members, including the secretaries of health and human services, labor, and the treasury, the commissioner of the Social Security Administration, and two public trustees appointed by the president. The administrator of the Health Care Financing Administration serves as secretary of the board. Similar actuarial reports are prepared in the Social Security Administration for the old-age, survivors, and disability insurance trust funds.

49. Of course, Medicare funds are not exhausted in the sense that the program has no revenues. The payroll taxes collected from current workers and their employers guarantee that Medicare receives annual income. Exhaustion means that these funds are not sufficient to cover costs—in other words, Medicare is in deficit.

50. George Buck, "Actuarial Soundness in Trusteed and Governmental Retirement Plans," *Proceedings of Panel Meeting: "What Is Actuarial Soundness in a Pension Plan?"* sponsored by the American Statistics Association, the American Association of University Teachers of Insurance, and the Industrial Relations Research Association, Chicago, December 29, 1952. Quoted in Myers, *Social Security,* 140.

51. Interview with Robert Myers, August 1, 1995.

52. These conservative assumptions were ended in 1971, and this change was partly responsible for the financing problems that developed in Social Security in the mid-1970s. See Martha Derthick, *Policymaking,* 228–51, 381–411.

53. The actuarial practices in Social Security are summarized in Myers, *Medicare,* 135–77.

54. Interview with Robert J. Myers, August 1, 1995.

55. However, Medicare continued to make forecasts for twenty-five-year periods. In 1984, Medicare actuaries began to make forecasts for seventy-five-year periods, in addition to the traditional twenty-five-year forecasts. This change came about despite the fact that federal actuaries had previously discounted the value of seventy-five-year forecasts for Medicare.

56. Myers, *Medicare,* 154–72, 185–218.

57. This stabilizing influence was present at the time of Medicare's enactment and remained as such until the early 1970s.

58. Myers interview, August 1, 1995. Robert Myers was chief actuary of the Social Security Administration from 1950 to 1970. On actuarial influence and Social Security, see Derthick, *Policymaking*, 170–82, 244–46.

59. Not only do actuaries set the parameters of funding debates, but their pronouncements on the fiscal consequences of proposed reforms are influential.

60. Nelson Polsby, *Political Innovation in America* (New Haven, Conn.: Yale University Press, 1984).

61. Paul Pierson, *Dismantling the Welfare State* (Cambridge: Cambridge University Press, 1994), 65–66.

62. Caroll Estes, "Social Security: The Social Construction of a Crisis," *Milbank Memorial Fund Quarterly* 61 (1983): 445–61. On the social construction of crises more generally, see Murray Edelman, *The Symbolic Uses of Politics* (Urbana: University of Illinois Press, 1964); and Joseph R. Gusfield, *The Culture of Public Problems* (Chicago: University of Chicago Press, 1981).

63. Interview with Jay Constantine, formerly of the staff of the Senate Finance Committee, October 27, 1994.

64. Review of the first thirty years of annual reports of the board of trustees of the hospitalization insurance trust fund produced not one reference to "crisis" in Medicare finances. See *Annual Reports of the Board of Trustees of the Hospitalization Insurance Trust Fund, 1966–95.*

65. There is a substantial literature on the psychology of decision making that analyzes how people think numerically. See Daniel Kahneman, Paul Slovic, and Amos Tversky, eds., *Judgment under Uncertainty: Heuristics and Biases* (New York: Cambridge University Press, 1982).

66. There were six such councils from 1937 to 1971; thereafter, they were required by law to be appointed every four years. The councils, which review Social Security and Medicare operations and make recommendations for program reforms, have traditionally been composed of representatives from labor, employers, and the public. In Social Security, they have served as a corporatist arena for contending political interests to reach consensus and as a mechanism for the executive leadership of the Social Security Administration to co-opt social interests in support of their own programmatic agenda. See Derthick, *Policymaking*, 89–109.

67. The role of the Social Security advisory councils is summarized in Derthick, *Policymaking*, 89–109.

68. Advisory Council on Social Security (1975), *Reports of the Advisory Council on Social Security* (Washington, D.C.: Government Printing Office, 1975), 60.

69. Ibid., 82.

70. Advisory Council on Social Security (1979), *Reports of the 1979 Advisory Council on Social Security* (Washington, D.C.: Government Printing Office 1979), and "Social Security Financing," *Social Security Bulletin* 43, no. 5 (May 1980): 18–29.

71. Unfortunately, polling on willingness to pay Medicare payroll taxes or support for additional general revenue financing has been sporadic, peaking in the early to mid-1980s and later dropping off. See Roper Public Opinion Online for a complete list of these polls.

72. National Commission on Social Security, Peter D. Hart Research Associates poll, November 1979; Opinion Research Corporation, September 1981.

73. Constantine interview.. On Social Security, see Derthick, *Policymaking*, 239.

74. The quote is taken from a dissenting statement on Medicare financing written by three members of the 1971 Social Security advisory council: Charles Siegfried of Metropolitan Life Insurance, Robert Tyson of U.S. Steel, and Dwight Wilbur, former president of the American Medical Association. See 1971 Advisory Council, 105.

75. Advisory Council on Social Security (1982), *Medicare: Benefits and Financing* (Washington, D.C.: Government Printing Office, 1984), 2.

76. Constantine interview.

77. In a 1981 Cambridge Reports poll, only 13% of the public selected raising payroll taxes as their "most favored" way of resolving programs' financial difficulties; in 1982 that number dropped to 10%, though in both cases majorities favored the introduction of general revenues. See Roper Public Opnion Online Archives.

78. Cambridge Reports, Research International, October 1984; Roper Public Opinion Online.

79. Benjamin I. Page and Robert Y. Shapiro, *The Rational Public* (Chicago: University of Chicago Press), 130–31; Robert J. Blendon and Mollyann Brodie, "Public Opinion and Health Policy," In Theodore J. Litman and Leonard S. Robins, eds., *Health Politics and Policy*, 3d ed. (Albany, N.Y.: Delmar, 1997), 205.

80. Employee Benefit Research Gallup Institute polls, 1990, 1992, 1993; Roper Public Opinion Online.

81. Ibid.

82. 1986 AMA survey; Roper Public Opinion Online.

83. On the influence of the wording of questions, see Page and Shapiro, *Rational Public*, 29–30, 39–40.

84. Fay Lomax Cook and Edith J. Barrett, *Support for the American Welfare State: The View of Congress and the Public* (New York: Columbia University Press, 1992), 90; see also 58–145.

85. For a discussion of intergenerational equity, see chap. 3.

86. This conclusion must remain tentative because of the lack of consistent public opinion studies on Medicare, though it is supported by existing work, as summarized in Cook and Barrett, *Support for the American Welfare State*.

87. In addition to the deductible for hospitalization coverage, beneficiaries also must pay coinsurance for hospital stays that are longer than sixty days.

88. Moon, *Medicare: Now and in the Future*, 82.

89. Ibid., 214.

90. It is difficult to attribute the limited reliance on increases in beneficiary cost sharing to the power of interest groups representing the elderly. The reason is that in Medicare physicians' insurance there have been quite substantial premium increases imposed on beneficiaries.

91. In five polls conducted between 1981 and 1995, support for cutting benefits or imposing higher costs on wealthier beneficiaries exceeded opposition in every poll, with a high of 70% of respondents to a 1990 NBC/Wall Street Journal poll favoring taxing or cutting benefits for Medicare beneficiaries with incomes over one hundred thousand dollars. See Roper Public Opinion Online.

92. See Moon, *Medicare: Now and in the Future*, 180–81.

93. On professional standard review organizations, see Karen Davis, Gerard E. Anderson, Diane Rowland, and Earl P. Steinberg, *Health Care Cost Containment* (Baltimore: Johns Hopkins University Press, 1990), pp. 20–22. On the prospective pay-

ment system, see David G. Smith, *Paying for Medicare: The Politics of Reform* (New York: Aldine de Gruyter, 1992). For a review of Medicare regulation that analyzes the significance of both PSROs and the PPS, see Lawrence Brown, "Technocratic Corporatism and Administrative Reform in American Medicine," *Journal of Health Politics, Policy and Law* 10, no. 3 (fall 1985): 579–99.

94. Actually, to the extent that regulatory reforms slow down the rate of increase in Medicare spending, they save beneficiaries money by reducing through cost-sharing provisions the total bill of which they will have to pay a share. This logic, however, is rarely acknowledged in the debate over Medicare spending.

95. For a discussion of these international efforts, and their implications for the United States, see Joseph White, *Competing Solutions: American Health Care Proposals and International Experience* (Washington, D.C.: Brookings Institution Press, 1995). See also William Glaser, *Health Insurance in Practice* (San Francisco: Jossey-Bass, 1991); and Theodore R. Marmor, *Understanding Health Care Reform* (New Haven, Conn.: Yale University Press, 1994).

96. Interviews with William Roper and Nancy-Ann Deparle, formerly chief administrators, Health Care Financing Administration.

97. John Kingdon, *Agendas, Alternatives, and Public Policies* (New York: Harper-Collins, 1984).

CHAPTER FIVE

1. Theodore Marmor, *Political Analysis and American Medical Care* (Cambridge: Cambridge University Press, 1983), 61–75.

2. *Medicare and Social Security Law* (Chicago: Commerce Clearing House, 1965), 2811.

3. Theodore Marmor, *The Politics of Medicare* (Chicago: Aldine, 1973), 15. On the opposition of the AMA to Medicare and the politics of Medicare's enactment, see also, Peter A. Corning, *The Evolution of Medicare: From Idea to Law* (Washington, D.C.: Government Printing Office, 1969); Sheri I. David, *With Dignity: The Search for Medicare and Medicaid* (Westport, Conn.: Greenwood, 1985); Eugene Feingold, *Medicare: Policy and Politics: A Case Study and Policy Analysis* (San Francisco: Chandler, 1966); Richard Harris, *A Sacred Trust* (New York: New American Library, 1966); Lawrence R. Jacobs, *The Health of Nations: Public Opinion and the Making of American and British Health Policy* (Ithaca, N.Y.: Cornell University Press, 1993); and Max J. Skidmore, *Medicare and the American Rhetoric of Reconciliation* (University: University of Alabama Press, 1970).

4. Marmor, *The Politics of Medicare*, 15–16.

5. *Medicare and Social Security Law*, 2815.

6. As private insurance for hospital services spread across the United States in the 1930s and 1940s, hospitals were typically paid by insurers according to what the hospitals charged patients. Insurers, the most important being the nonprofit Blue Cross associations, reimbursed hospitals for a percentage of charges determined in negotiations between the insurers and hospitals. Payment based on "reasonable costs" replaced negotiated reimbursement of charges in the 1950s as the prevailing method of hospital payment. Reasonable-cost reimbursement sought to measure actual hospital costs for treating patients and to define what constituted the "allowable costs" that hospitals could bill to insurers. In 1953, the American Hospital Association (AHA), the primary

organization representing the hospital industry, endorsed the use of reasonable-cost reimbursement and issued guidelines for its operation.

7. However, there had not been much attention to how the federal government would pay for physician services, since it had been assumed that these services would not be part of Medicare. From the initial drafting of Medicare in 1957 until 1964, proposals for federal health insurance for the aged were limited to hospitalization insurance.

8. *Medicare and Social Security Law*, 2820.

9. Interview with Theodore Marmor, formerly special assistant to Wilbur Cohen, April 17, 2002.

10. Ibid.

11. Interview with Arthur Hess, director of the Bureau of Health Insurance of the Social Security Administration (1966–67), December 19, 1994.

12. Medicare statute 1842(b).

13. Marmor, *The Politics of Medicare*, 85.

14. In addition, physicians retained the right to bill Medicare patients for amounts in excess of the "reasonable charges" for which they were reimbursed by the federal government.

15. *Medicare and Social Security Law*, 2816–17, 2827.

16. Blue Cross began in the 1930s as a nonprofit insurance company sponsored by hospitals during the depression in order to address financial shortfalls brought on by the inability of middle-class patients to pay for medical care. For accounts of its origins, and the subsequent development of Blue Shield insurance for physician services, see Sylvia A. Law, *Blue Cross: What Went Wrong?* (New Haven, Conn.: Yale University Press, 1974); and Paul Starr, *The Social Transformation of American Medicine* (New York: Basic Books, 1982).

17. The role of private intermediaries in Medicare administration is discussed in Law, *What Went Wrong?* 31–46.

18. See especially the special winter 1991 issue (vol. 16, no. 4) of the *Journal of Health Politics, Policy, and Law* on Blue Cross and Blue Shield; Law, *What Went Wrong?* 6–30; and Lawrence D. Brown, "Capture and Culture: Organizational Identity in New York Blue Cross," *Journal of Health Politics, Policy and Law* 16 (1991): 651–70.

19. On Blue Cross's self-promotion of the voluntary way as a bulwark against national health insurance, see David J. Rothman, *Beginnings Count: The Technological Imperative in American Health Care* (New York: Oxford University Press, 1997).

20. My thanks to Lawrence Brown for emphasizing this point.

21. Ibid., 34–40.

22. Jacobs, *Health of Nations*, 156.

23. Hess interview.

24. Hess interview. Physicians opposed disability insurance as a first step to "socialized medicine" because it would lead to federal involvement in medical determinations of eligibility. See Martha Derthick, *Policymaking for Social Security* (Washington, D.C.: Brookings Institution Press, 1979), 300–304.

25. Interview with Robert Ball.

26. Robert Ball, *A Report of the Implementation of the Social Security Amendments of 1965,* November 15, 1965. Reproduced in National Academy of Social In-

surance, *Reflections on Implementing Medicare* (Washington, D.C.: National Academy of Social Insurance, 1993).

27. Ibid.

28. Quoted in Law, *What Went Wrong?* 34.

29. Judith M. Feder, *Medicare: The Politics of Federal Hospital Insurance* (Lexington, Mass.: D. C. Heath, 1977).

30. Ibid.

31. The politics of Medicare's implementation are analyzed in Feder, *Medicare*. See also Law, *What Went Wrong?* and Herman M. Somers and Anne R. Somers, *Medicare and the Hospitals* (Washington, D.C.: Brookings Institution Press, 1967).

32. Feder, *Medicare*, 66.

33. Ibid.

34. Ibid., 134–35.

35. It was the Senate Finance Committee, rather than the House Committee on Ways and Means, that served as the primary source of congressional oversight on Medicare during the program's first decade of operation. This is somewhat puzzling given the predominance of Ways and Means in Medicare's enactment. One explanation of the reversal of roles may be that the Senate Finance Committee became active in Medicare's implementation *because* of its lack of influence over Medicare's enactment. Wilbur Mills, chair of Ways and Means, used his position to shape the 1965 Medicare statute to his specifications. Russell Long, chair of the Senate Finance Committee, was far less satisfied with the outcomes of 1965 and consequently became far more critical of its early implementation than Mills. The difference between the two committees' oversight of Medicare is exemplified by the fact that the Finance Committee hired a staffer for Medicare policy in 1966, while Ways and Means did not do so until 1970. This discrepancy in staff resources reinforced the predominance of Senate Finance Committee oversight of Medicare's early operation.

36. The report was officially requested by Senator John Williams, the senior Republican on the Senate Finance Committee, in 1969. Russell Long was intimately involved with the 1960–70 activities, and, in general, there was a bipartisan consensus on the committee that Medicare needed reform (interview with Jay Constantine, formerly of the staff of the Senate Finance Committee, October 27, 1994). Much of the actual work documenting the problems in Medicare and offering solutions was done by Jay Constantine, the committee's chief staff person for Medicare, working with Bill Fullerton, then of the Library of Congress Research Services, and Tom Vail, also on the Senate Finance Committee staff. Because of the key role played by the staff in these events and the level of support they received from Long and others, it is virtually impossible to distinguish the committee's preferences from the staff's. As a consequence, all references to the Senate Finance Committee in this section are meant to signify both senators and the staff as part of a bipartisan critique of Medicare. It should be noted that while the hearings and report were also concerned with Medicaid, I focus here only on their relevance for Medicare.

37. *Medicare and Medicaid: Problems, Issues, and Alternatives,* report of the staff to the Committee on Finance, U.S. Senate, 91st Cong. (Washington, D.C.: Government Printing Office, 1970), 9, 62, 81–88. See also Senate Committee on Finance, *Medicare and Medicaid: Hearings before the Committee on Finance,* July 1–2, 1969 (Washington, D.C.: Government Printing Office, 1969), and *Medicare and Medicaid: Hearings*

before the Committee on Finance, February 25–26, 1970 (Washington, D.C.: Government Printing Office, 1970).

38. Senate Committee on Finance, *Medicare and Medicade Hearings,* February 25–26, 1970 113–20.

39. Constantine interview.

40. Starr, *Social Transformation,* 399–400.

41. Constantine interview.

42. Ibid.

43. Jay Constantine, statement for the Subcommittee on Health of the Senate Committee on Finance, March 23, 1981.

44. Bennett was influenced by the model of "medical care foundations," which reviewed the medical care received by Medicaid patients in twenty states in 1970. See Starr, *Social Transformation,* 400.

45. In addition to Medicare patients, PSROs were to review the care received by patients from the Medicaid and Maternal and Child Health programs.

46. *Floor Manager's Book, U.S. Senate, Medicare-Medicaid Amendments of 1972,* H.R. 1.

47. For a summary of the origins of PSROs and the 1970 Bennett proposal, see Wallace Bennett, *Congressional Record,* July 1, 1970; and *Social Security Amendments of 1972,* House of Representatives Report 92–1605, October 14, 1972.

48. Constantine interview.

49. See Starr, *Social Transformation,* 400.

50. The PSRO bill actually passed the Senate in 1971, but congressional enactment was delayed by continued debate over other features of the Social Security amendments, chiefly welfare.

51. Starr, *Social Transformation,* 400–401.

52. See Karen Davis, Gerard E. Anderson, Diane Rowland, and Earl P. Steinberg, *Health Care Cost Containment* (Baltimore: Johns Hopkins University Press, 1990), 22.

53. Congressional Budget Office, *The Effect of PSROs on Health Care Costs: Current Findings and Future Evaluations* (Washington, D.C.: Government Printing Office, 1979).

54. Spencer Rich, "Who Should Police Hospitals and Doctors? Senators Rescue Medical Review Program," *Washington Post,* November 29, 1983.

55. Rich, "Who Should Police Hospitals"; Spencer Rich, "Excess Profits for Monitoring Medicare," *Washington Post,* June 2, 1987; David Zimman, "Doctors Judging Doctors," *Newsday,* March 15, 1989.

56. On the politics of implementation, see Jeffrey L. Pressman and Aaron B. Wildavsky, *Implementation: How Great Expectations in Washington Are Dashed in Oakland* (Berkeley: University of California Press, 1993).

57. On this point, see Eliot Friedson, *Doctoring Together: A Study of Professional Social Control* (New York: Elsevier, 1975).

58. Senate Committee on Finance, *Social Security Amendments of 1972: Report of the Committee on Finance,* (Washington, D.C.: Government Printing Office, 1972). For a summary of the amendments, see Lawrence D. Brown, "Technocratic Corporatism and Administrative Reform in American Medicine," *Journal of Health Politics, Policy and Law* 10, no. 3 (fall 1985): 579–99; and Davis et al., *Cost Containment,* 17–25.

59. In 1970, Medicare expenditures accounted for 3.5% of the federal budget, and

by 1975 they had risen to 4.2% (House Committe on Ways and Means, *1994 Green Book* [Washington, D.C.: Government Printing Office, 1994]).

60. See Paul Starr's analysis of medical care inflation in the United States during the 1980s in *The Logic of Health Care Reform* (New York: Penguin, 1994).

61. The most comprehensive account of the adoption of the prospective payment system, as well as the Medicare fee schedule, is in David G. Smith, *Paying for Medicare: The Politics of Reform* (New York: Aldine de Gruyter, 1992).

62. *Medicare and Medicaid: Problems, Issues, and Alternatives*, 47–48, 89; Senate Committee on Finance, *Social Security Amendments of 1972.*

63. Davis et al., *Cost Containment*, 24.

64. Ibid. On subsequent problems and issues in state rate-setting experiments, see John E. McDonough, *Interests, Ideas, and Deregulation: The Fate of Hospital Rate Setting* (Ann Arbor: University of Michigan Press, 1997).

65. The New Jersey experience with DRGs and its influence on Medicare is elaborated in James Morone and Andrew Dunham, "Slouching to National Health Insurance," *Yale Journal on Regulation* 2, no. 2 (fall 1985), 263–91.

66. Smith, *Paying for Medicare*, 33. The DRG project was funded from a federal grant authorized by the 1972 Social Security Amendments.

67. Prospective payment means setting predetermined rates for hospital reimbursement. There are, however, multiple methodologies available for calculating prospective rates—DRGs represent just one of these methodologies.

68. According to David Smith, Richard Schweiker, secretary of health and human services, had a meeting with the president of the American Hospital Association, Jack Owen, in 1982, during the time when Schweiker was searching for a prospective payment methodology. Owen had been president of the New Jersey hospital association and recommended DRGs to the secretary. This led Schweiker to push for DRGs as the basis for the Medicare prospective payment, helping their supporters within the Health Care Financing Administration (which replaced the Bureau of Health Insurance as the administrative agency for Medicare in 1977) to overcome proponents of other payment methodologies. During the late 1970s and early 1980s, Health Care Financing Administration researchers had continued to work on refining the DRG methodology. See Smith, *Paying for Medicare*, 42–43.

69. Karen Davis and Diane Rowland, *Medicare Policy: New Directions for Health and Long-Term Care* (Baltimore: Johns Hopkins University Press, 1986), 41.

70. On the political battle over the Carter hospital cost containment proposals, see Nicholas Laham, *Why the United States Lacks a National Health Insurance Program* (Westport, Conn.: Praeger, 1993); and Davis et al., *Cost Containment*, 25–32.

71. Jeff Goldsmith, "Death of a Paradigm: The Challenge of Competition," *Health Affairs* 3, no. 3 (1984): 5–19.

72. Davis et al., *Cost Containment*, 30.

73. John Kingdon has identified the convergence between problems, alternatives, and politics as critical to explaining why policies are adopted. See John Kingdon, *Agendas, Alternatives, and Public Policies* (New York: HarperCollins, 1984).

74. On the ideology and budgetary goals of the Reagan administration, see David A. Stockman, *Triumph of Politics: How the Reagan Revolution Failed* (New York: Harper and Row, 1986).

75. For an account of the Reagan administration's flirtation with market-based

health reform, see Richard Sorian, *The Bitter Pill: Tough Choices in America's Health Policy* (New York: McGraw-Hill, 1988).

76. This question is analyzed in Thomas Oliver, "Health Care Market Reform in Congress: The Uncertain Path from Proposal to Policy," *Political Science Quarterly* 106 (fall): 453–77.

77. Ibid.; and Smith, *Paying for Medicare.*

78. This antigovernment ideology, however, ruled out so-called all-payer medical care regulation, such as the Carter hospital proposals, that would go beyond Medicare and Medicaid to regulate private patients.

79. Joseph White, "Budgeting and Health Policymaking," in *Intensive Care: How Congress Shapes Health Policy,* ed. Thomas E. Mann and Norman I. Ornstein (Washington, D.C.: American Enterprise Institute and Brookings Institution Press), 61. As White argues, when government is already paying for program expenditures, regulation is a more desirable alternative for conservatives than when it is to be imposed in new areas of policymaking.

80. Smith, *Paying for Medicare,* 37–47.

81. In other words, hospitalization episodes were classified according to the primary diagnosis of the patient and the government reimbursed hospitals according to the predetermined rate for that given diagnosis.

82. The dual political appeal of DRGs is analyzed in Morone and Dunham, "Slouching," 277. For a critique of prospective payment's efficiency aspirations, see David Frankford, "The Medicare DRGs: Efficiency and Organizational Rationality," *Yale Journal on Regulation* 10 (1993): 300–371.

83. The prospective payment reforms were attached to the 1983 Social Security amendments, which not only obscured their visibility, but also aided in their enactment by linking them to legislation that was viewed as "must-pass."

84. Davis et al., *Cost Containment,* 34–39.

85. Smith, *Paying for Medicare,* 28–31.

86. Brown, "Technocratic Corporatism," 593.

87. Morone and Dunham, "Slouching," 263. Most members of Congress outside the health subcommittees that were involved in Medicare policymaking understood little about the Medicare reforms. See Smith, *Paying for Medicare.*

88. Prospective Payment Assessment Commission, *Medicare and the American Health Care System: Report to Congress* (Washington, D.C.: Prospective Payment Assessment Commission, 1995), 20–22. The growing disparity between Medicare and private payers in the payment-to-cost ratio indicated cost shifting, efforts by medical providers to recoup their lost Medicare income from the private sector.

89. These are imperfect measures, since there is often a loose relationship between what hospitals spend on Medicare patients and what they define as "costs." Still, the measure does provide the basis for comparing trends in hospital margins and Medicare payments over time.

90. Medicare Payment Advisory Commission, *Report to the Congress: Medicare Payment Policy* (Washington, D.C.: Medicare Payment Advisory Commission, 1998), 54. On the cost savings of Medicare prospective payment, see Stuart Guterman, "Prospective Payment, Medicare Spending and Hospital Costs: The Impact of Medicare PPS" (paper presented at the Rutgers University Health Care Policy and Regulation Workshop, March 17, 1995); Judith Lave, "The Impact of the Medicare Prospective

Payment System and Recommendations for Change," *Yale Journal on Regulation* 7, no. 2 (1990) 499–528; Marilyn Moon, *Medicare: Now and in the Future* (Washington, D.C.: Urban Institute Press, 1993); and Louise B. Russell, *Medicare's New Hospital Payment System: Is It Working?* (Washington, D.C.: Brookings Institution Press, 1989).

91. On deficit politics in the 1980s, see Joseph White and Aaron Wildavsky, *The Deficit and the Public Interest* (Berkeley: University of California Press, 1989).

92. Brown, "Technocratic Corporatism."

93. Arnold Epstein and David Blumenthal, "Physician Payment Reform: Past and Future," *Milbank Quarterly* 71, no. 2 (1993): 195.

94. Thomas Oliver, "Analysis, Advice and Congressional Leadership: The Physician Payment Review Commission and the Politics of Medicare," *Journal of Health Politics, Policy and Law* 18, no. 1 (spring 1993): 117–21. Oliver argues that the success of Medicare prospective payment for hospitals persuaded policymakers that a similar regulatory approach might work as well for physician reimbursement.

95. Julie Rovner, "Doctor Bills Are Next Target for Cost-Control Efforts," *Congressional Quarterly*, February 25, 1989, 386. See also Thomas Rice and Jill Bernstein, "Volume Performance Standards: Can They Control Growth in Medicare Services," *Milbank Quarterly* 68, no. 3 (1990): 300–301; and Epstein and Blumenthal, "Physician Payment Reform," 193–215.

96. There was strong sentiment in the Reagan administration for capitation, which would prepay a fixed amount for all the physician care received by a beneficiary during the year. Others favored adapting DRGs for physician services. See Smith, *Paying for Medicare*, 138–53; and Sorian, *Bitter Pill*.

97. Smith, *Paying for Medicare*, 173–81.

98. The origins and subsequent role of the PPRC in Medicare policy are discussed in Oliver, "Analysis, Advice, and Congressional Leadership."

99. The research on RBRVS is summarized in William Hsiao et al., *A National Study of Resource-Based Relative Value Scales for Physician Services: Final Report* (Boston: Harvard School of Public Health, 1988). For an illuminating critique of the scientific pretensions of RBRVS, see William Glaser, "Designing Fee Schedules by Formulae, Politics and Negotiations," *American Journal of Public Health* 80, no. 7 (July 1990): 804–9. See also the exchange between Glaser and defenders of RBRVS in *Health Affairs:* William Glaser, "The Politics of Paying American Physicians," *Health Affairs* 8, no. 3 (fall 1989): 129–46; and Paul B. Ginsburg and Philip R. Lee, "Defending U.S. Physician Payment Reform," 61–71; William C. Hsiao, "Objective Research and Physician Payment: A Response from Harvard," 72–75; Victor Rodwin, "Physician Payment Reform: Lessons from Abroad," 76–83; and William Glaser, "The Author Responds," 87–96, all in *Health Affairs* 8, no. 4 (winter 1989).

100. See, generally, Smith, *Paying for Medicare*, 200–210. The prospects for the bill's passage were enhanced by the support of William Roper, President Bush's deputy assistant for domestic policy. In addition to Pete Stark, Senators David Durenburger, Lloyd Bentsen, and Jay Rockefeller, as well as Ways and Means chair Dan Rostenkowski and Representatives Bill Gradison and Henry Waxman, played a critical role in the legislation of the Medicare fee schedule. The volume controls were based, in part, on similar regulatory mechanisms used in the Canadian health system. On Medicare regulation of physician balance billing, see David C. Colby, Thomas Rice, Jill Bernstein, and Lyle Nelson, "Balance Billing under Medicare," *Journal of Health Politics, Policy*

and Law 20, no. 1 (spring 1995): 51–74. The right to balance bill patients had been part of Medicare since its enactment.

101. However, the AMA did mount a campaign against the volume controls—originally proposed as "expenditure targets," though they did not succeed in having them eliminated from the legislation.

102. See Brown, "Technocratic Corporatism," for the argument that Medicare regulation approximates European corporatism.

103. James A. Morone, "American Political Culture and the Search for Lessons from Abroad," *Journal of Health, Politics, Policy, and Law* 15 (spring 1990): 133.

104. Ibid.

105. Health Care Financing Administration, *Profile of Medicare: 1998* (Washington, D.C.: Health Care Financing Administration, 1998), 40.

106. Morone, "American Political Culture," 77.

107. In political science, an early version of capture theory is Marver Bernstein, *Regulating Business by Independent Commission* (Princeton, N.J.: Princeton University Press, 1955). Pluralist theories of American politics that emphasize the domination of public policy by private interests are also compatible with this vein of regulatory theory. See Theodore Lowi, *The End of Liberalism* (New York: Norton, 1969), and Grant McConnell, *Private Power and American Democracy* (New York: Knopf, 1966). In economics, see George Stigler, "The Theory of Economic Regulation," *Bell Journal of Economics and Management Science* 2 (spring 1971): 137–47; and, on concentrated interests, Mancur Olson, *The Logic of Collective Action* (Cambridge, Mass.: Harvard University Press, 1965). Capture theory is also very much connected to rational choice models of politics that argue that political behavior is fundamentally self-interested (e.g., "rent-seeking") and that the modern state has an inherent, and uncontrollable, tendency to expand: "government as Leviathan." For a summary of rational choice and regulation, see Dennis Mueller, *Public Choice II* (New York: Cambridge University Press, 1989), esp. 229–73, 320–42.

108. This is the argument in McConnell, *Private Power and American Democracy.*

109. See Alain Enthoven, *Health Plan* (Reading, Mass.: Addison-Wesley, 1980).

110. E. E. Schattschneider, *The Semisovereign People* (New York: Holt, Reinhart, and Winston, 1960).

111. For a legal perspective on the politics of regulation, see Timothy Jost, "Governing Medicare," *Administrative Law Review* 51 (1998): 39–116.

112. Murray Edelman, *The Symbolic Uses of Politics* (Urbana: University of Illinois Press, 1964).

113. The reassuring nature of Medicare's "scientific" reforms is a theme emphasized in Smith, *Paying for Medicare.*

114. The annual update factor for hospital reimbursement under prospective payment was supposed to be equal to increases in the hospital market basket—the goods and services that hospitals purchase—plus a supplement for changes in technology and medical practice. However, the update factor has, since the introduction of prospective payment in 1983, consistently fallen below the hospital market basket index. See the data presented in by the Prospective Payment Assessment Commission in *Medicare and the American Health Care System,* 41.

115. For similar conclusions about state-centered health care regulation, see, especially, Starr, *Social Transformation,* 400–401; Morone and Dunham, "Slouching," 284–91; and Brown, "Technocratic Corporatism."

116. For a summary of the debate in political science over bureaucratic or congressional dominance of regulation, see Terry Moe, "An Assessment of the Positive Theory of Congressional Dominance," *Legislative Studies Quarterly* 12 (November 1987): 475–520.

117. Morone and Dunham, "Slouching," 290.

118. David Smith, in *Paying for Medicare,* documents the importance of congressional bureaucracies but does not relate them to broader theoretical issues regarding Congress or regulation.

119. For discussions of the operation of the update and conversion factors, see *1995 Annual Report to Congress* of the Physician Payment Review Commission (Washington, D.C.: Physician Payment Review Commission, 1995); and the Prospective Payment Assessment Commission's June 1995 report, *Medicare and the American Health Care System.*

120. Of course, those members of Congress on health subcommittees experienced with Medicare, as well as their staffs, are experts in federal health regulation—possessing a sort of permanent expertise often ignored in academic accounts of Congress.

121. Smith, *Paying for Medicare,* 69–114.

122. David Mayhew, *Congress: The Electoral Connection* (New Haven, Conn.: Yale University Press,1974); and Morris P. Fiorina, *Congress: Keystone of the Washington Establishment* (New Haven, Conn.: Yale University Press. 1977).

123. Hugh Heclo, "Issue Networks and the Executive Establishment," in *The New American Political System,* ed. Anthony King (Washington, D.C.: American Enterprise Institute, 1978).

124. On deficit politics, see White and Wildavsky, *The Deficit and The Public Interest.*

125. Uwe E. Reinhardt, "Can America Afford Its Elderly Citizens?" in *Policy Options for Reforming the Medicare Program,* ed. Stuart H. Altman, Uwe Reinhardt, and David Schactman (Princeton, N.J.: Robert Wood Johnson Foundation, 1997).

126. Joseph White, *Competing Solutions: American Health Care Proposals and International Experience* (Washington, D.C.: Brookings Institution Press, 1995).

CHAPTER SIX

1. David Mayhew, *Congress: The Electoral Connection* (New Haven, Conn.: Yale University Press, 1974); R. Kent Weaver, "The Politics of Blame Avoidance," *Journal of Public Policy* 6 (1986): 371–98; R. Douglas Arnold, *The Logic of Congressional Action* (New Haven, Conn.: Yale University Press, 1990).

2. Walter Dean Burnham, *Critical Elections and the Mainsprings of American Government* (New York: Norton, 1970). On the application of electoral incentives to the politics of the welfare state, see Hugh Heclo, *Modern Social Politics in Britain and Sweden* (New Haven, Conn.: Yale University Press, 1964), 6–7.

3. This assumption is inherent in realignment theories of American politics. See James Sundquist, *The Dynamics of the Party System* (Washington, D.C.: Brookings Institution Press, 1983); and Burnham, *Critical Elections.* For a critical review of realignment models, see Richard L. McCormick, *The Party Period and Public Policy* (New York: Oxford University Press, 1986), 64–88.

4. There is a second caveat relating to the nature of American political parties. The Democratic Party has long been divided between a conservative, primarily Southern-

based wing and a more liberal, primarily Northern-based wing. Expectations of party divergence on public policies in the United States may be reduced, since a Democratic partisan majority cannot be automatically equated with a liberal majority.

5. Anthony Downs, *An Economic Theory of Democracy* (New York: Harper, 1957). See also Martha Derthick, *Policymaking for Social Security* (Washington, D.C.: Brookings Institution Press, 1979).

6. See Mayhew, *Congress: The Electoral Condition;* and Morris Fiorina, *Congress: Keystone of the Washington Establishment* (New Haven, Conn.: Yale University Press, 1977).

7. These conditions are borrowed from Heclo, *Modern Social Politics,* 288.

8. For an argument that electoral mandates are more media constructions than evidence of public approval, see Robert Dahl, "Myth of the Presidential Mandate," *Political Science Quarterly* 105, no. 3 (fall 1990): 355–72. A contrasting view of mandates is provided in Patricia Heidotting Conley, *Presidential Mandates* (Chicago: University of Chicago Press, 2001).

9. The closest Medicare has come to prominence in a presidential election since 1964 was in the 1984 contest between Ronald Reagan and Walter Mondale.

10. Lawrence R. Jacobs, *The Health of Nations: Public Opinion and the Making of American and British Health Policy* (Ithaca, N.Y.: Cornell University Press, 1993); Benjamin I. Page and Robert Y. Shapiro, *The Rational Public* (Chicago: University of Chicago Press, 1992), and "Effects of Public Opinion on Policy," *American Political Science Review* 77 (March 1983): 175–90; James A. Stimson, Michael B. MacKuen, and Robert S. Erickson, "Dynamic Representation," *American Political Science Review* 89 (1995): 543–65; and Paul J. Quirk and Joseph Hinchliffe, "The Rising Hegemony of Mass Opinion," *Journal of Policy History* 10, no. 1:19–50. On the impact of anticipated public opinion see Arnold, *Logic of Congressional Action;* and John R. Zaller, *The Nature and Origins of Mass Opinion* (New York: Cambridge University Press, 1992). For a revisionist view that politicians track public opinion not to follow but to influence it, see Lawrence R. Jacobs and Robert Y. Shaprio, *Politicians Don't Pander: Political Manipulation and the Loss of Democratic Responsiveness* (Chicago: University of Chicago Press, 2000).

11. Fay Lomax Cook and Edith J. Barrett, *Support for the American Welfare State: The Views of Congress and the Public* (New York: Columbia University Press, 1992).

12. Ibid., 60–63.

13. Page and Shapiro, *Rational Public.*

14. On the politics of targeting Medicare cuts, see Joseph White, "Budgeting and Health Policymaking," in *Intensive Care: How Congress Shapes Health Policy,* ed. Thomas E. Mann and Norman I. Ornstein (Washington, D.C.: American Enterprise Institute and Brookings Institution Press, 1995), 58–62. On public opinion on cost containment, see Mark. D. Smith, Drew E. Altman, Robert Leitman, et al., "Taking the Public's Pulse on Health System Reform," *Health Affairs* 11:125–33.

15. Here a crucial distinction between Medicare and Social Security emerges. In Medicare, costs can be controlled not only by cutting back program benefits, but by slashing payments to medical providers. This is not an option in Social Security, which directly provides cash benefits to the elderly, rather than purchasing services as Medicare does.

16. See Arnold, *Logic of Congressional Action.*

17. Derthick, *Policymaking,* 202.

18. Cook and Barrett, *Support for the American Welfare State*, 90–93.

19. See Jacobs and Shaprio, *Politicians Don't Pander*, for the argument that politicians use public opinion polls to sell their own policy goals and promote public acceptance of their political agendas through a strategy of "crafted talk."

20. See Jacobs, *Health of Nations*, 221–22, for an argument that public opinion is relatively autonomous of elite preferences.

21. On democratic responsiveness and the case for policymaking that responds to public opinion, see Page and Shapiro, *Rational Public*, 383–98; and Jacobs and Shapiro, *Politicians Don't Pander*, 295–324.

22. Jacobs, *Health of Nations*.

23. E. E. Schattschneider, *The Semisovereign People* (New York: Holt, Reinhart, and Winston, 1960).

24. Derthick, *Policymaking*, 12. See also 412–28 on "keeping society's options open."

25. Given the international trend of enacting social insurance programs and expanding pension benefits, it is questionable whether Social Security expansion can really be explained by the dominance of "program proprietors." My thanks to Ted Marmor for this observation.

26. On this point, see Page and Shapiro, *Rational Public*, 383–98; and Jacobs and Shapiro, *Politicians Don't Pander*, 295–324.

27. Mayhew, *Congress: The Electoral Connection*, 130. On interest groups and concentrated interests, see Mancur Olson, *The Logic of Collective Action* (Cambridge, Mass.: Harvard University Press, 1965); and James Q. Wilson, *American Government: Institutions and Policies* (Lexington, Mass.: D. C. Heath, 1980). On interest groups' provision of information to policymakers and its connection to electoral incentives, see John Mark Hansen, *Gaining Access: Congress and the Farm Lobby, 1919–1981* (Chicago: University of Chicago Press, 1991).

28. The policy subsystems model argues that public policy is carved up into a series of networks corresponding to individual policy areas. See Theodore Lowi, *The End of Liberalism* (New York: Norton, 1979); Grant McConnell, *Private Power and American Democracy* (New York: Knopf, 1966). For an application to health politics, see Theodore Marmor, "The Politics of Medical Inflation," in *Political Analysis and Medical Care* (Cambridge: Cambridge University Press, 1983).

29. On the influence of interest groups over public policy, see Lowi, *The End of Liberalism*; McConnell, *Private Power and American Democracy*; George Stigler, "The Theory of Economic Regulation," *Bell Journal of Economics and Management Science* 2 (spring 1971): 137–46; and David Truman, *The Governmental Process* (New York: Knopf, 1951). For analysis emphasizing the power of interest groups to determine health policy, see David R. Hyde et al., "AMA: Power, Purpose and Politics in Organized Medicine," *Yale Law Journal* 63, no. 7 (1954): 938–1022; Harry Eckstein, *Pressure Group Politics: The Case of the British Medical Association* (London: Allen and Unwin, 1960); Robert R. Alford, *Health Care Politics: Ideological and Interest Group Barriers to Reform* (Chicago: University of Chicago Press, 1975); Nicholas Laham, *Why the United States Lacks a National Health Insurance Program* (Westport, Conn.: Praeger, 1993). For more recent accounts of interest groups in American politics, see Beth L. Leech and Frank Baumgartner, *Basic Interests* (Princeton, N.J.: Princeton University Press, 1998); Jeffrey M. Berry, *The Interest Group Society*, 2d ed. (Glenville, Ill.: Scott, Foresman; Boston: Little, Brown, 1989); Paul S. Herrnson,

Ronald G. Shaiko, and Clyde Wilcox, eds. *The Interest Group Connection: Election-eering, Lobbying, and Policymaking in Washington* (Chatham, N.J.: Chatham House Publishers, 1997); John R. Wright, *Interest Groups and Congress* (Boston: Addison Wesley 1995); Jack Walker, *Mobilizing Interest Groups in America* (Ann Arbor: University of Michigan Press); and Kay Lehman Schlozman and John T. Tierney, *Organized Interests and American Democracy* (New York: HarperCollins, 1986).

30. A similar conclusion is reached by Robert H. Binstock in "The Old Age Lobby in a New Political Era," in *The Future of Age-Based Public Policy,* ed. Robert B. Hudson (Baltimore: Johns Hopkins University Press, 1997), 56–74.

31. Physicians have also lost much of their ability to bill Medicare beneficiaries for amounts beyond what they are paid by the government.

32. For instance, see Lowi, *The End of Liberalism;* McConnell, *Private Power and American Democracy;* and Truman, *The Governmental Process.*

33. Schattschneider, *Semisovereign People.*

34. For an exemplar of rational choice thinking about Medicare, see Ronald J. Vogel, *Medicare: Issues in Political Economy* (Ann Arbor: University of Michigan Press, 2000). See also Paul Feldstein, *Health Policy Issues: An Economic Perspective on Reform* (Ann Arbor: University of Michigan Press, 1994).

35. For a summary of rational choice theory, see Dennis Mueller, *Public Choice II* (New York: Cambridge University Press, 1989). For a critique, see Donald P. Green and Ian Shapiro, *Pathologies of Rational Choice Theory* (New Haven, Conn.: Yale University Press, 1994).

36. Bruce C. Vladeck, "The Political Economy of Medicare," *Health Affairs* 18, no. 1 (1999): 22–36.

37. Ibid., 26–27.

38. Ibid.

39. See, especially, Theda Skocpol, "Bringing the State Back In," in *Bringing the State Back In,* ed. Peter Evans, Dietrich Rueschemeyer, and Theda Skocpol (Cambridge: Cambridge University Press, 1985), 3–37. The state-centered model is applied to health politics in James Morone and Andrew Dunham, "Slouching to National Health Insurance," *Yale Journal on Regulation* 2 (1985): 263–91; and David Wilsford, *Doctors and the State* (Durham, N.C.: Duke University Press, 1991). The effect of political institutions on health policy is explored in Ellen N. Immergut, *Health Politics: Interests and Institutions in Western Europe* (Cambridge: Cambridge University Press, 1992).

40. For instance, see Wilsford, *Doctors and the State.*

41. This conclusion supports the findings of others about the strength of the American state in Medicare regulation. See Morone and Dunham, "Slouching"; and Lawrence D. Brown, "Technocratic Corporatism and Administrative Reform in American Medicine," *Journal of Health Politics, Policy, and Law* 10, no. 3 (fall 1985): 579–99.

42. See Joseph White, *Competing Solutions: American Health Care Proposals and International Experience* (Washington, D.C.: Brookings Institution Press, 1995).

43. On the obstacles to national health insurance, see Jonathan Oberlander and Theodore Marmor, "The Path to Universal Health Care," in *The Next Agenda,* ed. Robert. Boorsage and Roger Hickey (Boulder, Colo.: Westview Press, 2001): 93–125.

44. For an excellent statement of this position, see Lawrence D. Brown, *New Poli-*

cies, New Politics: Government's Response to Government's Growth (Washington, D.C.: Brookings Institution Press, 1983).

45. This has been argued, for example, by Morris Fiorina. See *Congress: Keystone of the Washington Establishment.*

46. These assumptions are exemplified by Wilsford, *Doctors and the State.*

47. On the low standing of American bureaucrats compared with their counterparts abroad and the implications for health policy, see Wilsford, *Doctors and the State,* 73–83; and Carol S. Weissert and William G. Weissert, *Governing Health: The Politics of Health Policy* (Baltimore: Johns Hopkins University Press, 1996): 144–81

48. On this point, see also David G. Smith, *Paying for Medicare: The Politics of Reform* (New York: Aldine de Gruyter, 1992).

49. Autonomy is defined by state-centered theorists as the ability of states to act independently of, and in opposition to, social interests. Capacity is defined as a precondition for autonomy; it is the expertise and resources that state actors need to formulate and implement independent policy goals. See Skocpol, "Bringing the State Back In."

50. For a similar conclusion about the "congressional state" in American politics, see Joseph White and Aaron Wildavsky, *The Deficit and the Public Interest* (Berkeley: University of California Press, 1989), 544–46.

51. For a review, see Paul Pierson, "Increasing Returns, Path Dependence, and the Study of Politics," *American Political Science Review* 94 (2000): 251–66.

52. I am drawing here on the work of Paul Pierson, *Dismantling the Welfare State* (Cambridge: Cambridge University Press, 1994).

53. Pierson, "Increasing Returns," 252.

54. Ibid., 251.

55. Ibid., 262.

56. Carolyn Hughes Tuohy provides an exception to this determinism in linking changes in health policy (and path dependence) to external political conditions. See *Accidental Logics: The Dynamics of Change in the Health Care Arena in the United States, Britain, and Canada* (New York: Oxford University Press, 1999).

57. Jacob Hacker, "A Tale of Two Editions: Marmor's *The Politics of Medicare* and the Study of Health Politics after Thirty Years," *Journal of Health Politics, Policy, and Law* 26, no. 1 (2001): 133.

58. Marc K. Landy and Martin A. Levin, eds., *The New Politics of Public Policy* (Baltimore: Johns Hopkins University Press, 1995); Robert B. Reich, ed., *The Power of Public Ideas* (Cambridge, Mass.: Harvard University Press, 1990); Martha Derthick and Paul J. Quirk, *The Politics of Deregulation* (Washington, D.C.: Brookings Institution Press, 1985); Peter Hall, *The Power of Economic Ideas* (Princeton, N.J.: Princeton University Press, 1989); Steven Kelman, *Making Public Policy* (New York: Basic Books, 1987); and Margaret Weir, *Politics and Jobs: The Boundaries of Employment Policies in the United States* (Princeton, N.J.: Princeton University Press, 1992).

59. Louis Hartz, *The Liberal Tradition* (New York: Harcourt Brace Jovanovich, 1955). See also Samuel P. Huntingon, *American Politics: The Promise of Disharmony* (Cambridge, Mass.: Harvard University Press, 1981). The classic statement of the impact of values on public policy is Anthony King, "Ideas, Institutions, and the Policies of Governments," pts. 1–3, *British Journal of Political Science* 3 (1973): 291–313, 409–23. For a critique that instead argues for the primacy of institutions, see Sven Steinmo,

"American Exceptionalism Reconsidered: Culture or Institutions," in *The Dynamics of American Politics,* ed. Lawrence C. Dodd and Calvin Jillson (Boulder, Colo.: Westview Press, 1994):106–31.

60. James Morone, "American Political Culture and the Search for Lessons from Abroad," *Journal of Health Politics, Policy and Law* 15 (spring 1990): 133.

61. See Heclo, *Modern Social Politics;* and Wilsford, *Doctors and the State.*

CHAPTER SEVEN

1. Eugene Feingold, *Medicare: Policy and Politics: A Case Study and Policy Analysis* (San Francisco: Chandler, 1966), 100–156. A plan to subsidize the purchase of private insurance by the elderly was introduced in 1962 by Representative Frank Bow (Republican, Ohio) and was supported by another Republican conservative, William Miller of New York, the chairman of the Republican National Committee. Other Republican bills, such as one introduced by John Lindsey, a moderate from New York, called for offering cash benefits that could be used to purchase private insurance. Jacob Javits was another prominent support of the private insurance approach.

2. Allen J. Matusow, *The Unraveling of America: A History of Liberalism in the 1960s* (New York: HarperCollins, 1985).

3. Portions of this chapter are based on Jonathan Oberlander, "Medicare: The End of Consensus" (paper presented at the meetings of the American Political Science Association, Boston, 1998.

4. For a fascinating account of the Clinton administration's early agenda on economic policy and the battles fought over these issues, see Bob Woodward, *The Agenda: Inside the Clinton White House* (New York: Pocket Books, 1994).

5. Bill Clinton and Al Gore, *Putting People First: How We Can All Change America* (New York: Random House, 1992).

6. Woodward, *The Agenda.*

7. Theda Skocpol, *Boomerang: Clinton's Health Security Effort and the Turn against Government in U.S. Politics* (New York: W. W. Norton, 1996); Haynes Johnson and David S. Broder, *The System: The American Way of Politics at the Breaking Point* (Boston: Little, Brown and Company, 1996); Jacob Hacker, *The Road to Nowhere* (Princeton, N.J.: Princeton University Press, 1997); Paul Starr, "What Happened to Health Care Reform," *American Prospect* 6 (winter 1995): 20–31.

8. This argument is made in Skocpol, *Boomerang.*

9. Johnson and Broder, *The System,* 563.

10. Ibid., 560.

11. Interview with Charles Kahn, formerly of the staff of the House Ways and Means Committee and president of the Health Insurance Association of America, February 13, 2002.

12. Charles N. Khan III and Hans Kuttner, "Budget Bills and Medicare Policy: The Politics of the BBA," *Health Affairs* 18 (1999): 39–42.

13. Anonymous interview.

14. See the analysis by Lawrence R. Jacobs and Robert Y. Shapiro in *Politicians Don't Pander: Political Manipulation and the Loss of Democratic Responsiveness* (Chicago: University of Chicago Press, 2000), 28–36.

15. Keith T. Poole and Howard Rosenthal, *Congress: A Political-Economic History of Roll Call Voting* (New York: Oxford University Press, 1997).

16. Jacobs and Shapiro, *Politicians Don't Pander,* 32.

17. Interview with Chris Jennings, formerly deputy assistant to President Clinton on health care policy, February 29, 2002; and interview with Bill Vaughan, formerly of the staff of the House Ways and Means Committee, February 11, 2002.

18. Vaughan interview.

19. Ibid.

20. Carolyn Hughes Tuohy, *Accidental Logics: The Dynamics of Change in the Health Care Arena in the United States, Britain, and Canada* (New York: Oxford University Press, 1999).

21. On the politics of Social Security, see Martha Derthick, *Policymaking for Social Security* (Washington, D.C.: Brookings Institution Press, 1979). On Wilbur Mills's attitude to social insurance, see Julian E. Zelizer, *Taxing America: Wilbur D. Mills, Congress, and the State, 1945–1975* (Cambridge: Cambridge University Press, 1998).

22. See Joseph White and Aaron Wildavsky, *The Deficit and the Public Interest* (Berkeley: University of California Press, 1989); and Aaron Wildavsky, *The New Politics of the Budgetary Process*, 2d ed. (New York: HarperCollins, 1992).

23. Theodore Marmor, *The Politics of Medicare* (Chicago: Aldine, 1973).

24. Robert H. Binstock, "Scapegoating the Old: Intergenerational Equity and Age-Based Health Care Rationing," in *The Generational Equity Debate,* ed. John B. Williamson, Diane M. Watts-Roy, and Eric R. Kingson (New York: Columbia University Press, 1999), 157–84.

25. Fay Lomax Cook and Edith J. Barrett, *Support for the American Welfare State: The Views of Congress and the Public* (New York: Columbia University Press, 1992); and Lawrence R. Jacobs and Robert Y. Shaprio, "Is Washington Disconnected from Public Thinking about Social Security?" *Public Perspective* (June/July 1998): 54–57.

26. Robert H. Binstock, "The Aged as Scapegoat," *The Gerontologist* 23 (1983): 136–43.

27. Robert B. Hudson, "The History and Place of Aged-Based Public Policy," in *The Future of Age Based Public Policy,* ed. Robert B. Hudson (Baltimore: Johns Hopkins University Press: 1997), 1–22.

28. Marilyn Moon and Janemarie Mulvey, *Entitlements and the Elderly* (Washington, D.C.: Urban Institute Press, 1996).

29. Robert H. Binstock, "The Old Age Lobby in a New Political Era," in Hudson, *The Future of Age-Based Public Policy,* 56–74.

30. Peter G. Peterson, *Will America Grow Up Before It Grows Old?* (New York: Random House, 1996).

31. Daniel Callahan, *Setting Limits: Medical Goals in An Aging Society* (New York: Simon and Schuster, 1987).

32. Ken Dychtwald, *Age Power* (New York: Putnam, 1999), 1, 226–27. For an example of critical attitudes towards the AARP, see Ronald J. Vogel, *Medicare: Issues in Political Economy* (Ann Arbor: University of Michigan Press, 1999).

33. Samuel H. Preston, "Children and the Elderly: Divergent Paths for America's Dependents." *Demography* 21 (1984): 450–52.

34. Joseph White, *False Alarm: Why the Greatest Threat to Social Security and Medicare Is the Campaign to "Save" Them* (Baltimore: Johns Hopkins University Press, 2001); Theodore R. Marmor and Jerry L. Mashaw, "The Great Social Security Scare," *American Prospect* 29 (1996): 30–37; Theodore R. Marmor and Jonathan

Oberlander, "Rethinking Medicare Reform," *Health Affairs* 17(1998): 52–68; Jill Quadagno, "Generational Equity and the Politics of the Welfare State," *Politics and Society* 17, no. 3 (1989): 353–76; John Palmer and Isabel Sawhill, eds., *The Vulnerable* (Washington, D.C.: Urban Institute Press, 1988); Carrol Estes, "Social Security: The Social Construction of a Crisis," *Milbank Memorial Fund Quarterly* 61 (1983): 445–61; and Binstock, "Scapegoating the Old," 157–84.

35. Uwe E. Reinhardt, "Can America Afford Its Elderly Citizens?" in *Policy Options for Reforming the Medicare Program*, ed. Stuart H. Altman, Uwe Reinhardt, and David Schactman (Princeton, N.J.: Robert Wood Johnson Foundation, 1997), 171–99.

36. Norman Daniels, *Am I My Parent's Keeper?* (New York: Oxford University Press, 1988).

37. Cook and Barrett, *Support for the American Welfare State;* Jacobs and Shaprio, *Politicians Don't Pander.*

38. Robert J. Blendon and John M. Blendon, "Americans' View on Health Policy: A 50 Year Historical Perspective," *Health Affairs* 20, no. 2 (2001): 42.

39. Robert J. Blendon et al., "The Public's View of the Future of Medicare," *JAMA* 274(1995): 1645–48; Robert J. Blendon et. al., "Voters and Health Care in the 1998 Election," *JAMA* 282, no. 2 (1999): 189–94; Jill Bernstein and Rosemary Stevens, "Public Opinion, Knowledge, and Medicare Reform," *Health Affairs* 18, no. 1 (1999): 180–93. One change the public was willing to support was charging wealthier beneficiaries more for their Medicare coverage.

40. Judith M. Feder, *Medicare: The Politics of Federal Hospital Insurance* (Lexington, Mass.: D..C Heath, 1977); and Mark Schlesinger and Pamela Brown Drumheller, "Medicare and Innovative Insurance Plans," in *Renewing the Promise: Medicare and Its Reform*, ed. David Blumenthal, Mark Schlesinger, and Pamela Brown Drumheller (New York: Oxford University Press, 1988), 133–59.

41. The classic analysis of the professional dominance of the medical profession is Paul Starr, *The Social Transformation of American Medicine* (New York: Basic Books, 1982).

42. As Ted Marmor and Jacob Hacker point out, the term "managed care" has been applied so broadly that its meaning is unclear; too often it is used as a term of "persuasive definition." Nevertheless, it remains a conventional term to describe a host of changes in American medicine, and so, while aware of its limitations, I use the term here. See Jacob S. Hacker and Theodore R. Marmor, "The Misleading Language of Managed Care," *Journal of Health Politics, Policy and Law* 24 (1999): 1033–43.

43. Thomas Bodenheimer, "The American Health Care System: Physicians and the Changing Medical Marketplace," *New England Journal of Medicine* 340 (1999): 584–88.

44. Mark Peterson, "Introduction: Health Care into the Next Century," *Journal of Health Politics, Policy, and Law* 22 (1997): 292–313.

45. Gail Jensen, Michael Morrisey, Sharon Gaffney, and Derek Liston, "The New Dominance of Managed Care," *Health Affairs* 16 (1997): 125–36; Jon Gabel, Paul Ginsburg, Heidi Whitmore, and Jeremy Pickreign, "Withering on the Vine: The Decline of Indemnity Health Insurance," *Health Affairs* 19 (2000): 152–57.

46. In the 1990s, Medicaid, adopted at the same time as Medicare and along the same insurance model, was moving aggressively towards managed care, as more and more states in search of cost savings mandated that program recipients join HMOs and other managed care arrangements.

47. Interview with William Roper and Peter Fox.

48. Jonathan Oberlander, "Managed Care and Medicare Reform," *Journal of Health Politics, Policy, and Law* 22, no. 2 (1997): 595–631; Health Care Financing Administration, *A Profile of Medicare* (Washington, D.C.: Department of Health and Human Services, 1998).

49. Robin Toner, "GOP Moves Health Debate to Medicare," *New York Times,* February 12, 1995.

50. Rudolf Klein, *The Politics of the National Health Service,* 2d ed. (London: Longman, 1989).

51. Kahn interview.

52. Henry Aaron and Robert Reischauer, "Rethinking Medicare Reform Needs Rethinking," *Health Affairs* 17 (1998): 69–71.

53. Interview with Bruce Vladeck, formerly chief administrator of the Health Care Financing Administration and member of the National Bipartisan Commission on the Future of Medicare, February 25, 2002; Vaughan interview.

54. Bill Gradison quoted in Johnson and Broder, *The System,* 591–92.

55. David Maraniss and Michael Weiskopf, *"Tell Newt to Shut Up!"* (New York: Simon and Schuster, 1996).

56. Kahn interview.

57. Ibid.

58. Ibid.

59. Joseph White, "Saving Medicare—from What?" (paper presented at the annual meetings of the American Political Science Association, Boston, 1998).

60. Marilyn Moon and Stephen Zuckerman, "Are Private Insurers Really Controlling Spending Better Than Medicare?" (Henry J. Kaiser Family Foundation discussion paper, July 1995).

61. Bill Thomas, "Medicare at a Crossroads," *Journal of the American Medical Association* 274 (1995): 276–78.

62. George Hager, "Medicare Is Targeted for Large Cuts," *Congressional Quarterly,* April 8, 1995, 1013.

63. Kahn interview.

64. Ibid.

65. Gingrich consciously tried to avoid the apparent mistakes of the Clinton administration in not consulting with affected interests. He managed to win AMA support for Medicare reform by promising to loosen antitrust rules that prevented physicians from forming their own health plans and by limiting malpractice awards. The AARP was also muted, in part due to the threat of congressional hearings into its tax-exempt status.

66. On public opinion and Medicare reform, see Jacobs and Shapiro, *Politicians Don't Pander,* 274–77.

67. Mark A. Peterson, "The Politics of Health Care Policy: Overreaching in an Age of Polarization," in *The Social Divide,* ed. Margaret Weir (Washington, D.C.: Brookings Institution Press, 1998), 181–229.

68. Linda Killian, *The Freshmen: What Happened to the Republican Revolution?* (Boulder, Colo.: Westview Press, 1998): 169–70.

69. Ibid., 169.

70. For another analysis of the Medicare "flip-flop" of 1995–97, see Theodore R. Marmor, *The Politics of Medicare,* 2d ed. (New York: Aldine de Gruyter, 2000).

71. Congressional Budget Office, *Budgetary Implication of the Balanced Budget Act of 1997* (Washington, D.C.: Government Printing Office, 1997).

72. Lynn Etheredge, "The Medicare Reforms of 1997: Headlines You Didn't Read," *Journal of Health Politics, Policy, and Law* 23 (1998): 573–79.

73. In one respect, the Senate's passage of a higher eligibility age and income-related premiums was a "free vote"; they could show their commitment to controlling entitlements and standing up to the elderly since they knew the bill would never pass the House. That perspective was aided by the fact that the senators come up for reelection every six years, while House members must face the political heat every two years. In any case, at a key conference meeting on the legislation, deputy whip Dennis Hastert declared flatly that the House would never consider the provisions, apparently reflecting the political calculus of much of the House leadership that after the wounds inflicted by the 1995 Medicare debate, this simply was not politically achievable for the Republican Party (Vaughan interview).

74. Charles N. Han III and Hans Kuttner, "Budget Bills and Medicare Policy," 37–47.

75. Ibid., 44.

76. Vaughan interview; Jennings interview.

77. Vaughan interview.

78. Jennings interview.

79. Kahn interview.

80. Jennings interview; Vaughan interview. In part, as explained by Jennings, from the administration's perspective this reflected a lesson from political analysis of the history of entitlement reform: entitlement reform would not work politically if the public perceived reform as taking away benefits they were comfortable with or forcing them into something new they were uncertain about.

81. Vaughan interview.

82. Jennings interview.

83. Ibid.

84. Etheredge, "Medicare Reforms," 573, 575–76.

85. Ibid., 577.

86. Jennifer O'Sullivan et al., *Medicare Provisions in the Balanced Budget Act of 1997* (Washington, D.C.: Congressional Research Service, 1997); Sandra Christensen, "Medicare + Choice Provisions in the Balanced Budget Act of 1997," *Health Affairs* 17 (1998): 224–31.

87. Ibid. The BBA waived the 50/50 rule that required at least half of a Medicare HMO's enrollees to be from commercial insurance.

88. Alain C. Enthoven, *Health Plan: The Only Practical Solution to the Soaring Cost of Medical Care* (Reading, Mass.: Addison-Wesley, 1980).

89. Henry Aaron and Robert Reischauer, "The Medicare Reform Debate: What Is the Next Step?" *Health Affairs* 14 (1995): 8–30; Stuart M. Butler and Robert E. Moffit, "The FEHBP as a Model for a New Medicare Program," *Health Affairs* 14 (1995): 47–61; Congressional Budget Office, *Reducing the Deficit: Spending and Revenue Options* (Washington, D.C.: Government Printing Office, 1996).

90. O'Sullivan et al., *Medicare Provisions*.

91. O'Sullivan et al., *Medicare Provisions;* and Congressional Budget Office, *Budgetary Implications*.

92. I thank Larry Brown for this formulation.

93. The Social Security commission is described in Paul Light, *Artful Work: The Politics of Social Security Reform* (New York: Random House, 1985).

94. Ibid., 163–76.

95. Vladeck interview.

96. However, the defined contribution in premium support plans was based on a percentage of the average plan premium—the bipartisan commission recommended 88%—that offered beneficiaries more financial protection than other defined-contribution plans, since the federal government's share of beneficiary costs would rise automatically as health plan premiums reflected inflation in the cost of medical care.

97. Vladeck interview.

98. Democrats' appointment of Bob Kerrey to the commission was curious in that it was predictable that he would defect and support Republican premium support plans. His appointment apparently was due to internal Democratic politics in the Senate. He demanded a place on the commission, in the context of his previous work on entitlement reform.

99. Indeed, Aaron and Reischauer authored the most talked-about premium support proposal, an act that itself was taken as a sign of the shifting politics of Medicare reform. There were, however, notable exceptions to health economists aboard the premium support train, including Marilyn Moon and Tom Rice.

100. For an incisive analysis of the problems associated with conventional health economics, see Thomas Rice, *The Economics of Health Reconsidered* (Chicago: Health Administration Press, 1998).

101. John Kingdon has written in *Agendas, Alternatives, and Public Policies* (New York: HarperCollins, 1984) that policy change results from the convergence of three separate streams: problems, politics, and solutions. Implicit is the notion that policy ideas are developed in a world independent of political circumstances and enter the agenda when political developments enable their emergence. The Medicare case, though, shows convincingly that these streams are not as separate as Kingdon suggests. In the aftermath of Republican victory in 1994, a flood of proposals for remaking Medicare into a managed competition system emerged. This reflected in no small measure the need for policy analysts to remain relevant in the political game. In brief, policy analysts are subject to political pressures; they are not at liberty to ignore politics if their goal, or the goal of their institution, is influence. Consequently, policy proposals on Medicare after 1994 embodied a political calculus that belied any notion of separate processes of political change and policy development.

102. The retirement age of sixty-seven was to be phased in over a twenty-four-year period, making Medicare eligibility consistent with that for Social Security.

103. As noted by many observers, this ratio does not take into account the overall dependence ratio, which, since the number of children as a proportion of the population will drop as well, is much more favorable in terms of social spending than the worker/retiree numbers suggest.

104. John Breaux, "Medicare Reform: Its Time Has Come," March 4, 1999, National Bipartisan Commission on the Future of Medicare op-ed.

105. Another influential model for the commission was CalPERS, a defined-contribution health insurance system for California state employees.

106. Phil Gramm quoted in Amy Goldstein, "Impasse over Medicare Reform Looks Likely," *Washington Post*, February 26, 1999.

107. For similar reasons, in 2001 the Bush administration renamed HCFA the Centers for Medicare and Medicaid Services, or CMS.

108. The quote comes from commission member Stuart Altman in Michael Weinstein, "For Medicare: A Rocky Road to Competition," *New York Times,* January 1, 1999.

109. Transcript of the final meeting of the National Bipartisan Commission on the Future of Medicare, March 19, 1999, Washington, D.C.

110. Thomas Bodenheimer et al., *Rebuilding Medicare for the Twenty-first Century* (San Francisco: Health Access Foundation, 1999)

111. Vladeck interview.

112. Ibid.

113. Jennings interview.

114. Vladeck interview; Vaughan interview.

115. Weinstein, "A Rocky Road to Competition."

116. Vladeck interview.

117. Ibid.

118. Jennings interview.

119. Vladeck interview.

120. Thomas, however, dropped his sponsorship of the legislation and Breaux was joined by another Republican member of the commission, Senator Bill First, formerly a physician.

121. Congressional Budget Office, *Economic and Budget Outlook: Fiscal Years 2000–2009* (Washington, D.C.: Government Printing Office, 1999).

122. Data on trust fund provided by the Office of the Actuary of HCFA.

123. Kaiser Family Foundation, *Prescription Drug Trends* (Menlo Park, Calif.: September 2000).

124. See William Schwartz, *Life without Disease: The Pursuit of Medical Utopia* (Berkeley: University of California Press, 1998).

125. Ibid., 1.

126. Breaux, "Medicare Reform."

127. Kaiser Family Foundation, *Medicare and Prescription Drugs* (Menlo Park, Calif.: March 2000).

128. Kaiser Family Foundation, *National Survey on Prescription Drugs* (Menlo Park, Calif.: September 2000), 2.

129. President Clinton had actually proposed Medicare drug coverage as part of his 1994 health care reform plan, as part of a package to reassure seniors about the impact of reform, though the issue received scant attention at the time.

130. Health Policy Alternatives, *Health Issues in the 2000 Presidential Election* (Melo Park, Ca: Kaiser Family Foundation, 2000).

131. Without mandatory enrollment, the danger was that sicker and high-utilization patients in the Medicare population would select prescription drug coverage, yielding higher per capita costs than anticipated and producing an insurance pool unable to effectively cross-subsidize more expensive enrollees.

132. William M. Welch, "Older Voters' Issues May Be Key in Election," *USA Today,* May 1, 2002. Bush's performance among seniors in the 2000 election and the success of the Republican Party in maintaining its House and Senate majorities in 1996 after the controversial debate over Medicare reform contravene the myth that seniors

vote as a single bloc on issues relating to public programs for the aged, and that all seniors think alike on these issues.

133. Office of the Actuary of HCFA.

134. Marmor, *The Politics of Medicare,* 2d ed., 147.

135. Lori Achman and Marsha Gold, "Medicare + Choice 1999–2001," Commonwealth Fund, February 2002.

136. The managed care industry was also distracted by an enormous fight with physicians over permitting physician-organized health plans to participate in Medicare, a fight that diverted both their resources and attention (Jennings interview).

BIBLIOGRAPHY

INTERVIEWS

Robert Ball, formerly commissioner of the Social Security Administration, October 26, 1994, and March 25, 2002.

Otis Bowen, formerly secretary of health and human services, May 15, 1995.

Kenneth Bowler, formerly of the staff of the House Ways and Means Committee, April 8, 1991.

Tom Burke, formerly chief of staff at the Department of Health and Human Services, May 10, 1995.

Hale Champion, formerly undersecretary at the Department of Health, Education, and Welfare, October 18, 1994.

Jay Constantine, formerly of the staff of the Senate Finance Committee, October 27, 1994.

Nancy-Ann DeParle Minh, formerly administrator of the Health Care Financing Administration, March 1, 2001.

Robert Derzon, formerly administrator of the Health Care Financing Administration, December 15, 1994.

Peter Fox, formerly of the staff of the Health Care Financing Administration, 2001.

Bill Frenzel, formerly member of Congress and the House Ways and Means Committee, May 1, 1995.

Bill Fullerton, formerly of the staff of the House Ways and Means Committee, December 20, 1994.

Bill Gradison, formerly member of Congress and the House Ways and Means Committee and president of the Health Insurance Association of America, May 15, 1995.

George Greenberg, Department of Health and Human Services, June 20, 1995.

Stuart Gutterman, deputy executive director of the staff of the Prospective Payment Assessment Commission, June 10, 1995.

Arthur Hess, formerly director of the Bureau of Health Insurance of the Social Security Administration, December 19, 1994.

Chris Jennings, formerly deputy assistant to President Clinton on health care policy, February 29, 2002

Charles Kahn, formerly staff director of the House Ways and Means Committee and president of the Health Insurance Association of America, February 13, 2002.

Theodore Marmor, formerly special assistant to Wilbur Cohen, assistant secretary at the Department of Health, Education, and Welfare, April 17, 2002.

Robert Myers, formerly chief actuary of the Social Security Administration, July 8, 1995, August 1, 1995, and March 25, 2002.

Howard Newman, formerly administrator of the Medical Services Administration, December 15, 1994.

William Roper, formerly chief administrator of the Health Care Financing Administration, 2001.

John Rother, director of legislative affairs of the American Association for Retired Persons, May 11, 1995.

Bill Vaughan, formerly of the staff of the House Ways and Means Committee, February 11, 2002.

Bruce Vladeck, formerly chief administrator of the Health Care Financing Administration, February 25, 2002.

Don Wortman, formerly director of the reorganization group of the Department of Health, Education, and Welfare, November 9, 1994.

WORKS CITED

Aaron, Henry, ed. 1996. *The Problem That Won't Go Away: Reforming U.S. Health Care Financing.* Washington, D.C.: Brookings Institution Press.

Aaron, Henry, Barry Bosworth, and Gary Burtless. 1989. *Can America Afford to Grow Old?* Washington, D.C.: Brookings Institution Press.

Aaron, Henry, and Robert Reischauer. 1998. *Countdown to Reform.* New York: Century Foundation Press.

Aaron, Henry, and William B. Schwartz. 1984. *The Painful Prescription.* Washington, D.C.: Brookings Institution Press.

Aberbach, Joel D., Robert D. Putnam, and Bert A. Rockman. 1981. *Bureaucrats and Politicians in Western Democracies.* Cambridge, Mass.: Harvard University Press.

Alford, Robert. 1975. *Health Care Politics: Ideological and Interest Group Barriers to Reform.* Chicago: University of Chicago Press.

Allison, Graham. 1971. *The Essence of Decision.* Boston: Little, Brown.

Altman, Stuart H., Uwe Reinhardt, and David Schactman, eds. 1997. *Policy Options for Reforming the Medicare Program.* Princeton, N.J.: Robert Wood Johnson Foundation.

Arnold, R. Douglas. 1990. *The Logic of Congressional Action.* New Haven, Conn.: Yale University Press.

Ball, Robert. 1995. "Perspectives on Medicare: What Medicare's Architects Had in Mind." *Health Affairs* 14, no. 4:62–72.

Bardach, Eugene. 1977. *The Implementation Game: What Happens after a Bill Becomes Law.* Cambridge, Mass.: MIT Press.

Bauer, Raymond A., Itiel de Sola Pool, and Lewis A. Dexter. 1963. *American Business and Public Policy.* New York: Atherton.

Baumgartner, Frank R., and Bryan D. Jones. 1993. *Agendas and Instability in American Politics.* Chicago: University of Chicago Press.

Berger, Suzanne, ed. 1981. *Organizing Interests in Western Europe: Pluralism, Corporatism and the Transformation of Politics.* Cambridge: Cambridge University Press.

Berkowitz, Edward D. 1991. *America's Welfare State.* Baltimore: Johns Hopkins University Press.

————. 1995. *Mr. Social Security.* Lawrence: University Press of Kansas.

Bernstein, Jill, and Rosemary Stevens. 1999. "Public Opinion, Knowledge, and Medicare Reform." *Health Affairs* 18, no. 1:180–93.

Bernstein, Marver H. 1955. *Regulating Business by Independent Commission.* Princeton, N.J.: Princeton University Press.

Berry, Jeffrey M. 1997. *The Interest Group Society,* 3d ed. New York: Addison Wesley Longman.

Binstock, Robert H. 1983. "The Aged as Scapegoat." *Gerontologist* 23:136–43.

————. 1995. "A New Era in the Politics of Aging: How Will Older Voters Respond?" *Generations* 19, no. 3 (fall): 68–74.

————. 1997. "The Old Age Lobby in a New Political Era." In *The Future of Age-Based Public Policy,* edited by Robert B. Hudson, 56–74. Baltimore: Johns Hopkins University Press.

————. 1999. "Scapegoating the Old: Intergenerational Equity and Age-Based Health Care Rationing." In *The Generational Equity Debate,* edited by John B. Williamson, Diane M. Watts-Roy, and Eric R. Kingson, 157–84. New York: Columbia University Press.

————. 2000. "Older People and Voting Participation: Past and Future." *Gerontologist* 40, no. 1:18–31.

Binstock, Robert H., and Linda George, eds. 1996. *Handbook of Aging and Social Sciences.* 4th ed. New York: Academy Press.

Blendon, Robert. 1998. "Public Opinion and Medicare Restructuring." In *Medicare: Preparing for the Challenges of the Twenty-first Century,* edited by Robert D. Reischauer, Stuart Butler, and Judith R. Lave, 288–93. Washington, D.C.: Brookings Institution Press.

Blendon, Robert J., and John M. Benson. 2001. "Americans' View on Health Policy: A Fifty Year Historical Perspective." *Health Affairs* 20, no. 2:33–46.

Blendon, Robert J., et al. 1999. "Voters and Health Care in the 1998 Election." *Journal of the American Medical Association* 282, no. 2:189–94.

Blumenthal, David, Mark Schlesinger, and Pamela Brown Drumheller, eds. 1988. *Renewing the Promise: Medicare and Its Reform.* New York: Oxford University Press.

Bodenheimer, Thomas S., and Kevin Grumbach. 1995. *Understanding Health Policy.* Appleton and Lange.

Bodenheimer, Thomas S., Kevin Grumbach, Bruce Lee Livingston, Don R McCanne, Jonathan Oberlander, Dorothy Rice, and Pauline Vaillancourt Rosenau. 1999. *Rebuilding Medicare for the Twenty-first Century.* San Francisco: Health Access Foundation.

Brown, Lawrence D. 1983. *New Policies, New Politics: Government's Response to Government's Growth.* Washington, D.C.: Brookings Institution Press.

———. 1983. *Politics and Health Care Organization: HMOs as Federal Policy.* Washington, D.C.: Brookings Institution Press.

———. 1985. "Technocratic Corporatism and Administrative Reform in American Medicine." *Journal of Health Politics, Policy, and Law* 10, no. 3 (fall): 579–99.

———. 1992. "Political Evolution of Federal Health Regulation." *Health Affairs* 11 (winter): 17–37.

Burke, Sheila, Eric Kingson, and Uwe Reinhardt, eds. *Social Security and Medicare.* 2000. Washington, D.C.: National Academy of Social Insurance.

Callahan, Daniel. 1987. *Setting Limits: Medical Goals in an Aging Society.* New York: Simon and Schuster.

———. 1990. *What Kind of Life: The Limits of Medical Progress.* New York: Simon and Schuster.

Century Foundation Task Force on Medicare Reform. 2002. *Medicare Tomorrow: The Report of the Century Foundation Task Force on Medicare Reform.* New York: Century Foundation Press.

Christensen, Sandra. 1998. "Medicare + Choice Provisions in the Balanced Budget Act of 1997." *Health Affairs* 17, no. 4:224–31.

Chubb, John E., and Paul E. Peterson, eds. 1985. *The New Direction in American Politics.* Washington, D.C.: Brookings Institution Press.

Cobb, Roger, and Charles Elder. 1972. *Participation in American Politics.* Boston: Allyn and Bacon.

Conley, Patricia Heidotting. 2001. *Presidential Mandates.* Chicago: University of Chicago Press.

Cook, Fay Lomax, and Edith J. Barrett. 1992. *Support for the American Welfare State: The Views of Congress and the Public.* New York: Columbia University Press.

Cooper, Barbara S., and Bruce C. Vladeck. 2000. "Bringing Competitive Pricing to Medicare." *Health Affairs* 19, no. 5:49–54.

Corning, Peter A. 1969. *The Evolution of Medicare: From Idea to Law.* Washington, D.C.: U.S. Government Printing Office.

Daniels, Norman. 1988. *Am I My Parent's Keeper?* New York: Oxford University Press.

David, Sheri I. 1985. *With Dignity: The Search for Medicare and Medicaid.* Westport, Conn.: Greenwood.

Davis, Karen, Gerard E. Anderson, Diane Rowland, and Earl P. Steinberg. 1990. *Health Care Cost Containment.* Baltimore: Johns Hopkins University Press.

Davis, Karen, and Diane Rowland. 1986. *Medicare Policy: New Directions for Health and Long-Term Care.* Baltimore: Johns Hopkins University Press.

Davis, Karen, and Cathy Schoen. 1978. *Health and the War on Poverty: A Ten Year Appraisal.* Washington, D.C.: Brookings Institution Press.

Day, Christine. 1990. *What Older Americans Think: Interest Groups and Aging Policy.* Princeton, N.J.: Princeton University Press.

Derthick, Martha. 1979. *Policymaking for Social Security.* Washington, D.C.: Brookings Institution Press.

———. 1990. *Agency under Stress.* Washington, D.C.: Brookings Institution Press.

Derthick, Martha, and Paul J. Quirk. 1985. *The Politics of Deregulation.* Washington, D.C.: Brookings Institution Press.

Dodd, Lawrence C., and Calvin Jillson, eds. 1994. *The Dynamics of American Politics.* Boulder, Colo.: Westview Press.

Dowd, Bryan. 1999. "An Unusual View of Health Economics." *Health Affairs* 18, no. 1:266–69.

Downs, Anthony. 1957. *An Economic Theory of Democracy.* New York: Harper and Row.

Dychtwald, Ken. 1999. *Age Power: How the Twenty-first Century Will Be Ruled by the New Old.* New York: Putnam.

Eckstein, Harry. 1960. *Pressure Group Politics: The Case of the British Medical Association.* London: Allen and Unwin.

Edelman, Murray. 1964. *The Symbolic Uses of Politics.* Urbana: University of Illinois Press.

Enthoven, Alain C. 1980. *Health Plan: The Only Practical Solution to the Soaring Cost of Medical Care.* Reading, Mass.: Addison-Wesley.

Epstein, Leon. 1967. *Political Parties in Western Democracies.* New York: Praeger.

———. 1986. *Political Parties in the American Mold.* Madison: University of Wisconsin Press.

Etheredge, Lynn. 1998. "The Medicare Reforms of 1997: Headlines You Didn't Read." *Journal of Health Politics, Policy, and Law* 23, no. 3:573–79.

Evans, Peter, Dietrich Rueschemeyer, and Theda Skocpol. 1985. *Bringing the State Back In.* Cambridge: Cambridge University Press.

Evans, Robert. 1984. *Strained Mercy: The Economics of Canadian Health Care.* Toronto: Butterworths.

Feder, Judith M. 1977. *Medicare: The Politics of Federal Hospital Insurance.* Lexington, Mass.: D. C. Heath.

Feder, Judith M., John Holahan, and Theodore Marmor, eds. 1980. *National Health Insurance: Conflicting Goals and Policy Choices.* Washington, D.C.: Urban Institute.

Fein, Rashi. 1989. *Medical Care, Medical Costs.* Cambridge, Mass.: Harvard University Press.

Feingold, Eugene. 1966. *Medicare: Policy and Politics: A Case Study and Policy Analysis.* San Francisco: Chandler.

Feldman, Roger, and Mark Pauly. 2000. *American Health Care: Government, Market Processes, and the Public Interest.* New Brunswick, N.J.: Transaction Publications.

Feldstein, Paul J. 1994. *Health Policy Issues: An Economic Perspective on Reform.* Ann Arbor: University of Michigan Press.

———. 1996. *The Politics of Health Legislation: An Economic Perspective.* Ann Arbor, Mich.: Health Administration Press.

Fiorina, Morris P. 1977. *Congress: Keystone of the Washington Establishment.* New Haven, Conn.: Yale University Press.

Flora, Peter, and Jens Abler, eds. 1981. *The Development of Welfare States in Europe and America.* New Brunswick, N.J.: Transaction Books.

Foner, Eric. 1984. "Why Is There No Socialism in the United States?" *History Workshop* 17:57–80.

Fox, Daniel. 1986. *Health Policies, Health Politics: The British and American Experience, 1911–1965.* Princeton, N.J.: Princeton University Press.

———. 1993. *Power and Illness: The Failure and Future of American Health Policy.* Berkeley: University of California Press.

Frankford, David. 1993. "The Complexity of Medicare's Hospital Reimbursement System: Paradoxes of Averaging." *Iowa Law Review* 78:517–668.

———. 1993. "The Medicare DRGs: Efficiency and Organizational Rationality." *Yale Journal on Regulation* 10:300–371.

Fraser, Steven, and Gary Gerstle, eds. 1989. *The Rise and Fall of the New Deal Order.* Princeton, N.J.: Princeton University Press.

Friedson, Eliot. 1970. *Professional Dominance: The Social Structure of Medical Care.* New York: Atherton Press

———. 1975. *Doctoring Together: A Study of Professional Social Control.* New York: Elsevier.

Garceau, Oliver. 1941. *The Political Life of the American Medical Association.* Cambridge, Mass.: Harvard University Press.

Geer, John G. 1996. *From Tea Leaves to Opinion Polls.* New York: Random House.

Glaser, William. 1990. "Designing Fee Schedules by Formulae, Politics and Negotiations." *American Journal of Public Health* 80:804–9.

———. 1991. *Health Insurance in Practice.* San Francisco: Jossey-Bass.

Graetz, Michael J., and Jerry L. Mashaw. 1999. *True Security: Rethinking American Social Insurance.* New Haven, Conn.: Yale University Press.

Greenberg, Stanley B., and Theda Skocpol, eds. 1997. *The New Majoirty.* New Haven, Conn.: Yale University Press.

Gusfield, Joseph. 1981. *The Culture of Public Problems.* Chicago: University of Chicago Press.

Hacker, Jacob. 1997. *The Road to Nowhere.* Princeton, N.J.: Princeton University Press.

———. 2001. "A Tale of Two Editions: Marmor's *The Politics of Medicare* and the Study of Health Politics after Thirty Years." *Journal of Health Politics, Policy, and Law* 26, no. 1:120–38.

Harris, Richard. 1966. *A Sacred Trust.* New York: New American Library.

Hartz, Louis. 1955. *The Liberal Tradition in America.* New York: Harcourt Brace Jovanovich.

Heclo, Hugh. 1974. *Modern Social Politics in Britain and Sweden.* New Haven, Conn.: Yale University Press.

———. 1977. *A Government of Strangers.* Washington, D.C.: Brookings Institution Press.

Heidenheimer, Arnold, Hugh Heclo, and Carolyn Adams. 1983. *Comparative Public Policy.* 2d ed. New York: St. Martin's Press.

Herrnson, Paul S., Ronald G. Shaiko, and Clyde Wilcox, eds. 1997. *The Interest Group Connection : Electioneering, Lobbying, and Policymaking in Washington.* Chatham, N.J.: Chatham House Publishers.

Himmelfarb, Richard. 1995. *Catastrophic Politics: The Rise and Fall of the Medicare Catastrophic Coverage Act of 1988.* University Park: Pennsylvania State University Press, 1995.

Hirschman, Albert O. 1970. *Exit, Voice and Loyalty.* Cambridge, Mass.: Harvard University Press.

Hirshfield, Daniel S. 1970. *The Lost Reform: The Campaign for Compulsory Health Insurance in the United States from 1932 to 1943.* Cambridge, Mass.: Harvard University Press.

Hoffman, Beatrix. 2001. *The Wages of Sickness: The Politics of Health Insurance in Progressive America.* Chapel Hill: University of North Carolina Press.

Hudson, Robert B. 1997. "The History and Place of Aged-Based Public Policy." In *The*

Future of Age-Based Public Policy, edited by Robert B. Hudson, 1–22. Baltimore: Johns Hopkins University Press.

Huntington, Samuel P. 1981. *American Politics: The Promise of Disharmony.* Cambridge, Mass.: Harvard University Press.

Hyde, David R., Payson Wolff, Ann Gross, and Elliott Lee Hifman. 1954. "AMA: Power, Purpose, and Politics in Organized Medicine." *Yale Law Journal* 63, no. 7:938–1022.

Immergut, Ellen M. 1992. *Health Politics: Interests and Institutions in Western Europe.* Cambridge: Cambridge University Press.

Jacobs, Lawrence R. 1993. *The Health of Nations: Public Opinion and the Making of American and British Health Policy.* Ithaca, N.Y.: Cornell University Press.

Jacobs, Lawrence R., and Robert Y. Shapiro. 1998. "Is Washington Disconnected from Public Thinking about Social Security?" *Public Perspective,* June/July, 54–57.

———. 2000. *Politicians Don't Pander: Political Manipulation and the Loss of Democratic Responsiveness.* Chicago: University of Chicago Press.

Johnson, Haynes, and David S. Broder. 1996. *The System: The American Way of Politics at the Breaking Point.* Little, Brown.

Kahn, Charles N., III, and Hans Kuttner. 1999. "Budget Bills and Medicare Policy: The Politics of the BBA." *Health Affairs* 18, no. 1:37–47.

Katz, Michael. 1986. *In the Shadow of the Poorhouse: A Social History of Welfare in America.* New York: Basic Books.

Kernell, Samuel. 1986. *Going Public: New Strategies of Presidential Leadership.* Washington, D.C.: Congressional Quarterly Press.

Key, V. O. 1961. *Public Opinion and American Democracy.* New York: Alfred A. Knopf.

Killian, Linda. 1998. *The Freshmen: What Happened to the Republican Revolution?* Boulder, Colo.: Westview Press.

King, Anthony, ed. 1978. *The New American Political System.* Washington, D.C.: American Enterprise Institute.

King, Gary, Robert Keohane, and Sidney Verba. 1994. *Designing Social Inquiry: Scientific Inference in Qualitative Research.* Princeton, N.J.: Princeton University Press.

Kingdon, John. 1984. *Agendas, Alternatives, and Public Policies.* New York: Harper-Collins.

Kingson, Eric, and Edward Berkowitz. 1993. *Social Security and Medicare: A Policy Primer.* Westport, Conn.: Auburn House.

Kingson, Eric, and James Schulz, eds. 1997. *Social Security in the Twenty-first Century.* New York: Oxford University Press.

Klein, Rudolf. 1989. *The Politics of the National Health Service,* 2d ed. London: Longman.

Krasner, Stephen. 1978. *Defending the National Interest.* Princeton, N.J.: Princeton University Press.

Laham, Nicholas. 1993. *Why the United States Lacks a National Health Insurance Program.* Westport, Conn.: Praeger.

Landy, Marc K., and Martin A. Levin, eds. 1995. *The New Politics of Public Policy.* Baltimore: Johns Hopkins University Press.

Law, Sylvia A. 1974. *Blue Cross: What Went Wrong?* New Haven, Conn.: Yale University Press.

Leech, Beth L., and Frank Baumgartner. 1998. *Basic Interests*. Princeton, N.J.: Princeton University Press.

Light, Paul. 1985. *Artful Work: The Politics of Social Security Reform*. New York: Random House.

Lipset, Seymour Martin. 1990. *Continental Divide: The Values and Institutions of the United States and Canada*. New York: Routledge.

Litman, Theodore J., and Leonard S. Robins, eds. 1997. *Health Politics and Policy*. Albany, N.Y.: Delmar.

Lowi, Theodore. 1964. "American Business, Public Policy, Case Studies and Political Theory." *World Politis* 16:677–715.

———. 1979. *The End of Liberalism*. New York: W. W. Norton.

Lubove, Roy. 1968. *The Struggle for Social Security, 1900–1935*. Cambridge, Mass.: Harvard University Press.

Maas, Arthur. 1983. *Congress and the Common Good*. New York: Basic Books.

Majone, Guandomenico. 1989. *Evidence, Argument, and Persuasion in the Policy Process*. New Haven, Conn.: Yale University Press.

Mann, Thomas E., and Norman Ornstein, eds. 1995. *Intensive Care: How Congress Shapes Health Policy*. Washington, D.C.: AEI and Brookings Institution Press.

Mansbridge, James J. 1990. *Beyond Self-Interest*. Chicago: University of Chicago Press.

Maraniss, David, and Michael Weisskopf. 1996. *"Tell Newt to Shut Up!"* New York: Simon and Schuster.

March, James, and Johan Olsen. 1989. *Rediscovering Institutions: The Organizational Basis of Politics*. New York: Free Press.

Marmor, Theodore R. 1973. *The Politics of Medicare*. Chicago: Aldine.

———. 1983. *Political Analysis and American Medical Care*. New York: Cambridge University Press.

———. 1987. "Entrepreneurship in Public Management: Wilbur Cohen and Robert Ball." In *Leadership and Innovation: A Biographical Perspective on Entrepreneurs in Government*, edited by Jameson W. Doig and Erwin C. Hargrove, 246–81. Baltimore: Johns Hopkins University Press.

———. 1994. *Understanding Health Care Reform*. New Haven, Conn.: Yale University Press.

———. 2000. *The Politics of Medicare*. 2d ed. New York: Aldine de Gruyter.

Marmor, Theodore R., and Jerry L. Mashaw, eds. 1988. *Social Security: Beyond the Rhetoric of Crisis*. Princeton, N.J.: Princeton University Press.

———. 1997. "The Case for Social Insurance." In *The New Majority*, edited by Stanley Greenberg and Theda Skocpol, 78–103. New Haven, Conn.: Yale University Press.

Marmor, Theodore R., Jerry L. Mashaw, and Philip L. Harvey. 1990. *America's Misunderstood Welfare State*. New York: Basic Books.

Matusow, Allen J. 1985. *The Unraveling of America: A History of Liberalism in the 1960s*. New York: HarperCollins.

Mayhew, David. 1974. *Congress: The Electoral Connection*. New Haven, Conn.: Yale University Press.

———. 1991. *Divided We Govern*. New Haven, Conn.: Yale University Press.

McConnell, Grant. 1966. *Private Power and American Democracy*. New York: Knopf.

McDonough, John E. 1977. *Interests, Ideas, and Deregulation: The Fate of Hospital Rate Setting*. Ann Arbor: University of Michigan Press, 1997.

Mitchell, Daniel J. B. 2000. *Pensions and the Elderly*. Armonk, N.Y.: M. E. Sharpe.

Moon Marilyn. 1993. *Medicare: Now and in the Future*. Washington, D.C.: Urban Institute Press.

———. 1996. *Medicare: Now and in the Future*. 2d ed. Washington, D.C.: Urban Institute Press.

Moon, Marilyn, and Janemarie Mulvey. 1996. *Entitlements and the Elderly*. Washington, D.C.: Urban Institute Press.

Moon, Marilyn, and Stephen Zuckerman. 1995. "Are Private Insurers Really Controlling Spending Better Than Medicare?" Henry J. Kaiser Family Foundation discussion paper.

Morone, James A. 1994. "The Bureaucracy Empowered." In *The Politics of Health Care Reform*, edited by James A. Morone and Gary S. Belkin, 148–64. Durham, N.C.: Duke University Press

———. 1990. "American Political Culture and the Search for Lessons from Abroad." *Journal of Health Politics, Policy, and Law* 15 (spring 1990), 129–43.

———. 1990. *The Democratic Wish: Popular Participation and the Limits of American Government*. New York: Basic Books.

Morone, James, and Andrew Dunham. 1985. "Slouching to National Health Insurance." *Yale Journal on Regulation* 2:263–91.

Mueller, Dennis. 1989. *Public Choice II*. New York: Cambridge University Press.

Myers, Robert J. 1970. *Medicare*. Bryn Mawr, Pa: McCahan Foundation.

———. 1975. *Social Security*. Bryn Mawr, Pa: McCahan Foundation.

Myles, John. 1989. *Old Age in the Welfare State*. Lawrence: University Press of Kansas.

Navarro, Vincente. 1994. *The Politics of Health Policy*. Cambridge: Blackwell.

Neustadt, Richard. 1960. *Presidential Power*. New York: John Wiley.

Numbers, Ronald. 1978. *Almost Persuaded: American Physicians and Compulsory Health Insurance*. Baltimore: Johns Hopkins University Press.

Oberlander, Jonathan. 1995. "Medicare and the American State: The Politics of Federal Health Insurance" Ph.D. diss.,, Yale University.

———. 1997. "Managed Care and Medicare Reform." *Journal of Health Politics, Policy and Law* 22, no. 2:595–31.

———. 1998. "Medicare: The End of Consensus." Paper presented at the annual meetings of the American Political Science Association, Boston, Mass.

———. 1998. "Reforming Medicare: The Voucher Myth." *International Journal of Health Services* 28 (January/February): 29–46.

———. 2000. "Is Premium Support the Right Medicine for Medicare?" *Health Affairs* 19, no. 5:84–99.

Offe, Claus. 1984. *Contradictions of the Welfare State*. Cambridge, Mass.: MIT Press.

Oliver, Thomas. 1991. "Health Care Market Reform in Congress: The Uncertain Path from Proposal to Policy." *Political Science Quarterly* 106, no. 3:453–77.

———. 1993. "Analysis, Advice, and Congressional Leadership: The Physician Payment Review Commission and the Politics of Medicare." *Journal of Health Politics, Policy, and Law* 18 (spring): 113–74.

Olson, Mancur. 1965. *The Logic of Collective Action*. Cambridge, Mass.: Harvard University Press.

Page, Benjamin I., and Robert Y. Shapiro. 1983. "Effects of Public Opinion on Policy." *American Political Science Review* 77 (March): 175–90.

———. 1992. *The Rational Public.* Chicago: University of Chicago Press.

Palmer, John, and Isabel Sawhill, eds. 1988. *The Vulnerable.* Washington, D.C.: Urban Institute.

Patashnik, Eric. 2000. *Putting Trust in the U.S. Budget: Federal Trust Funds and the Politics of Commitment.* Cambridge: Cambridge University Press.

Pauly, Mark, and William Kissick, eds. 1988. *Lessons from the First Twenty Years of Medicare.* Philadelphia: University of Pennsylvania Press.

Peterson, Mark A. 1998. "The Politics of Health Care Policy: Overreaching in an Age of Polarization." In *The Social Divide,* edited by Margaret Weir, 181–229. Washington, D.C.: Brookings Institution Press.

———, ed. 1998. *Healthy Markets? The New Competition in Medical Care.* Durham, N.C.: Duke University Press.

Peterson, Peter G. 1999. *Gray Dawn: How the Coming Age Wave Will Transform America—and The World.* New York: Times Books.

———. 1996. *Will America Grow Up Before It Grows Old?* New York: Random House.

Pierson, Paul. 1994. *Dismantling the Welfare State.* Cambridge: Cambridge University Press.

———. 2000. "Path Dependence and the Study of Politics." *American Political Science Review* 94, 2:251–67.

Poen, Monty M. 1979. *Harry S. Truman versus the Medical Lobby.* Columbia: University of Missouri Press.

Polsby, Nelson. 1975. "Legislatures." In *Handbook of Political Science,* edited by Nelson Polsby and Fred Greenstein, vol. 5, 257–319. Reading, Mass.: Addison-Wesley.

———. 1984. *Political Innovation in America.* New Haven, Conn.: Yale University Press.

Powell, Walter W., and Paul J. Dimaggio, eds. 1991. *The New Institutionalism in Organizational Analysis.* Chicago: University of Chicago Press.

Pratt, Henry J. 1976. *The Gray Lobby.* Chicago: University of Chicago Press.

———. 1993. *Gray Agendas: Interest Groups and Public Pensions in Canada, Britain, and the United States.* Ann Arbor: University of Michigan Press.

Pressman, Jeffrey L., and Aaron B. Wildavsky. 1973. *Implementation: How Great Expectations in Washington Are Dashed in Oakland.* Berkeley: University of California Press.

Preston, Samuel H. 1984. "Children and the Elderly: Divergent Paths for America's Dependents." *Demography* 21:435–57.

Quadagno, Jill. 1988. *The Transformation of Old Age Security.* Chicago: University of Chicago Press.

———. 1989. "Generational Equity and the Politics of the Welfare State." *Politics and Society* 17, no. 3:353–76.

Reinhardt, Uwe E. 1997. "Can America Afford Its Elderly Citizens?" In *Policy Options for Reforming the Medicare Program,* edited by Stuart H. Altman, Uwe Reinhardt, and David Schactman, 171–99. Princeton, N.J.: Robert Wood Johnson Foundation.

———. 1993. "Reforming the Health Care System: The Universal Dilemma." *American Journal of Law and Medicine* 19, nos. 1 and 2:21–36.

Reischauer, Robert D., ed. 1997. *Setting National Priorities: Budget Choices for the Next Century.* Washington, D.C.: Brookings Institution Press.

Reischauer, Robert D., Stuart Butler, and Judith R. Lave, eds. 1998. *Medicare: Preparing for the Challenges of the Twenty-first Century.* Washington, D.C.: Brookings Institution Press.

Rettenmaier, Andrew J., and Thomas R. Saving, eds. 1999. *Medicare Reform: Issues and Answers.* Chicago: University of Chicago Press.

Rice, Thomas. 1998. *The Economics of Health Reconsidered.* Chicago: Health Administration Press.

Rivlin, Alice M., and Joshua M. Wiener. 1988. *Caring for the Disabled Elderly: Who Will Pay?* Washington, D.C.: Brookings Institution Press.

Rodgers, Daniel T. 1998. *Atlantic Crossings: Social Politics in a Progressive Age.* Cambridge, Mass.: Harvard University Press.

Rosenberg, Charles. 1987. *The Care of Strangers: The Rise of America's Hospital System.* New York: Basic Books.

Rothman, David J. 1997. *Beginnings Count: The Technological Imperative in American Health Care.* New York: Oxford University Press.

Rubinow, I. M. 1916. *Social Insurance.* New York: Henry Holt and Company.

Russell, Louise B. 1989. *Medicare's New Hospital Payment System—Is It Working?* Washington, D.C.: Brookings Institution Press.

Schattschneider, E. E. 1960. *The Semisovereign People.* New York: Holt, Reinhart, and Winston.

Schiltz, Michael. 1970. *Public Attitudes toward Social Security, 1935–1965.* Washington, D.C.: U.S. Government Printing Office.

Schlesinger, Mark, and Pamela Brown Drumheller. 1988. "Medicare and Innovative Insurance Plans." In *Renewing the Promise: Medicare and Its Reform,* edited by David Blumenthal, Mark Schlesinger, and Pamela Brown Drumheller, 133–59. New York: Oxford University Press.

Schlesinger, Mark, and Terrie Wetle. 1988. "Medicare's Coverage of Health Services." In *Renewing the Promise: Medicare and Its Reform,* edited by David Blumenthal, Mark Schlesinger, and Pamela Brown Drumheller, 58–89. New York: Oxford University Press.

Schlozman, Kay Lehman, and John T. Tierney. 1986. *Organized Interests and American Democracy* New York: HarperCollins.

Skidmore, Max J. 1970. *Medicare and the American Rhetoric of Reconciliation.* University: University of Alabama Press.

———. 1999. *Social Security and Its Enemies.* Boulder, Colo.: Westview Press.

Skocpol, Theda. 1992. *Protecting Soldiers and Mothers.* Cambridge, Mass.: Harvard University Press.

———. 1996. *Boomerang: Clinton's Health Security Effort and the Turn against Government in U.S. Politics.* New York: W. W. Norton.

Skowronek, Stephen. 1982. *Building a New American State: The Expansion of National Administrative Capacities.* New York: Cambridge University Press.

Smith, David G. 1992. *Paying for Medicare: The Politics of Reform.* New York: Aldine de Gruyter.

Somers, Herman M., and Anne R. Somers. 1967. *Medicare and the Hospitals.* Washington, D.C.: Brookings Institution Press.

Sorian, Richard. 1988. *The Bitter Pill.* New York: McGraw-Hill.

Sparer, Michael S. 1996. *Medicaid and the Limits of State Health Reform.* Philadelphia: Temple University Press.

Starr, Paul. 1982. *The Social Transformation of American Medicine.* New York: Basic Books.

———. 1994. *The Logic of Health Care Reform.* New York: Penguin.

———. 1995. "What Happened to Health Care Reform?" *American Prospect* 20:20–31.

Steinmo, Sven, Kathleen Thelen, and Frank Longstreth, eds. 1992. *Structuring Politics: Historical Institutionalism in Comparative Analysis.* New York: Cambridge University Press.

Steinmo, Sven, and Jon Watts. 1995. "It's the Institutions Stupid! Why Comprehensive National Health Insurance Always Fails in America." *Journal of Health Politics, Policy, and Law* 20, no. 2 (summer): 329–72.

Stevens, Rosemary. 1971. *American Medicine and the Public Interest.* New Haven, Conn.: Yale University Press.

Stimson, James A., Michael B. MacKuen, and Robert S. Erickson. 1995. "Dynamic Representation." *American Political Science Review* 89 (September): 543–65.

Stone, Deborah A. 1980. *The Limits of Professional Power.* Chicago: University of Chicago Press.

———. 1984. *The Disabled State.* Philadelphia: Temple University Press.

———. 1997. *Policy Paradox and Political Reason.* New York: W. W. Norton.

Sundquist, James. 1968. *Politics and Policy: The Eisenhower, Kennedy, and Johnson Years.* Washington, D.C.: Brookings Institution Press.

Truman, David. 1951. *The Governmental Process.* New York: Knopf.

Tuohy, Carolyn Hughes. 1999. *Accidental Logics: The Dynamics of Change in the Health Care Arena in the United States, Britain, and Canada.* New York: Oxford University Press.

Vladeck, Bruce C. 1980. *Unloving Care: The Nursing Home Tragedy.* New York: Basic Books.

———. 1999. "The Political Economy of Medicare." *Health Affairs* 18, no. 1:22–36.

Vogel, Ronald J. 1999. *Medicare: Issues in Political Economy.* Ann Arbor: University of Michigan Press.

Weaver, R. Kent. 1986. "The Politics of Blame Avoidance." *Journal of Public Policy* 6:371–98.

———. 1988. *Automatic Government: The Politics of Indexation.* Washington, D.C.: Brookings Institution Press.

———. 2000. *Ending Welfare as We Know It.* Washington, D.C.: Brookings Institution Press.

Weaver, R. Kent, and Bert Rockman, eds. 1993. *Do Institutions Matter?* Washington, D.C.: Brookings Institution Press.

Weir, Margaret. 1992. *Politics and Jobs: The Boundaries of Employment Policies in the United States.* Princeton, N.J.: Princeton University Press.

———, ed. 1998. *The Social Divide: Political Parties and the Future of Activist Government.* Washington, D.C.: Brookings Institution Press.

Weir, Margaret, Ann Shola Orloff, and Theda Skocpol, eds. 1988. *The Politics of Social Policy in the United States.* Princeton, N.J.: Princeton University Press.

Weissert, Carol S., and William G. Weissert. 1996. *Governing Health: The Politics of Health Policy.* Baltimore: Johns Hopkins University Press.

White, Joseph. 1995. "Budgeting and Health Policymaking." In *Intensive Care: How Congress Shapes Health Policy,* edited by Thomas E. Mann and Norman I. Ornstein, 53–78. Washington, D.C.: American Enterprise Institute and Brookings Institution Press.

———. 1995. *Competing Solutions: American Health Care Proposals and International Experience.* Washington, D.C.: Brookings Institution Press.

———. 2001. *False Alarm: Why the Greatest Threat to Social Security and Medicare Is the Campaign to "Save" Them.* Baltimore: Johns Hopkins University Press.

White, Joseph, and Aaron Wildavsky. 1989. *The Deficit and the Public Interest.* Berkeley: University of California Press.

Wiener, Joshua M., Laurel Hixon Illston, and Raymond J. Hanley. 1994. *Sharing the Burden: Strategies for Public and Private Long-Term Care Insurance.* Washington, D.C.: Brookings Institution Press.

Wildavsky, Aaron. 1992. *The New Politics of the Budgetary Process.* 2d ed. New York: HarperCollins.

Williamson, John B., Diane M. Watts-Roy, and Eric R. Kingson, eds. 1999. *The Generational Equity Reform Debate.* New York: Columbia University Press.

Wilsford, David. 1991. *Doctors and the State.* Durham, N.C.: Duke University Press.

Wilson, James Q. 1973. *Political Organizations.* New York: Basic Books.

———, ed. 1980. *The Politics of Regulation.* New York: Basic Books.

———. 1989. *Bureaucracy: What Government Agencies Do and Why They Do It.* New York: Basic Books.

Witte, Edwin. 1963. *The Development of the Social Security Act.* Madison: University of Wisconsin Press.

Woodward, Bob. 1994. *The Agenda: Inside the Clinton White House.* New York: Pocket Books.

Zaller, John R. 1992. *The Nature and Origins of Mass Opinion.* New York: Cambridge University Press.

Zelizer, Julian E. 1998. *Taxing America: Wilbur D. Mills, Congress, and the State, 1945–1975.* Cambridge: Cambridge University Press.

INDEX